Religion and Illness

Religion and Illness

Edited by
ANNETTE WEISSENRIEDER
and
GREGOR ETZELMÜLLER

CASCADE *Books* · Eugene, Oregon

RELIGION AND ILLNESS

Copyright © 2016 Wipf and Stock Publishers. All rights reserved. Except for brief quotations in critical publications or reviews, no part of this book may be reproduced in any manner without prior written permission from the publisher. Write: Permissions, Wipf and Stock Publishers, 199 W. 8th Ave., Suite 3, Eugene, OR 97401.

Completely revised and expanded translation of *Religion und Krankheit*, published by WBG (Wissenschaftliche Buchgesellschaft) Darmstadt, Germany, 2010.

Cascade Books
An Imprint of Wipf and Stock Publishers
199 W. 8th Ave., Suite 3
Eugene, OR 97401

www.wipfandstock.com

PAPERBACK ISBN: 978-1-4982-9351-8
HARDCOVER ISBN: 978-1-4982-9353-2
EBOOK ISBN: 978-1-4982-9352-5

Cataloguing-in-Publication data:

Names: Weissenrieder, Annette, 1967–. | Etzelmüller, Gregor, 1971–.

Title: Religion and illness / edited by Annette Weissenrieder and Gregor Etzelmüller.

Description: Eugene, OR: Cascade Books, 2016 | Includes bibliographical references and index.

Identifiers: ISBN 978-1-4982-9351-8 (paperback) | ISBN 978-1-4982-9353-2 (hardcover) | ISBN 978-1-4982-9352-5 (ebook)

Subjects: LCSH: Medicine—Religious aspects—Congresses. | Health—Religious aspects—Congresses. | Religion and medicine—History. | Diseases—Religious aspects—Congresses. | Healing—Religious aspects—Congresses. | Mediterranean Region.

Classification: BL65 M4 R474 2016 (print) | BL65 M4 (ebook)

Manufactured in the U.S.A.   10/31/16

Contents

List of Contributors | vii

Religion and Illness: An Introduction | 1
—Annette Weissenrieder and Gregor Etzelmüller

Part 1: Religion, Illness, and Care of the Sick in Galen and in Islam

1 Religion and Therapy in Galen | 15
—Teun Tieleman

2 Galenism Caught between Faith in God and "Prophetic Medicine" in Islam | 32
—Gotthard Strohmaier

3 Medicine in Islam: Contested Autonomy | 44
—Lutz Richter-Bernburg

4 Medical Concepts and Therapeutic Networks among Tamasheq Nomads in Mali | 58
—Anna K. Münch

Part 2: Religion, Illness, and Care of the Sick in Asiatic Health Care

5 A Focus on the Law or on the Individual? The Uncoupling of Religion and Health Care and the Emergence of Medical Science in Ancient China | 77
—Paul U. Unschuld

6 Buddhist Principles of Tibetan Medicine? The Buddhist Understanding of Illness and Healing and the Medical Ethics of the *rGyud-bzhi* | 90
—Jens Schlieter

7 Emotional Affliction and Mental Illness: From a Tibetan Vajrayana Buddhist Perspective | 114
—Martina E. Dannecker

Part 3: Religion, Illness, and Care of the Sick in the Old Testament and Judaism

8 Written on the Body: Body and Illness in the Physiognomic Tradition of the Ancient Near East and the Old Testament | 137
   —Angelika Berlejung

9 "Heal me, for I have sinned against you!" (Psalm 41:5 MT): On the Concept of Illness and Healing in the Old Testament | 173
   —Bernd Janowski

10 "Let This House Be Healed" (Psalm 51) | 198
   —Robert B. Coote

11 The Medical Interpretation of Jewish Religious Rites in the Nineteenth Century | 215
   —Klaus Hödl

12 "Whoever Saves a Soul Saves an Entire World": *Pikuah Nefesh* in Rabbinic Literature | 235
   —Lieve Teugels

Part 4: Religion, Illness, and Care of the Sick in Greco-Roman Antiquity and Christianity

13 Illness and Healing in Christian Traditions | 263
   —Gregor Etzelmüller and Annette Weissenrieder

14 Becoming a Doctor, Becoming a God: Religion and Medicine in Aelius Aristides' *Hieroi Logoi* | 306
   —Georgia Petridou

15 Interior Views of a Patient: Illness and Rhetoric in "Autobiographical" Texts (L. Annaeus Seneca, Marcus Cornelius Fronto and the Apostle Paul) | 336
   —Annette Weissenrieder

16 The Numinous Dimension in New Testament Narratives: Reorienting Miracle Research | 358
   —Werner Kahl

17 Word and Touch: Ritualizing Experiences of Illness and Healing in Christian Liturgical Traditions | 396
   —Andrea Bieler

18 Holistic Medicine in Late Modernity: Some Theses on the Efficacy of Spiritual Healing | 413
   —Anne Koch and Karin Meissner

Contributors

Angelika Berlejung is Professor of Old Testament (history and history of religion of ancient Israel and its environment) at the Theological Faculty of Leipzig University and extraordinary Professor at the Department of Ancient Studies at Stellenbosch University (South Africa); main areas of research: history and religious history of Israel and its environment, ancient Near Eastern iconography, Semitic epigraphy, archeology of Palestine, cultural anthropology.

Andrea Bieler is Professor for Practical Theology at the Kirchliche Hochschule Wuppertal/Bethel; main areas of research: theories of vulnerability, phenomenology of the body, practical theology in intercultural contexts.

Robert B. Coote is Senior Research Professor of Hebrew Exegesis and Old Testament at the San Francisco Theological Seminary and the Graduate Theological Union; main areas of research: history of early Israel; formation of the Hebrew Scriptures; use of Scripture in the New Testament.

Martina E. Dannecker has taught at the University of California Berkeley, the Institute of Transpersonal Psychology, Laney College, and California Institute of Integral Studies.

Gregor Etzelmüller is Professor of Systematic Theology at the Institute for Protestant Theology of Osnabrück University; main areas of research: interdisciplinary anthropology; dogmatics, especially election, providence and eschatology; ecumenical theoloy; science and religion.

Klaus Hödl is University Lecturer at the Centrum for Jewish Studies at Graz University; main areas of research: Jewish history in the nineteenth century, body images in medical discourse, culture and memory.

Contributors

Bernd Janowski is Professor emeritus of Old Testament at the Protestant Faculty of the Eberhard Karls University Tübingen; main areas of research: theology and anthropology of the Old Testament, religious history of Israel, Psalms, creation theology, biblical theology.

Werner Kahl is Professor of New Testament and Ancient Church History at the Theological Faculty at Frankfurt University and Director of the Academy of Mission at the University of Hamburg; main areas of research: miracles, Synoptic Gospels, African Bible interpretation, intercultural hermeneutics, Qur'an.

Anne Koch is Professor for the Study of Religions and Head of Department "Religious Study" at the University of Salzburg; main areas of research: method and theory of cultural studies; contemporary spirituality, economics of religion, aesthetics of religion (embodied cognition).

Karin Meissner is Professor for Integrative Medicine at the University of Applied Sciences Coburg, Germany and Adjunct Professor of Complementary Medicine at the Ludwigs Maximillians University, Munich; main area of research: Placebo and nocebo effects, complementary treatments, psychoneuroimmunology, time perception.

Anna Katharina Münch is Postdoctoral Associate at the Emerging Pathogens Institute (EPI) University of Florida; main areas of research: nomadic women's health practice; local interpretations of life-worlds in social networks.

Georgia Petridou is Lecturer of Ancient Greek History at the Department of Archaeology, Classics, and Egyptology at the University of Liverpool; main areas of research: Greek literature; religion and history of Graeco-Roman medicine in its socio-political contexts; divine epiphany in Greek literature and culture; the correlations of medicine, rhetoric and religion in Aelius Aristides' *Sacred Discourses*.

Lutz Richter-Bernburg is Professor emeritus for Islamic Studies at the Eberhard Karls University Tübingen; main areas of research: transmission and appropriation of classical learning (primarily medicine, with forays into philosophy) in Arabic and Persian; geographical and travel writing in Arabic and Persian, 3rd–7th/9th–13th centuries; Zengid and Ayyubid history; Nāṣer-e Khosrow and contemporaneous Ismailism.

Jens Schlieter is extraordinary Professor for the Systematic Study of Religion at the University of Berne, Institute for the Science of Religion; Director of the Center for Global Studies, University of Berne; main areas of research: Indian and Tibetan Buddhism, theory of religion, bioethics of religion—especially Buddhist bioethics, and religion/philosophy in comparative perspective.

Gotthard Strohmaier is Professor emeritus of Islamic Studies at the Freie Universität Berlin; main areas of research: Greek heritage in Islam, Koranic studies.

Lieve M. Teugels is University lecturer at Utrecht University; main areas of research: midrash, rabbinic literature.

Teun Tieleman is Associate Professor of Ancient Philosophy; Department of Philosophy and Religious Studies, Utrecht University; main research areas: ancient medicine (Galen) and philosophy (Stoicism).

Paul Unschuld, M.P.H., is Professor of the Theory, History, and Ethics of Chinese Life Sciences, and Director of the Horst-Goertz-Institute for the Theory, History, and Ethics of Chinese Life Sciences, Charité—Medical University Berlin; main areas of research: comparative history of Chinese and European medical history, comparative history of Chinese and Western medical ethics/bioethics, public health issues associated with heterogenous health care systems in contemporary Western and non-Western societies.

Annette Weissenrieder is Professor of New Testament at the San Francisco Theological Seminary and the Graduate Theological Union Berkeley; main areas of research: anthropology, ancient medicine, New Testament ecclesiology, Pneumatology, the interface between the Greco-Roman world and the New Testament, ancient visual art and architecture, ancient numismatics, methodology of ancient visual art.

Religion and Illness
An Introduction

TODAY ILLNESS CONTINUES TO be a paradigmatic symbol of insecurity that provokes varied interpretations. Especially when medical expertise fails, people draw on different interpretive perspectives—including religious ones. This realities of everyday life contrast, however, with the medical ideal of identifying and treating diseases dispassionately. From this perspective, illness appears as a phenomenon devoid of deeper meaning. Even if patients experience illness as a disaster, modern medicine merely sees the organism accidentally swamped by microorganisms. However, in the case of a specific individual who is ill, the model of illness as a biological accident fails. It would seem that a medical diagnosis creates a vacuum of interpretation. For the person in question, the illness demands an explanation. In the fundamental scenario of the physician-patient dialogue the medical system depends de facto on socially-acceptable patterns of interpretation. This raises the question of whether all interpretations of illness are equally valid from a medical point of view.

Given such an interpretive vacuum, the archaic explanation of illness as caused by individual guilt reemerges. Widespread psychological theories of illness attribute the ultimate responsibility to the unfortunate patient. Sick persons are plagued by the notion of their own guilt. A standard religious interpretation of sickness thus seems to come back to life: illness is understood as divine punishment. The experience of clinicians shows that religious interpretations and attitudes play a role in understanding illnesses and therapeutic processes—but these attitudes are usually not made explicit, which harms the patient. The constructive potential of religious attitudes is neither fully tapped, nor are those religious attitudes taken fully into account which contribute to depression and may hamper therapy.

It is the task of theology to identify such religious background assumptions and to elucidate the way they function. Furthermore, the dialogue between theology and medicine needs to raise questions about which religious interpretations are helpful in therapy. This question forces medicine to relinquish the interpretive parsimony that it seeks, and challenges theology to overcome the "silence on sickness" that is so pervasive at the moment. Both partners in dialogue can benefit from the fact that a conversation between medicine and theology on appropriate interpretations of illness has already been underway for 2,500 years, reflecting the experiences of different ages and regions. Yet even today, drawing conclusions jointly through this dialogue remains elusive: which interconnections of religion and therapy will indeed prove constructive in the long run in supporting the healing process?

While the discussion of "religion and health" often directs attention primarily to Christianity, the present volume begins with perspectives on "Religion, Illness, and Care of the Sick in Galen and Islam." This shows that in Islam ancient notions of disease continue to be influential today, although they have been passed on not as beliefs from the ancient world but as genuinely Muslim traditions.

In his article "Religion and Therapy in Galen," Teun Tieleman considers the religious dimensions of Galen's work and self-understanding as a medical practitioner and theorist, in particular his relation to the healing god Asclepius. He distinguishes between personal, traditional and philosophical aspects and asks: How does Galen reconcile his "rational" approach to medicine with his belief in therapeutic interventions by Asclepius? Why is Asclepius so important to him? He argues that Galen assimilates God as a creative power into Asclepius: God maintains the world, which "includes a healing influence, which however does not go against nature." So Galen is able to reconcile his religious beliefs and his rational medical praxis. Furthermore, his attitude to Asclepius reveals the need to impose his authority as a practitioner and to find psychological confirmation. The positive result is a personal religion enriched by philosophy, notably the Platonic ideal of "assimilation to God." Religion and rational medicine go hand in hand because "what god does or orders is always and in principle in full arcordance with what can be scientifically demonstrated to be true."

In his contribution, "Galenism Caught between Faith and 'Prophetic Medicine' in Islam," Gotthard Strohmaier demonstrates that Galen's physiology and humoral pathology continue to be influential still in current presentations of "Islamic Medicine." From its Hippocratic beginnings, Ancient Greek medicine had a distinct materialist character by rejecting divine or demonic causes of disease. Its impact on Muslim culture is to be seen in various instances, e.g., in the encounters with therapeutic procedures of other cultures as that of the Hindus or the Frankish crusaders. This attitude was in line with Mohammed's beliefs, which, according to tradition, rejected various kinds of magic. This included, unfortunately, also the denial of the possibility of contagion. Unimpeded by the authority of the Prophet, the Christian author Qusṭā ibn Lūqā ventured the idea that the transfer of a disease between individuals was caused by a material "spark."

In his essay, "Medicine in Islam: Contested Autonomy," Lutz Richter-Bernburg also discusses the integration of the medical authorities, which primarily include Galen and Hippocrates, into Muslim medicine, which he sees thus becoming obliged to—and profiting from—a "basic naturalism." However, the picture is not complete without medical classics in Sanskrit, which had been translated under the caliphs, and the unbroken popularity of folk methods of healing, according to Richter-Bernburg. He remarks critically that the "subsumption under the ideal of Mohammed" robbed Galen's medicine "of any positive perspective of change."

By contrast, the essay attributes a positive effect to the coupling of medicine and religion in the hospital system, which "unambiguously served the well-being of potential patients." Under Abassid rule the development of hospitals benefited from the institutional tradition established among Nestorian Christians in Mesopotamia. Since both Christian and Muslim traditions had developed an ethos of care for the sick and destitute, Muslims were able to continue the work begun by Christians in laying a religious groundwork for this ethos.

Given her own research in this field, Anna K. Münch discusses the understanding of illness among Tamasheq nomads in Mali, which constitutes limitations on what any international medical help can achieve in the area. Kel Alhafra nomads in the North of Mali understand human health as a physical and psychic equilibrium dependent on conditions in the natural surroundings and the individual's relationship to a supernatural power. If this fragile balance breaks down, or if the believer deviates from the righteous path, the individual ends up in disharmony and diseased. The Kel Alhafra not only associate illness directly with the divine creative power, but also believe in the miraculous nature of healing. In every disease, they think there is an element of divine wisdom, not always comprehensible to humans. Thus, a total cure requires and comprises not only a physical healing but also an inner spiritual cleansing in order to regain inner equilibrium and good health. For them, religious attitudes to illness and healing are more important than choosing the right treatment. Therefore, the Kel Alhafra feel much closer to a *marabout* or traditional healer, who is endowed with the divinely inspired power of blessing, than to biomedically-trained physicians or state-trained health personnel.

In order to avoid a focus only on the so-called Abrahamic religions, the second section juxtaposes Muslim tradition with understandings of "Religion, Illness, and Care of the Sick in Asiatic Health Care."

In his contribution, "A Focus on the Law or on the Individual? The Uncoupling of Religion and Health Care and the Emergence of Medical Science in Ancient China," Paul U. Unschuld points out the parallel development of rational medicine in ancient Greece and in ancient China. A unique type of cultural revolution has taken place in world history: first, in the eastern Mediterranean and then just a few centuries later in China. In both cases, the naturalization of all earthly processes liberated individuals from the caprice of deities and bondage to one's ancestors, creating "the notion of a right to health." In ancient China this cultural revolution took place in the second century BCE. "From now on, therapy is directed to the disease, no longer just to the individual case." No one other than the sick person is responsible for the illness. By violating the order of the laws of nature—which is not conceived in moral terms—the individual has caused the disease. Medicine places "its adherents into a position of self-responsibility." This understanding of medicine, which also understands the human organism as analogous to a unified empire, was met with resistance—and not only in China: "The ideological counterpart of the new medicine was articulated in the pharmaceutical art of healing—which went hand in hand with a continued individualism."

In the next chapter, Jens Schlieter provides a comprehensive introduction to Tibetan medicine. The fundamental axiom of Buddhist ethics is the universal "preference to avoid suffering." This is the reason for a positive attitude towards the physician's work. However, "a tension between the ideal of the codified ethics of religious specialists and the professional ethos of the physicians" can be discerned at the same time, because the physician's ethos is influenced especially by the desire to protect his socio-economic interest. The physician is not obliged to help and heal all the time. Accordingly, the ethics of compassion of the Bodhisattva does not figure prominently in the texts of the physicians. Tibetan medicine thus represents the social differentiation of a practice of medicine oriented towards professional interests and a religion that bolsters an ethics of compassion. This social differentiation becomes manifest in the understanding of the causes of a disease: while religious texts attribute disease to negative karma, medical texts refer to other factors. For a "karmic determinism ... would subvert the basics of medical practice as a whole."

Next, Martina E. Dannecker's essay demonstrates the potential of Buddhist teachings for dealing with emotional problems and mental instability. These call into question modern dualisms—body and mind, person and world, individual and environment, rationality and emotions—thus moving towards a holistic image of the human person. While Western cultures often isolate a medical therapy oriented towards the laws of nature from the sick person's attempt to understand the illness, Buddhism reunites these factors: "In Tibetan Buddhism there is no conflict between the two therapeutic approaches, be it cognitive-behavioral or catharsis." After highlighting the overall positive effects of the practice of meditation, Dannecker also points out specific dangers in meditation techniques. Since past things are experienced once again in meditation, and people come in touch again with that which is generally repressed, experiences bordering on the psychotic may occur, which the technical literature calls a "religious or spiritual problem." "Meditation as a technique for spiritual growth can trigger the actualization of a person's potentialities which . . . commonly includes going through one's emotional difficulties and personal estrangement so that one can gain greater emotional maturity and awareness. It becomes a matter of learning how to tolerate the intensities of pleasure and pain. By being present to that which is in the moment, one becomes less and less emotionally affected by the ups and downs of life."

The third section focuses on "Religion, Illness, and Care of the Sick in the Old Testament and Judaism," while also looking at the contexts of the ancient Near East.

Angelika Berlejung's contribution discusses the Mesopotamian notion of physiognomic omens, which use the human body as the basis and medium for divinatory practices. She thus demonstrates how the ancient Near East (and the Old Testament by implication) treats the body. Reading the body allows one to draw conclusions about a person's fate and his or her morality, for the gods inscribed a person's fate onto his or her human body. By examining male and female bodies separately, physiognomy contributed to a "dichotomous view of being male or female. This included gender ideals and roles established in conformity to the wider system," which was cemented as "natural and 'inscribed onto the body' accordingly by the gods" and influenced the understanding of sickness. The Old Testament transforms the deterministic notion of fate inscribed onto the body into a more dynamic view, thus overcoming it. Sickness is thought of within the connection between deeds and consequences, "which keeps new courses of action continuously open both for humans and God, as for example conversion, remorse, forgiveness, and a reconstitution of the relation to God."

In his contribution, Bernd Janowski demonstrates that there is a religious and a social dimension to the Old Testament concept of sickness and healing. The *religious dimension* interprets sin as upsetting life-supporting forms of balance. Since the individual person is always part of a wider social network, illness affects the social context of the person. This social dimension appears in the correlation of the sphere of the body and the social sphere. The social space is characterized by a conflict structure that requires resolution, so that healing can take place and justice be re-established.

Bob Coote's contribution, "Let This House Be Healed," concentrates on a crucial text, Psalm 51. Psalm 51 is the most intensely repentant of the psalms, written in the form of complaint about affliction. As originally conceived, the primary affliction was the plaintiff's illness. Through reinterpretation, revision, and repositioning in the post-Exilic period, composers construed the psalm's voice corporately to refer to the Jerusalem temple and the destruction of its sacrificial cult, i.e., as a plea for the healing of a social illness with supreme collective religious significance. What made this construal possible was that the plaintiff's illness was not just that of a person, but also of a house, because the plaintiff had likened himself to a sick house. The homology of individual and body politics rests on two related uses of a correspondence, both common in ancient Near Eastern conceptuality: between person and house and between house and temple.

Klaus Hödl shows that since the Middle Ages, and increasingly since the onset of pseudo-scientific anti-Semitism, the bodies of Jews have been the object of scientific research. The crucial point has been to demonstrate that Jewish bodies are "different" from the non-Jewish population. This went hand-in-hand with a medical interpretation of Jewish rites, which can be traced back to the last quarter of the eighteenth century. At that time, "Jewish religious life was to be brought into harmony with values considered normative for the broader community as a whole. Of central importance in this connection were medical standards." By pointing out the positive effects of Jewish rites (circumcision, ritual slaughter, funeral rites, Sabbath rest), Jewish scientists wanted to replace widespread anti-Semitic stereotypes with a positive image of Judaism. In the course of the nineteenth century, "there was at least a tendency among a growing number of Jews to abandon the religious interpretation of Jewish ceremonies in favor of their medical interpretation instead. From this perspective, Judaism appeared to be in keeping with the central social values of broader society. It was thus possible to convey an image of Judaism that non-Jews perceived as positive. For a certain period of time, it seemed as though as a result, Judaism was now viewed in a positive light among broad segments of society. However, in retrospect, it is necessary to note that this development did not have a long-term impact.

Lieve Teugel's paper, which deals with several foundational texts of Jewish thought, explores the religious-anthropological background of Jewish thinking about the value of human life. The texts from the Mishnah, and the Babylonian and Palestinian Talmuds discussed in this paper demonstrate that the rabbinic sages believed that observing religious commandments only makes sense if they enhance life, not when they diminish it. Some case studies are presented dealing with the breaking of the Sabbath laws in order to save a human life, e.g., by administering medicine to a patient when this involves "working" on the Sabbath. In other texts the rabbis state that under certain circumstances the dietary laws may be abrogated for a patient who has even a remote chance of not surviving by not eating non-kosher food. These ideas form the ideological background behind later, even contemporary, Jewish decision-making on specific medical end-of-life issues, such as organ donation, abortion, and euthanasia.

The concluding section addresses "Religion, Illness, and Care of the Sick in Greco-Roman Antiquity and Christianity". It starts with an essay by the editors of the collection on "Illness and Healing in Christian Traditions." Inspired by Teun Tieleman's work, in this essay we argue that to a large extent even the so-called rational medicine of antiquity does not stop being religious, although it does fundamentally reject the notion of a divine cause for illness. This cultural revolution resonates even in the New Testament and the early church: the Gospel of Luke in particular depicts Jesus's healings in such a way that they are comprehensible against the backdrop of antique rational medicine. Precisely in this context they can be understood as miracles that point to God as their ultimate source. In addition, the New Testament contradicts the notion that illness is a consequence of sin. Drawing on a demonological interpretation of illness, the New Testament texts clarify that at a minimum not every sick person should attribute the disease to his or her own guilt. One can be subject to purely external causes of illness. This New Testament line of reasoning figures prominently throughout the Reformed tradition from Calvin via Schleiermacher to Barth. These thinkers make a case both for coupling religion and science-based medicine and for distinguishing between them. Certainly, today the churches of the Reformation are challenged by the worldwide growth of the Pentecostal movement, which sees its own practice of religious healings as in continuity with the depiction of Jesus as a healer in the Gospel of Mark. The essay concludes by asking how Christianity can present itself, within such tensions, as a religion that, given its own origins, is dedicated to serving the ill.

The contributions that follow elaborate on this approach by addressing the context within the ancient world (Georgia Petridou), reconstructing Paul's understanding of illness within this context (Annette Weissenrieder), bringing the New Testament miracle narratives into dialogue with the contemporary Pentecostal movement (Werner Kahl) and, finally, asking about the potential liturgical consequences (Andrea Bieler).

The study by Georgia Petridou offers a close reading of a selection of passages from Aelius Aristides' *Hieroi Logoi*, which results in a new perspective on Aristides. Far from being a submissive patient who idly resided in the Pergamene Asclepieion and relied exclusively on the therapeutic powers of divine healers, Aristides is shown here as an active agent in the medical encounter, and a patient who is not only in possession of the basics of the medical discourse, but who also takes his own life and the lives of others into his hands. In particular, Aristides not only appropriates the healing powers of his earthly healers (thus becoming a physician of sorts), but he also appropriates the healing powers of Asclepius, the divine healer (thus becoming a god of sorts). He achieves the latter status via further appropriation, this time of the religious roles of the temple's priestly personnel (priests and dream-interpreters) and the traditional ritual schemata of supplication and incubation. In short, by tackling successfully both aspects of Asclepian healing (medical and religious), the author of the *Hieroi Logoi* reinvents himself as both a physician and a god.

Annette Weissenrieder's contribution "Interior Views of a Patient: Illness and Rhetoric in 'Autobiographical' Texts" offers a close reading of selected passages from letters written by L. Annaeus Seneca, Marcus Aurelius Fronto, and Paul. It can be seen that the depiction of illness varies according to the choice of literary genre: the letters range from reports to an individual person—the friendship letter—to the stylized and functionalized genre of the teaching letter and the genre of the tearful letter. In each of these the senders describe illness from the perspective of the person who is affected. However, despite their clearly high level of education, they largely avoid using any specialized terminology. Instead, they describe and reflect rhetorically on the condition, which in some cases is life-threatening, using generally comprehensible terms. Even if they are all sick, the message is that they are far from being submissive patients. However, the writings of the three authors are not homogeneous, neither in their choice of genre nor in the way they deal with physical weakness. The diverse literary genres also reflect a non-homogeneous relationship to illness. While Seneca's teaching letters are intended to communicate something about existence and the philosophy of positive thinking, Fronto and Marcus Aurelius communicate a deep bond in their friendship letters that goes beyond the power of the physical as well as the ephemeral nature of human life; finally, Paul attempts to show that his physical weakness is a visible sign that God's power is fulfilled in his physical existence.

Werner Kahl's article, "Miracles as Merciful Acts of Divine Liberation: Understanding References to Numinous Activity in New Testament Healing Narratives," is an attempt to transform the exegetical approach to New

Testament miracle traditions. Kahl radically opts for an emic perspective on New Testament references to miracles by taking seriously the conventionalized knowledge of the world in Mediterranean antiquity as it was essentially shared in Early Christianity. This leads him to a deconstruction of both the categories "miracle story" and "miracle worker." It is problematic to isolate particular "miracle stories" in the macro-narratives about Jesus as presented in the Gospels since the presence of numinous power is constantly experienced through encounters with Jesus, even in his teachings. Kahl rediscovers the value of the theological insights in Karl Barth's exegetical analyses of Jesus' miracles in an extensive section of volume IV/2 of the *Church Dogmatics*. Surprisingly, New Testament exegesis has paid scant attention to these very dense and convincing deliberations. Here Barth exhibits a deep sense for often overlooked but essential dimensions of meaning in these miracle traditions. Barth grasps the distinct significance of New Testament traditions vis-à-vis other miracle traditions past and present, by describing them as "miracles as merciful acts of divine liberation." On the one hand, such an understanding is an alternative to the usual elimination or disregard of the miraculous in common exegetical discourse, and to a preoccupation with miracle power in popular traditions, as, for example, in much of present day neo-Pentecostalism in, and from, the Global South.

Andrea Bieler shows that Christian liturgical traditions and emerging practices have the potential to create liminal spaces in which illness narratives and body images can be reordered before God in life-enhancing ways. This argument is developed in three steps. Bieler first highlights crucial points in liturgical history when rituals of healing developed. What follows are some insights from a survey of about a hundred contemporary liturgical texts drawn from North American Protestant liberal mainline resources. "Regarding the understanding of illness and health in relation to the divine we can recognize a vital interest in overcoming a dualism that privileges the soul and the mind over the body by identifying the first with the spiritual realm and the latter with the somewhat devalued material world. By contrast the stress is on God's presence to all kinds of bodily, mental, and spiritual crises. Most of these liturgical texts are based on the distinction between cure and healing. While the cure pertains to the transformation of physical illness in scientifically measurable terms, the term healing is used to describe a sense of holistic integration." Finally, the essay introduces a case study in which narrative, metaphor, and ritual enter into a powerful synergy that reshapes the body image and the interpretation of self for a person who lives with an HIV infection.

The concluding contribution by Anne Koch and Karin Meissner, "Holistic Medicine in Late Modernity: Some Theses on the Efficacy of Spiritual

Healing," takes an interdisciplinary perspective that bridges the boundaries between cultural studies and the sciences. The authors return to the question about the conditions in which spiritual healing has a positive influence on subjective well-being. They confirm an increased interest in holistic medicine in various late modern traditions. "Holistic medicine or mind-body-medicine is not only a trend in the complementary and alternative medicine sector but also in the fields of alternative spirituality and Christian revivalism, where spiritual healing is very common ... On the one hand, holistic medicine encompasses complex complementary medical systems like homeopathy, Ayurveda, traditional Western medicines, and anthroposophical medicine as well as secularist treatments on the other." Instead of describing these approaches individually from a hermeneutical cultural studies perspective—as the other contributions to this volume do—this concluding contribution seeks to overcome the difference between understanding in a cultural studies perspective and explaining in the scientific perspective. In light of two empirical pilot studies the authors describe different factors at work in processes of spiritual healing. Processes of spiritual healing, which result in improved wellbeing, intensify embodied emotions, train the body knowledge, offer meaning, and reframe worldviews. "They rely on the effect of afferent emotionality and gain efficacy mediated by the regulating circuits of the reframing of emotions, cognitive evaluation and the emotional body-image. Efficacy depends to some degree on repeated and even regular practice, which can be followed by behavioral change (for example on work load, relationships, sportive profile)." The authors draw attention to "the resources that lay within holistic medicine and spiritual especially for public health-care." As a conclusion to the present collection, they thus raise awareness of the great potential of the individual religious traditions, which this volume presented and interpreted individually.

The present volume is a version of the book *Religion und Krankheit*, published 2010 by Wissenschaftliche Buchgesellschaft, Germany, which has been completely revised and expanded by several new contributions for this edition. Some contributions that are less relevant in English-speaking contexts, and in the United States especially, have been left out of the English edition. During our time as research associates in Heidelberg, we already worked on the subject "Illness and Healing in New Testament and Theological Perspectives." As a result of winning the Klaus-Georg and Sigrid Hengstberger Prize for Promising Scientists at the University of Heidelberg in 2006, we had the opportunity to host an interdisciplinary and international symposium on the subject "Religion and Medicine: Which Forms of Relationship are Life-Enhancing?" (Heidelberg 2008).

At the symposium, medical experts, historians of medicine, physicians, psychologists, gerontologists, historians of religion and of Islam especially, as well as theologians entered into dialogue. The present volume shares the goals of the symposium: (1) to discuss the fundamental relationship between medical and religious interpretations of disease in different cultures and (2) to gain criteria for a life-enhancing coupling of religion and the interpretation of illness.

Several people contributed to the development of this work, and we want to thank them here:

First, Klaus-Georg and Sigrid Hengstberger, who generously funded the Hengstberger Award for Heidelberg's up-and-coming academics, which enabled us to host the symposium. They also supported the present English translation of the conference volume with a considerable financial contribution. Our heartfelt thanks go out to both of them.

The production of this collection of essays is the result of close cooperative, multi-lateral research between various disciplines ranging across the spectrum from religion to medicine.

Our special thanks go to the translator of several essays, Emily Banwell, Berkeley and to Alexander Massmann, Heidelberg. We are particularly grateful to Prof. Dr. Polly Coote for proofreading every article and we thank especially the doctoral students Philip Erwin and Eric Sias (Berkeley, GTU) and Corinna Klodt (Osnabrück University) for their consistent assistance.

We also offer our gratitude to Wipf & Stock and Cascade Books for their support, and especially to Dr. K. C. Hanson, the editor in chief, for his competent guiding of this work to publication, their trust in the final product, and their readiness to publish an unusual volume. Please accept our deepest gratitude!

Annette Weissenrieder and Gregor Etzelmüller
San Anselmo/Max Weber Kolleg Erfurt and Osnabrück August 2014

PART 1

Religion, Illness, and Care of the Sick in Galen and in Islam

1

Religion and Therapy in Galen[1]

—Teun Tieleman

INTRODUCTION: GALEN AND "RATIONAL" MEDICINE

IT COULD BE SAID that rational medicine originated in Greece in the fifth century BCE, i.e. the time when the first treatises of the Hippocratic corpus were written. But this is no longer the simple statement of fact it used to be until, say, fifty years ago. Historical scholarship has become not only more anxious to avoid any Eurocentric bias but also more sensitive to the fuzziness of the appellation "rational." Today one is under the obligation to do more by way of specification of what one means when using the term with reference to the ancient Greek doctors.[2] But this having been noted, it does seem to be the case that in Greek medicine we see the beginning of rational thought most clearly in the discovery of disease as a *natural process*: a

---

1. This chapter is a slightly reworked version of Tieleman, "Religion und Therapie in Galen." I have taken the opportunity to add references to von Staden, "Galen's Daimon: Reflections on 'Irrational' and 'Rational,'" which had escaped my notice, and Brockmann, "Galen und Asklepios." In Tieleman, "Miracle and Natural Cause in Galen," I further explore the cosmological context of Galen's view on divine interventions.

2. Cf. the judicious observations by von Staden, "Galen's Daimon," 15–17. Among the studies that deal with the theme of rationality in Greek philosophy and science see e.g., the collection of studies in Frede and Striker, *Rationality in Greek Thought*. Longrigg, *Greek Rational Medicine*, despite its title, pays insufficient attention to the notion as applied to Greek medicine or at least its intellectually respectable echelons.

particular type of cause produces *as a rule* a particular type of effect, which drastically reduces the scope for divine intervention. This insight (which has a parallel in the thought of the earliest natural philosophers) was applied both to the occurrence of disease and to the healing process. A well-known early example is the explanation of epilepsy offered by the Hippocratic author of the *On the Sacred Disease* (later fifth century BCE), viz. that this affliction despite its name does not occur through any divine agency but occurs when the veins leading to the brain are blocked by a surplus of phlegm, thus depriving the brain of the necessary supply of air (ch. VII, pp. 14–16 Jouanna). The author stresses that each disease has a natural cause and delivers a critique of certain religious healers. Yet it would be rash to conclude that the author wishes to ban all religious thinking from medicine; rather he seems concerned to reject particular uses of religion in the theory and practice of medicine. Further, it is not certain whether individual gods are ruled out as *healers*, since the text is silent on this point.[3]

The reference to phlegm here attests to the Hippocratic doctors' bid to arrive at a general explanatory schema, viz. a physiological theory such as that of the four bodily humours (or the elementary qualities corresponding to them) whose imbalance is taken to cause particular diseases. To provide an explanation along these lines one has to reason from visible symptoms to unseen causes. Therapy, then, is directed at the causes in the sense that it is aimed at restoring the balance between the substances that are assumed to be causally involved in the diseased condition. It would be rash to conclude that this scientific spirit in its incipient stage must have entailed the abandonment of religion, at least in the minds of these pioneering scientists. Again as in the case of the earliest philosophers, the notion of the divine often is not abolished but rather purged of certain traditional and irrational elements, most notably anthropomorphism with its belief in emotionally motivated interventions by the gods in human affairs. But generalization in this area remains precarious since there are exceptions.[4] In sum, we should be wary of projecting present-day secularized ideals back on to the scientists and philosophers of classical Greece.

The explanatory schema we have just attributed to mainstream Hippocratic medicine can be described as an empirically based speculative theory about hidden causes. In Hellenistic times (from roughly the third century BCE onwards) this came to be seen as distinctive of the so-called "rational"

---

3. On the treatise and its author's attitude toward religious forms of healing see Lloyd, *Magic, Reason and Experience*, 15–29; cf. van der Eijk, "The 'Theology' of the Author of the Hippocratic Treatise *On the Sacred Disease*."

4. See the observations made by van der Eijk, "The 'Theology' of the Author of the Hippocratic Treatise *On the Sacred Disease*," 70–73, with further references.

or "rationalistic" (*logikos*) or "dogmatist" (*dogmatikos*) school of medicine. Its method presupposes the belief that human reason, if properly trained, is capable of discovering truths about the unseen. The same period—in which medical knowledge expanded considerably through the work of great anatomists such as Herophilus and Erasistratus—also saw the emergence of the Empiricist school of medicine which claimed that theory-formation involving hidden factors was not indispensable for, or even conducive to, therapeutic success. For the successful doctor experience suffices—experience, that is, of a rather passive kind in that it consists of the accumulation of clinical data: for a particular disease *x* cure *a* has repeatedly been observed to be effective, etc. Some though not all Empiricist physicians accepted the legitimacy of trying out cures of proven efficacy on patients struck by *similar* diseases (the "transition to the similar"). But for all of them dissection and anatomical experimentation (notably, vivisection) were useless for improving therapeutic prospects. Their attitude may seem striking after the advances in anatomical knowledge made by the great pioneers of anatomy, Herophilus and Erasistratus, such as the discovery of the nervous system and its workings. These scientists had profited from the exceptionally favourable circumstances offered by the Hellenistic kings at Alexandria (and perhaps, in Erasistratus' case, Antioch). Their path-breaking work reflects an intellectual atmosphere in which theoretical curiosity was given free rein—so much so that the inveterate taboo on dissecting human bodies was temporarily lifted—with impressive results. But their achievements seem to have been less compelling when it came to showing their *therapeutic* relevance. After all, it was argued by Empiricists, facts discovered about the dead body do not warrant any conclusions about the living organism. Likewise, interventions in the functioning of living bodies through vivisection experiments do not yield reliable information about their unmanipulated functioning. So the old taboo on human dissection received a methodological justification. In consequence, it remained limited to a brief span of time (first half third century) and one location (Alexandria). This is not to say that their work lacked influence. For one thing, the practice of dissection was continued by others, albeit on animal material. Furthermore, it must have contributed to a further demythologization of the human body and the rise of a human biology in a more modern sense. Yet any conclusions about the disappearance of religion from medicine would be rash.[5]

---

5. Cf. von Staden, *Herophilus*, 7–8, 25–26. On whether Herophilus' statement that "drugs are the hands of the gods" (T 248a–c) can be taken as an expression of the belief in the gods' healing powers cf. von Staden, *Herophilus*, 8, 400. Note that Herophilus, like Galen, accepted the belief in god-inspired dreams: see von Staden, *Herophilus*, 306ff.

In the second century ce an influential compromise was struck by Galen of Pergamon (129–c. 213), who alongside Hippocrates may count as one of the two towering figures of ancient medicine in view of his voluminous writings and their later influence on western medicine. Galen wanted to practise the art of medicine in the Hippocratic tradition. But he had to adopt a position in the *methodological controversy* among the medical schools, including that between Rationalist and Empiricist medicine, that had been going on since Hellenistic times. His compromise consists of an attempt to establish a method which combines "reason" and "experience" as much as possible. Galen is hostile to dogmatist speculation of the kind that is ill-founded, i.e. unsupported by experiential data. But if checked by experience, theorizing about unseen causes is permissible and indeed indispensable. Experience for Galen includes the procedures of dissection and anatomical experimentation (performed on animals), which of course is a Rationalist feature. Likewise the use of "reason" as required by Galen refers not merely to the sound mind's ability to grasp what is obvious or to logical consistency but to "technical" or trained reason, i.e. to the use of logical methods such as definition and the method of division (diaeresis) that had been developed in the philosophical tradition and require extensive training on the part of the aspiring physician.[6] Galen recognized that the scientist can study sensible phenomena only by bringing to them conceptual tools for ordering them; sensible reality can only be explained on the basis of questions preconceived by the trained mind. In his own researches a logical stage of formulating assumptions is typically followed by one of testing these assumptions in the light of empirical data, whether provided by simple perception or by dissection and complicated experimental procedures. When such testing is impossible, then it is preferable to abstain from pronouncing upon the matter at issue or at least to qualify one's view as at best more plausible than others. But in fact the issues that belong to this category are precisely those that are not useful to know for scientific progress anyway, that is to say, in the case of medicine, for improving people's physical health, nor are they useful for moral improvement. Thus Galen's rejection of dogmatist speculation comes with an insistence on practical utility. In this connection he notes that it is precisely issues of the speculative kind which have caused doctors and philosophers alike to become divided into different "sects" (*haireseis*) or schools: for example, the substance of the soul, or God, or whether the world has been created or is eternal.

It is typical of the sectarian attitude to cling to the dogmas of one's school regardless of evidence that points to the contrary. Adherents of

---

6. On Galen's methodology see now Tieleman, "Methodology."

schools do so because they rely on the authority of the head or founder. This can be seen to apply to the attitude of many scientists and philosophers—a situation which constitutes a serious obstacle to scientific and moral progress.[7] This phenomenon can also be observed in religion and in particular among Jews and Christians, who, likewise, accept their laws and tenets on the authority of Moses or Christ.[8] Instead one should follow the "school of Nature." For Galen, there is a divine aspect to Nature—in this light it would be misleading to call Galen's position naturalistic in any modern sense. Thus in his *On the Use of Parts* Galen sets out to sing the praises of divine Nature by revealing its wondrous works, all of which display beauty and purposefulness down to the smallest details. Dissection thus becomes an act of piety, as he makes clear at the end of book III of this work (*UP* III. 10, p. 237 Kühn, vol. I, p. 174 Helmreich).

But there is also another side to Galen's religiosity, which is more personal and less philosophical. It is a side more closely connected with his native city of Pergamon and his ancestors, viz. the cult of the healing god Asclepius.[9] It is also a dimension that belongs in therapeutic contexts, i.e. those passages that do not deal with infallible and purposeful Nature but on the contrary with those cases where Nature seems to reveal imperfection. Even so, we are not dealing with two unrelated and irreconcilable sets of passages. In what follows I hope to show how and why this is the case with reference to a number of passages that illustrate the relation between therapy and religion in Galen.

GALEN'S ATTITUDE TOWARDS RELIGION: A KEY PASSAGE FROM *ON MY OWN OPINIONS*

The first passage to be considered is from Galen's treatise *On My Own Opinions*, a complete Greek text of which has been discovered only recently.[10] This work of Galen's old age has been described as his philosophical testament.[11] Looking back at his career Galen informs his readers about his latest

---

7. For Galen's attitude to arguments from authority see e.g., *PHP* II, 3.8–11; II, 4.3–4, III, 8.35; V, 7.83–84 De Lacy.

8. See Walzer, *Galen on Jews and Christians*; and Tieleman, "Galen and Genesis," and *infra*, p. 26.

9. The standard collection remains that of Edelstein and Edelstein, *Asclepius*.

10. Edited by Boudon-Millot and Pietrobelli, "Galien ressuscité: Édition princeps du texte Grec du *De propriis placitis*"; see further *infra*, n. 14.

11. Nutton, "Galen's Philosophical Testament."

thoughts on a number of key issues in the philosophy and medicine of his day. In chapter 2 we read what he has to say on the subject of God:

> I declare I do not know whether the universe is uncreated or created and whether or not there is anything outside it. Since I disclaim knowledge of such things, it will be clear that I do so also with regard to the nature of the creator (*dêmiourgos*) of everything in the universe, i.e. whether he is corporeal or incorporeal, and still more with regard to the place in which he resides. So about the gods, too, I profess doubt (*aporein*), as Protagoras did,[12] or I say also in their case that I do not know what their substance is like but that I do know that they exist from their actions. They are the designers of the constitution of all animals. They warn us about future events through significant utterances,[13] omens and dreams. The god who is revered in my own birthplace Pergamon [scil. Asclepius] showed his power and providence on many occasions but also by curing me once. I know from experience both the providence and the power of the Dioscuri at sea.[14] However, people are in my opinion in no way hindered by the fact that they are ignorant of the substance of the gods, but I decided to honour them following ancestral tradition and in line with the advice given by Socrates to obey the orders of the Pythian one [scil. Apollo]. This is the attitude I take towards religious matters.[15]

Quite in line with his theory of science Galen withholds judgement on theological questions such as God's substance that cannot be resolved through

---

12. Cf. Protagoras fr. B 4 Diels-Kranz. But Protagoras here expresses doubt about the *existence* of the gods, which Galen accepts as certain in what follows. This could explain why Galen goes on to make his point more precise: it is the divine substance one cannot know.

13. *Klēdonōn*: viz. something said by people which turns out to be of a significance they had not intended and which therefore is attributed to a divine source; cf. *infra*, n. 20.

14. The divine Dioscuri ("sons of Zeus") were "saviors" of humans in a variety of spheres and in particular at sea where their presence in storm was visible in the electric discharge known as St Elmo's fire.

15. This translation is based upon the new edition by Boudon-Millot and Pietrobelli, "Galien ressuscité: Édition princeps du texte Grec du De propriis placitis," which profits from the find in 2005 of the first Greek text of this treatise in MS Vlatadon 14 in Thessaloniki. So far only a fragment in Greek was available and the treatise had to be reconstructed on the basis of Latin, Hebrew and Arabic versions on which V. Nutton's 1999 edition in the *CMG*-series (*Galen: On My Own Opinions*) is based. In the case of our passage the differences between the non-Greek versions and what is offered by Vlatadon 14 are from our perspective crucial due to the tendency of Arabic and Christian translators to suppress references to polytheism.

empirical means. But then, he adds a little further on, we do not *need* to know such things anyway—an equally typical point.[16] Yet, his is what may be called a regionalized skepticism. It is clear that he has no doubt about the existence of God, or the gods, which can be inferred from their observable[17] *actions*. Galen refers to three types of actions: (1) the creation of living things; (2) the disclosure of what lies in store for us through signs and dreams; (3) life-saving interventions. Apart from proving their existence, these actions reveal the power and providence of the gods. It is worth noting that Galen thinks only of benevolent influence coming from the gods. This may seem less obvious with regard to (1), but Galen's point seems to be that the beautiful and purposeful design displayed by living beings (note the term "constitution") can only be explained by reference to a divine creator. What he indicates here briefly is what he sets out extensively and in great detail in his *On the Use of Parts* and elsewhere.[18] The idea of the divine creator as a craftsman (*dêmiourgos*), as we have noticed, derives from the Platonic *Timaeus* with which Galen was intimately familiar (although he also reflects its later reception in those passages where he presents Nature itself as craftsman-like.) Indeed, Galen's agnostic attitude to the Creator's nature had also been anticipated by Plato.[19] The fact that Galen goes on to speak of gods in the plural as having created all living beings does not necessarily mean that he moves away from the *Timaeus* and its divine Craftsman. In the Platonic account the Demiurge does not create mankind directly but entrusts the lesser gods (i.e. the traditional Homeric pantheon) with this task (41d).[20] The switches between the singular and the plural reflect a more common ("henotheistic") way of referring to the divine in Galen as in so many other ancient authors, for whom it was possible to think both of an all-encompassing deity and of its many concretizations that are reconcilable with traditional polytheism. Galen expresses his acceptance of traditional

16. The distinction drawn by Galen between speculative and non-speculative parts of theology in the first half of the passage echoes *PHP* IX 7. 15–16 De Lacy, where too it is argued that divine providence is both rationally acceptable and useful to know. In this context Galen also appeals to the Platonic *Timaeus* as well as to Socrates with reference to Xenophon, *Memorabilia* I, 1,11–16.

17. Note the reference to personal *experience* in regard to the intervention of the Dioscuri.

18. The text strongly recalls passages such as *UP* VII, 14.1, pp. 418.19—419.8 Helmreich (= III. 576–77 K.) where Galen argues that his anatomical researches reveal the power, providence and wisdom of the creator of animals.

19. *Tim.* 28c, 40d; cf. 29c.

20. Out of humans the other animals will come into being in the cycle of reincarnation. Similarly Sen. *Ep.* 44.4 refers to the creation of the earliest human by gods in the plural in a passage that may reflect the *Timaeus* as well (cf. esp. 40d).

religious worship at the end of the passage: this is motivated both by personal experience of divine agency and by the authority of the arch-philosopher Socrates who "followed the orders of Apollo."[21] To my knowledge Galen's experience of the intervention by the Dioscuri in life-threatening circumstances at sea has no parallel in the extant work, whereas the reference to the cure performed on him by Asclepius does occur elsewhere. In fact, further passages show it was not the only instance of the intervention of this god at a crucial moment in Galen's life. To this group of testimonies I will turn now.

GALEN AND ASCLEPIUS

In two passages Galen informs us that while he was studying philosophy in Pergamon his father was told in dreams to have his son study medicine as well:

> When I was sixteen, my father was prompted by clear dreams to make me study medicine alongside philosophy (*On the Order of My Books* 4, *SM* II, p.88 Müller). And: [Eudemus][22] had also heard that when my father was introducing me to philosophy, he had been commanded by unambiguous dreams to educate me thoroughly in medicine, not just as a hobby. (*On Prognosis* 2, 12 Nutton)

We are meant to understand that these dreams came from Asclepius, the god of medicine whose main cultic centre was in Pergamon, although one may speculate why Galen does not name him.[23] But clearly, so we are given

---

21. The reference must be to *Apology* 23b–c; cf. 21b. Cf. the parallel reference at *Adhortatio* ch. 9, I. 22 K. = 9.7, pp. 101.21–102.1 Boudon; for examples of the value attached by Galen to Apollo's oracular pronouncements cf. *Prop. an dign cur.* V, p. 4 K., *MM* XIV, X, p.11 K. At *Praen.* 3.17, p.88.2–7 Nutton the philosopher Eudemus, who is successfully treated by Galen, praises the latter's powers of prognosis by exclaiming that "Apollo deigned to prophesy to the sick through Galen's mouth, and then to treat them and to cure them completely on the day predicted." On the context cf. Nutton *ad loc.*, Schlange-Schöningen, *Die römische Gesellschaft bei Galen*, 225. For Galen the significance of Eudemus' statement may have gone beyond that of a simple compliment; cf. *supra*, n.10 with text thereto. The cult of Apollo the healer (*iatros*) was widespread. Galen often links him with Asclepius: see e.g., *Praen.* 10.16 p.124.19–20 Nutton (medicine worthy of Apollo and Asclepius); similarly *Protr.* 1.12.

22. Eudemus was a family friend and Peripatetic philosopher who helped Galen find his way in Rome during the latter's first Roman period, see. *Praen.* 2.1, p. 74.12–17 Nutton and prev. n. It has been plausibly suggested that he is identical to the Peripatetic philosopher who taught young Galen Aristotelian philosophy in Pergamon: cf. *Aff. Dign.* V, p.41 K. (= *CMG* V 4.1.1.28) and Tieleman, "Galen and the Stoics."

23. See Schlange-Schöningen, *Die römische Gesellschaft bei Galen*, 73 ff. who

to understand, Galen's career as a medical theorist and practitioner was divinely sanctioned from the start. Thus these passages bear out what Galen says in the above passage from *On My Own Opinions* about prophetic dreams as one of the means by which the gods help humans.[24]

During his first Roman sojourn (162–166 CE) Galen had performed a series of spectacular cures and anatomical demonstrations, through which he had drawn upon himself the attention of the Roman élite. Although he had abruptly left Rome for Pergamon in the summer of 166, the reputation he had earned for himself led to his being summoned by the emperors Marcus Aurelius and Lucius Verus to come their headquarters in Aquileia in Northern Italy, where they were preparing a military campaign against the Germans along the Danube in the winter of 168/9.[25] Thus Galen was added to the team of court-physicians. The preparations for war were delayed by the sudden illness and death of Lucius Verus. The emperor and his court returned to Rome for the funeral. After that Marcus Aurelius took up again his preparations for his campaign. The following conversation between him and Galen took place:

> [The emperor] occupied himself with the campaign against the Germans, considering it of the utmost importance that I should accompany him. But he let himself be persuaded to exempt me when I told him that the opposite had been ordained by my ancestral god, Asclepius, whose servant[26] I had declared myself ever since the day he saved me from a fatal disease, viz. an ulcer. Out of reverence for the god he ordered me to wait for his return ... (*On My Own Books* XIX 18–19 K = *SM* II, p. 99 Müller)

---

suggests that Galen's father's decision was motivated by the Emperor Hadrian's religious policy. In Pergamon this led to the building of a new temple for Asclepius whose cult may have been connected with that of the Emperor himself. Schlange-Schöningen further suggests that by not naming Asclepius Galen in the passages at issue avoids association with the more magical aspects of the Asclepius cult in Pergamon, but this is speculation. Galen has no qualms about invoking dreams of his father when explaining this turning point in his life. Cf. Boudon, "Galien et le sacré," and Boudon-Millot, *Galien de Pergame*, 19–21.

24. See on the ancient belief in prophetic dreams as shared by Galen also Nutton, *Galen On Prognosis*, 135–40; cf. also *UP* X, 12: III 812–13 K. = II, 93.5–10 Helmreich.

25. Galen's life and career are comparatively well documented by passages in his own voluminous writings in particular—save for the last two decades. For a survey of the most important facts see now Hankinson, "The Man and His Work."

26. This term is used in a general sense; we need not infer that Galen fulfilled any specific cultic function: see Schlange-Schöningen, *Die römische Gesellschaft bei Galen*, 78–79; cf. Brockmann, "Galen und Asklepios," 55.

That Galen did not accompany the emperor to the Danube provided Galen's professional rivals with a welcome opportunity to accuse him of cowardice. A few modern historians too have spoken of a clever move on Galen's part.[27] But the very fact that Galen has no qualms about telling this suggests that he was sincere about his experience of divine guidance, just as Marcus Aurelius took him seriously.[28] To be sure, part of the reason why he tells it may precisely be to justify himself in the face of the charge of cowardice, but this too does not necessarily imply any insincerity. We may note that he refers to his close and long-standing relationship with Asclepius, which is related not only to his Pergamenian family background but also to what appears to be the same cure he ascribes to the god in the passage from *On My Own Opinions* we have just discussed (see above, p. 20) and which is here specified as the curing of a ulcer.[29] So Asclepius not only destined him for a medical career in his service but also watched over him so that he lived to continue that service. But Asclepius is also credited with guiding the way Galen treated his patients:

> I was led by two clear dreams I received to the artery between the thumb and index finger of my right hand and I let the blood flow until it stopped of itself, just as the dream had ordered ...
> (*How to Cure People through Bloodletting* 23, XI pp. 314–15 K.)

Again we come across the important role of divine dream-communication, which is by no means peculiar to Galen but quite in line with widespread Graeco-Roman religious belief.[30] Most intellectuals too ascribed prophetic significance at least to certain kinds of dream. We must note the recurring emphasis upon the required clarity of the dream; moreover, the dream repeated itself, just as Galen's father was visited by the same dream-message more than once.

It would be mistaken to see Galen here as the mere instrument of Asclepius; the latter's influence enhances rather than reduces Galen's merit.

---

27. Nutton, *Galen: On Prognosis*, 211–12; Hankinson, "The Man and His Work," 15; more empathically Boudon-Millot, *Galien*, vol. 1, *Introduction Générale*, 196.

28. For Marcus' reverence for Asclepius see his *Meditations* V 8.1 and 3; cf. VI 43.1; *Ep. ad Front.* III,9 (p. 43 van Hout). Cf. Boudon-Millot, *Galien de Pergame*, 19.

29. Cf. *On the Juices in Foodstuffs* (*Bon. Mal. Suc.* VI, p. 755–57 K.), where Galen reports on a health problem he suffered from when he was 18 and 19 years of age and which culminated in an ulcer. Galen recovered by drastically reducing the kinds of fruit he ate but here he does not attribute this therapeutic measure to the inspiration of Asclepius. Yet the gravity of his condition as reported here does suggest that we are dealing with the same illness as is referred to in the passages from *On My Own Opinons* and *On My Own Books*.

30. Oberhelman, "Dreams in Graeco-Roman Medicine."

Further, the cure suggested by the god is not of the irrational or paradoxical kind (as they often are in stories of miraculous healings by the same god from other sources) but follows from Galen's own system of medicine in which blood-letting played a considerable role.[31] The agreement between "rational" medical science and Asclepian inspiration can further be illustrated by passages such as the following:

> Another wealthy man, this one not a native but from the interior of Thrace, came to Pergamon because a dream had prompted him to do so. The dream appeared to him, the god prescribing that he should drink every day of the drug produced from the vipers and should anoint the body from the outside. The disease [i.e. elephantiasis] after a few days turned into leprosy; and this disease, in turn, was cured by the drugs which the god commanded (*Outline of Empiricism* 10, p.78 Deichgräber).[32]

From the context (where similar cases are reported) it is clear that it is Galen and his team who cure the disease into which the first, incurable disease has turned by following the instructions from the divine world. The procedure of effecting such a change was part of the doctor's therapeutic repertoire too. So it turns out that, at least in the pages of Galen, the god has studied medicine. Accordingly, it also constitutes an example of the god and the doctor working in concert.

That the god was also acquainted with Platonic psychology, to which Galen subscribed, appears from the following passage, which is concerned with the treatment of mental and psychosomatic disorders:

> A very important witness is also our ancestral god, Asclepius, who often prescribed the composition of poems, mimes and songs to people in whom the movements of the spirited part [scil. of the soul] had become too vehement and had made their bodily temperament hotter than it should be. (*On the Preservation of Health* 1, 8, 20 = *CMG* V, 4, 2, p. 20; K VI, 40)

Here the "spirited (*thymoeides*) part" of the soul is a distinctively Platonic feature, belonging as it does to the theory of the tripartition and trilocation of the soul as set out in the *Republic*, *Phaedrus* and (adding the trilocation) the *Timaeus*: reason in the brain, will-power (i.e. the "spirited part") in the heart, appetite in the belly (further specified by Galen as the liver)—a schema which is defended by Galen on the basis of post-Platonic physiological

---

31. See Brain, *Galen on Blood-Letting*.
32. Similarly *Simpl. med. temp. et fac.* 11, 1,1, XII, pp. 313 ff. K.

and anatomical observations in works such as *On the Doctrines of Hippocrates and Plato*.³³

The Jewish-Christian notion of divine omnipotence and miracles should not be allowed to obscure the basis for this striking relationship between "rational" medicine and divine intervention, viz. the fact that God, or the gods, are subject to the natural laws; or put in a more positive way, the gods are part of Nature, or in yet another way, the gods represent the divine aspect of Nature. Consider the following passage:

> Some constitutions are right from birth so weak that they cannot reach the age of sixty even if Asclepius himself were to attend them. (*On the Preservation of Health* 1, 12, 15 = CMG V, 4, 2, p. 29; K. VI, 63)

Certain things are impossible by nature and so with God. But this should not be construed as a statement of his irrelevance. Galen was sensitive to the fact that this constituted a crucial difference between his position, which had been informed by Greek intellectual tradition starting from the Platonic *Timaeus* in particular, on the one hand, and Jewish-Christian beliefs on the other. This is attested by the following passage:

> It is precisely this point in which our own opinion and that of Plato and the other Greeks who follow the right method in science differ from the position taken by Moses. For the latter it seems enough to say that God simply willed the arrangement of matter and instantaneously it was arranged; for he believes everything to be possible with God, even should he wish to make a bull or a horse out of ashes. We however do not hold this; we say that certain things are impossible by nature and that God does not attempt such things at all but that he chooses the best out of the possibilities of becoming. (*On the Usefulness of Parts* XI, ch. 14 = Vol. II, pp. 158–60 Helmreich).³⁴

So too in the case of people who are very weak by constitution, we may infer, Asclepius would not even attempt to cure them. Obviously, there is a tension between Galen's view of the world as marked by intelligent design, his rather robust brand of teleology, on the one hand, and his experience as a doctor of diseases and disabilities, on the other. The two above passages

---

33. For a full discussion see Tieleman, *Galen and Chrysippus on the Soul*, Part I.

34. For a full recent discussion of this passage see Tieleman, "Galen and Genesis." The evidence for Galen's response to Jewish-Christian beliefs and practices has been assembled and discussed by Walzer, *Galen on Jews and Christians*; cf. also Schlange-Schöningen, *Die römische Gesellschaft bei Galen*, 247–49.

however suggest how Galen could accommodate both design and imperfection within a predominantly Platonic framework.[35]

But, we may wonder, what was Galen's attitude towards the fact that the temple medicine as practised in Pergamon and elsewhere could hardly be reconciled with the medical tradition on which he drew and from which he had constructed his own system of medicine? The belief in divine prescriptions that are paradoxical and at odds with "regular" medicine appears to be at issue in the following passage that has given rise to diverging interpretations:

> We see that those who put themselves under the care of the god obey him when he prescribes that they should not drink for fifteen days and drink nothing whatsoever while refusing to obey any doctor. (*Commentary on the Sixth Book of Hippocrates' Epidemics* 4,8, p.199 Wenkebach)

The remarkable thing about this passage is that Galen does not seem to distance himself from the seemingly paradoxical and indeed, it would seem, fatal prescription not to drink for such a long period. But it has been pointed out that the prescription does not exclude the taking of food rich in juices. Galen suppresses the irrational manifestations of the Asclepius cult as much as possible and the above passage cannot be taken as offering a critique of it. As Schlange-Schöningen has observed, what is at stake here is rather Galen's wish to underline the importance of the doctor's authority.[36] His example of the prescription given by Asclepius is intended to show that patients are obedient if the authority of the one who gives the prescription is above question. They turned out to be quite capable of restraining natural desires, as this drastic but (at least for Galen) not harmful and eventually salutary prescription is meant to demonstrate.

In this connection it is worth noting a psychological and social aspect, viz. that of (medical) authority.[37] Asclepius initiates Galen's therapy, I submit, because Galen feels the need for divine backing. Ancient doctors had always faced the problem of authority and legitimacy, given the way the study and practice of medicine was organized or rather was unorganized, without officially recognized requirements, qualifications and degrees. Asclepius' authority, as we have seen, is above suspicion, so the doctor has to

---

35. On Galen's teleology see Hankinson, "Galen and the Best of All Possible Worlds"; on "failing nature" and Galen's concept of medicine see Vegetti, "L'immagine del medico," 1714–16.

36. Schlange-Schöningen, *Die römische Gesellschaft bei Galen*, 227–29; cf. Kudlien, "Galen's Religious Belief," 124–25.

37. On this aspect see also Brockmann, "Galen und Asklepios," 31.

become like him in this respect also. So the god turns doctor and operates in line with Galenic medicine on the one hand and the human doctor develops a special and close relationship with the god on the other. This is why Galen stresses the god's role at crucial points in his biography. I do not mean to detract from his sincerity by suggesting a psychological perspective. From such a perspective Galen's attitude may reveal a deep need for confirmation, especially in therapeutic contexts. It is true that Galen is known for his rejection of the reliance upon authority (witness, e.g., his criticism of the Mosaic account of creation which has to be accepted on his authority alone: see above, p. 26), but for him there is no contradiction because, as we have seen, what the god does or orders is always and in principle in full accordance with what can be scientifically demonstrated to be true.

Galen's identification with Asclepius also had philosophical legitimation and respectability. The standard formula of the Platonic end (telos) of life, which became prominent in later antiquity, was that of the assimilation to god (homoiōsis tōi theōi). For Galen, Plato was the greatest philosopher—although he refused to become an adherent of any philosophical school including the Platonist one. But this view of the telos was of significance to him also, as a few passages from his work indicate.[38] In this connection we must note that its meaning is not confined to the assimilation to the divine cosmos in the way that was stipulated by the Platonic Timaeus[39] but that in the famous Phaedrus myth, with its image of the procession of individual Olympian gods and human souls on the edge of the cosmic sphere: at 252c–253c, the souls in the procession are portrayed as aspiring to become more and more like the particular gods whom they revere, by adopting their particular customs, habits and ways of living. Each of the souls that follows a particular god in the procession "lives, so far as he is able, honouring and imitating that god"—which is precisely what Galen did in his relationship with Asclepius. Thus Galen in his *Exhortation to Medicine* 3.3, p.87.13–18

---

38. See esp. *Aff. Dign.* V, p.11 K., where he mentions the Platonist *telos* while stressing that one does not become similar to a god overnight. Even so, there is by no means an unbridgeable gap between man and god: see, e.g., *Protr.* 9,6, p. 101.17–21 Boudon (I, pp. 22 K.), where Galen leaves open the possibility that Asclepius himself was human before becoming deified.

39. Of course, the relevant passages from the *Timaeus*, most notably 90a2–c2, cited by Galen, *On Habits* (*De consuetudinibus*), pp. 26–27 Müller, SM II, where Plato introduces the idea of the human intellect as the divine part of our soul and so as the "inner *daimōn*," i.e. —an idea that was taken over and further developed by the Stoics: see, e.g., Diog. Laert. 7.88 (*SVF* III, 4, based on Chrysippus' *On Ends*); Posidonius *ap.* Gal. *PHP* V, 6.4–6, pp. 326 De Lacy (= Posid. F 187, p. 170, 3–9 E.-K.). See Von Staden, "Galen's daimon," 32–38, whose observations converge with what I have to say on Galen's tendency towards identification with Asclepius in particular.

Boudon (I, p.5 Kühn) echoes the Phaedrus passage in contrasting devotion to a provident deity with a life dedicated to following Fortune:

> You could see his devotees being as cheerful as the god who leads them and never complaining about him as the adherents of Fortune do, and never being left behind or separated [scil. from him], but following him and constantly enjoying his providence.[40]

CONCLUDING REMARKS

Galen assimilates God as the all-encompassing cosmic and creative power with Asclepius, the healing god, in line with the contemporary rise in importance of Asclepius, as evident from the title and worship of Zeus Asclepius. The act of creation is not limited to the beginning of the cosmos (in fact, as we have noticed, Galen adopts an agnostic stance on this traditional issue in the interpretation of the Platonic Timaeus), but God continues the creative process, that is to say, continues to exert his influence so as to maintain the world and the creatures in it. This appears to include a healing influence, which however does not go against nature.[41] In fact, the divine is assimilated to if not identified with nature. This explains why Galen is able to reconcile his belief in Asclepius with a system of medicine that is based on the notion of natural processes and so natural laws. Moreover, the idea of divine Nature (which is indebted to mainstream Greek philosophy: Plato, Aristotle, the Stoics) does not preclude concrete instantiations of the divine that are more compatible with traditional religion and more personal forms of religious experience and reverence. This puts Galen in a position to espouse and take part in the Asclepius cult of his native city and his ancestors. Moreover, we have found indications of a strong personal devotion linked to a need for confirmation Galen felt in making therapeutic choices and exercising authority as a medical practitioner.

---

40. On Galen's familiarity with, and use of, the Platonic *Phaedrus* see also De Lacy, "Galen's Platonism," 30, 37; on its role in second-century CE culture in general see Trapp, "Plato's Phaedrus in Second-century Greek Literature."

41. On healing as (re-creation) and Galen's notion of God see further Tieleman, "Miracle and Natural Cause in Galen," 108–9.

BIBLIOGRAPHY

Boudon-Millot, Véronique, ed. and trans. *Galien*. Vol. 1, *Introduction Générale; Sur l'ordre de ses propres livres; Sur ses propres Livres; Que l'excellent médecin est aussi philosophe*. Collection des universités de France, Série grecque 402. Paris: Les Belles Lettres, 2003.

———. *Galien de Pergame: Un médecin grec à Rome*. Histoire 117. Paris: Les Belles Lettres, 2012.

———. "Galien et le sacré." *Bulletin de l'Association Guillaume Budé*, n° 4 (Lettres d'Humanité XLVII) (1988) 327–37.

Boudon-Millot, Véronique, and Antoine Pietrobelli. "Galien ressuscité: Édition princeps du texte Grec du *De propriis placitis*." *Revue des Études Grecques* 118 (2005) 168–213.

Brain. Peter. *Galen on Blood-Letting: A Study of the Origins, Development and Validity of His Opinions, with a Translation of the Three Works*. Cambridge: Cambridge University Press, 1986.

Brockmann, Christian. "Galen und Asklepios." *ZAC* 17.1 (2013) 51–67.

De Lacy, Phillip H. "Galen's Platonism." *American Journal of Philology* 93 (Studies in Honor of Henry T. Rowell) (1972) 27–39.

Edelstein, Emma Jeannette, and Ludwig Edelstein. *Asclepius: A Collection and Interpretation of the Testimonies*. 2 vols. Baltimore: John Hopkins University Press, 1975.

Eijk, Philip J. van der. "The 'Theology' of the Author of the Hippocratic Treatise *On the Sacred Disease*." In *Medicine and Philosophy in Classical Antiquity: Doctors and Philosophers on Nature, Soul, Health and Disease*, edited by Philip J. van der Eijk, 45–74. Cambridge: Cambridge University Press, 2005. Reprinted with postscript from an article published in *Apeiron* 23 (1990) 87–119.

Frede, Michael. "Galen's Theology." In *Galien et la philosophie*, edited by J. Barnes and J. Jouanna, 73–129. Entretiens sur l'antiquité classique 49. Geneva: Fondation Hardt, 2003.

Frede, Michael, and Gisela Striker. *Rationality in Greek Thought*. Oxford: Clarendon, 1996.

Hankinson, R. J., ed. *The Cambridge Companion to Galen*. Cambridge Companions. Cambridge: Cambridge University Press, 2008.

———. "Galen and the Best of All Possible Worlds." *Classical Quarterly* 39 (1989) 206–27.

———. "The Man and His Work." In *The Cambridge Companion to Galen*, edited by R. J. Hankinson, 1–33. Cambridge: Cambridge University Press, 2008.

Kudlien, Fridolf. "Galen's Religious Belief." In *Galen: Problems and Prospects. A Collection of Papers Submitted at the 1979 Cambridge Conference*, edited by Vivian Nutton, 117–30. London: Wellcome Institute, 1981.

Lloyd, G. E. R. *Magic, Reason and Experience: Studies in the Origins and Development of Greek Science*. Cambridge: Cambridge University Press, 1979.

Longrigg, James. *Greek Rational Medicine: Philosophy and Medicine from Alcmaeon to the Alexandrians*. London: Routledge, 1993.

Nutton, Vivian. *Ancient Medicine*. Sciences of Antiquity. London: Routledge, 2004.

———, ed. and trans. *Galen: On My Own Opinions*. CMG V 3,2. Berlin: Akademie, 1999.

———, ed. and trans. *Galen: On Prognosis*. CMG V 8,1. Berlin: Akademie, 1979.

―――. "Galen's Philosophical Testament." In *Aristoteles—Werk und Wirkung 2: Kommentierung, Überlieferung, Nachleben*, edited by J. Wiesner, 2:27–51. Berlin: de Gruyter, 1987.
Oberhelman, Steven M. "Dreams in Graeco-Roman Medicine." In *ANRW* II, 37, 1 (1993) 121–56.
Schlange-Schöningen, Heinrich. *Die römische Gesellschaft bei Galen*. Untersuchungen zur antiken Literatur und Geschichte 65. Berlin: de Gruyter, 2003.
Staden, Heinrich von. "Galen's Daimon: Reflections on 'Irrational' and 'Rational.'" In *Rationnel et irrationel dans la médicine ancienne et médiévale: Aspects historiques, scientifiques et culturels*, edited by N. Palimieri, 15–44. Centre Jean Palerne Mémoires 26. Saint-Étienne: Publications de l'université de Saint-Étienne, 2003.
―――. *Herophilus: The Art of Medicine in Early Alexandria. Edition, Translation, and Essays*. Cambridge: Cambridge University Press, 1989.
Strohmaier, Gotthard. "Galen als Vertreter der Gebildetenreligion seiner Zeit." In *Neue Beiträge zur Geschichte der alten Welt*. Vol. 2, *Römisches Reich*, edited by Elisabeth Charlotte Welskopf, 375–80. Berlin: Akademie, 1965.
Tieleman, Teun. *Galen and Chrysippus on the Soul: Argument and Refutation in the De Placitis Books II–III*. Philosophia antiqua 68. Leiden: Brill, 1996.
―――. "Galen and Genesis." In *The Creation of Heaven and Earth: Re-interpretations of Genesis I in the Context of Judaism, Ancient Philosophy, Christianity, and Modern Physics*, edited by George H. van Kooten, 125–45. Themes in Biblical Narrative 8. Leiden: Brill, 2005.
―――. "Galen and the Stoics. Or: The Art of not Naming." In *Galen and the World of Knowledge*, edited by Christopher Gill, Tim Whitmarsh, and John Wilkins, 282–99. Greek Culture in the Roman World. Cambridge: Cambridge University Press, 2009.
―――. "Methodology." In *The Cambridge Companion to Galen*, edited by R. J. Hankinson, 49–65. Cambridge Companions. Cambridge: Cambridge University Press, 2008.
―――. "Miracle and Natural Cause in Galen." In *Miracles Revisited: New Testament Miracle Stories and Their Concepts of Reality*, edited by Stefan Alkier and Annette Weissenrieder, 101–15. Studies on the Bible and Its Reception 1. Berlin: de Gruyter, 2013.
―――. "Religion und Therapie in Galen." In *Religion und Krankheit*, edited by Annette Weissenrieder and Gregor Etzelmüller, 83–95. Darmstadt: Wissenschaftliche Buchgesellschaft, 2010.
Trapp, Michael B. "Plato's Phaedrus in Second-century Greek Literature." In *Antonine Literature*, edited by D. A. Russell, 141–73. Oxford: Clarendon, 1990.
Vegetti, Mario. "L'immagine del medico e lo statuto epistemologico della medicina in Galeno." In *ANRW* II.37.2 (1994) 1672–717. Reprinted in *Dialoghi con gli antichi*, 227–78. Berlin: Akademia 2007.
Walzer, Richard. *Galen on Jews and Christians*. Oxford Classical & Philosophical Monographs. London: Oxford University Press, 1949.

2

Galenism Caught between Faith in God and "Prophetic Medicine" in Islam[1]

—Gotthard Strohmaier

In 1986, a slim volume appeared from well-known publishers Routledge & Kegan Paul, titled *Islamic Medicine*;[2] the author, Muhammad Salim Khan, is a Muslim physician living in England. A prospective buyer might expect the book to contain alternative healing practices, in the style of Chinese acupuncture, that a conventional physician could include in his therapeutic offerings. However, the author's ambitions are greater than that; his *Islamic Medicine*, "the medicine of the future," is contrasted with the over-technologized and super-specialized form of European medicine that no longer considers the patient as a whole person. Like food restrictions, he sees it as part of Sharia law. He describes the general state of health in the original community of Medina, which he says was "wonderful" thanks to the instructions of the Prophet, and he criticizes Arab governments that—corrupted by Western influence—have denied the traditional healing arts their right to exist. This backward-looking utopia is also part of the ideology of terrorists; therefore the historical research showing how things really were is of strategic significance.[3]

What are the basic features of this "medicine of the future"? According to this philosophy, the world consists of four elements: earth, water, air and

1. See Strohmaier, *Zwischen Islamismus und Eurozentrismus*, 67–76.
2. Khan, *Islamic Medicine*.
3. Strohmaier, "Medizin- und Wissenschaftsgeschichte der Islamisten," 23–30.

fire; these elements are combined within the body to create the uniform body parts that have no internal structure—bones, muscles, membranes, tendons, etc. The human body is ruled by the four humors: phlegm, yellow and black bile and blood, which is formed in the liver. The left ventricle of the heart houses a life spirit, both a flame and the bearer of intellectual capacity. The "inner senses" are found in the brain ventricles, not the brain mass; these are the imagination, the power of thought and the memory, at the back of the head. There are warm, cold, moist and dry medicines, each with four degrees of effectiveness. They act as a counterbalance when the humors fall out of balance. In short, what we have here is a brief, slightly imprecise compendium of the physiology and humoral pathology propounded by Galen of Pergamon (129–216 CE),[4] enriched with a few modern elements.

Greek medicine had already been focused on natural science, even to the extent of materialism. Health was understood to be a balance of extremes that could be upset by the blind actions of natural forces, such as the weather, or by an imprudent lifestyle. Physicians were called upon to restore this balance by applying suitable medicines and dietary rules. Even from its Hippocratic beginnings, this form of medicine was in direct opposition to popular ideas that still contained religious and ethical motives. A papyrus fragment, presumably from a comedy, shows the heroes—that is, the spirits of the dead—threatening robbers with punishments such as swelling of the spleen, coughing, dropsy, colds, itching, gout, insanity, rashes, glandular swelling, chills and fever. The robbers are then given something else that is not included in the fragment.[5] The Hippocratic text "On the Sacred Disease" explicitly rejects the notion that the heroes or gods could be the source of an illness.[6] Even epilepsy, with its conspicuous symptoms, is no longer considered a form of demonic possession by the Hippocratic author. He explains it through mechanical causes, in that the air passages are temporarily blocked by mucus—a type of infarction. The author of "Airs, Waters, Places" even traces the cause of the mysterious "eunuch illness" among the barbaric Scythians, which the natives believe to be a punishment from their gods, back to their constant horseback riding; as support, he offers the observation that those affected are mainly the rich, who can afford horses. Otherwise, he says, it would be more common among the poor, who are able to make fewer sacrifices to the gods.[7]

---

4. On the date of death, which was previously assumed to be AD 199, cf. Strohmaier, "La longévité," 393–403.

5. Merkelbach, *Heroen*, 97–99.

6. Hippocrates, *De morbo sacro* 1,38.

7. Hippocrates, *De aere aquis locis* 22,8–12.

The gods and heroes, thus removed from the medical picture, nonetheless still kept watch over the observance of purely ethical norms. In the Hippocratic oath, Apollo and his son Asclepius are called upon in this capacity. In fact, Asclepius was originally merely a hero; his symbol, the staff and snake, is a reminder of his chthonic origins.[8] Among the common people, the connection between religion and teachings about illness persisted, as can be seen from the bustling trade at the Asclepius shrines and particularly the inscriptions of Epidaurus. The Christian pilgrimage sites with their votive offerings are more or less a continuation of this practice,[9] and it is the first area where a conflict appeared with scientific medicine, something that had not been documented in the pagan era. After the incubation practice at the Isis shrine in Abukir, Egypt, had been transformed into a Christian rite—with the martyrs Cyrus and John appearing in a dream to those who slept there, in place of the goddess—Gessius of Petra, a professor of medicine at the nearby Alexandrian school, made fun of it. Legend has it that he was punished by the saints when he became gravely ill and was forced to seek help at the shrine himself.[10]

Gessius was one of the so-called iatrosophists, whose teachings played a key role in communicating Galenic medicine to the Syrians and thus ultimately to the Muslims.[11] With its detailed and rationally grounded humoral pathology, the philosophy then became a fixed part of Arabic-Islamic culture from Córdoba to Bukhara.[12] In an indirect way, this can also be seen in the surprise with which educated persons spoke of their encounters with medicine from other cultures. There are two examples of this, the first from India and the other from the Palestine of the Crusader era. At the eastern edge of the Islamic world, the universally trained scholar al-Bīrūnī (973–1048) records the following observations in his large monograph on India:

> "Most of their charms are intended for those who have been bitten by serpents. Their excessive confidence in them is shown by this, which I heard a man say, that he had seen a dead man who had died from the bite of a serpent, but after the charm had been applied he had been restored to life, and remained alive, moving about like all others.

---

8. Strohmaier, "Zur Herkunft des Äskulapstabes," 503–4; Strohmaier, "Asklepios und das Ei," 143–53, 448–54.
9. Leipoldt, *Von Epidauros bis Lourdes*.
10. Migne, *Patrologia Graeca* 87,3, 3513–20.
11. Strohmaier, "Der syrische und der arabische Galen," 1987–2017.
12. Pormann and Savage-Smith, *Medieval Islamic Medicine*.

Another man I heard as he told the following story: 'He had seen a man who had died from the bite of a serpent. A charm was applied, and in consequence he rose, spoke, made his will, showed where he had deposited his treasures, and gave all necessary information about them. But when he inhaled the smell of a dish, he fell down dead, life being completely extinct.'

It is a Hindu custom that when a man has been bitten by a venomous serpent, and they have no charmer at hand, they bind the bitten man on a bundle of reeds, and place on him a leaf on which is written a blessing for that person who will accidentally light upon him, and save him by a charm from destruction.

I, for my part, do not know what I am to say about these things, since I do not believe in them. Once a man who had very little belief in reality, and much less in the tricks of jugglers, told me that he had been poisoned, and that people had sent him some Hindus possessing the knowledge of charms. They sang their charms before him, and this had a quieting effect upon him, and soon he felt that he became better and better, whilst they were drawing lines in the air with their hands and with twigs."[13]

The educated Arab knight Usāma ibn Munqidh, who lived from 1095 to 1188, reports in his often-cited memoirs that at the time of the Third Crusade (1189–1192) the Frankish lord of a castle in northern Lebanon sent a messenger to the author's uncle and asked him to send a physician. This was willingly done, but after ten days the physician returned and said he had been given two patients: a knight with an abscess on his foot and a woman suffering from "desiccation," which he had tried to treat with a "moist" diet. Then, however, a Frankish doctor intervened and had the foot amputated with an axe, which led to the knight's death. For the woman, the Frankish colleague's diagnosis was that she had a demon living in her head that was in love with her. He ordered her hair to be cut short, but it did not help—particularly since, as the Arab doctor disapprovingly noted, the woman immediately went back to her usual diet with plenty of garlic and mustard. Her "desiccation" increased, and following the instructions of the Frankish doctor, a cross-shaped cut was made in her scalp and her bare skull was rubbed with salt. This, too, had a lethal outcome. The Arab's gentler treatment was completely in keeping with Galenic medicine. In the female patient's case, mustard and garlic were exactly the wrong things to eat; according to Galen's teachings as laid out in his work on simple medicines,

---

13. Al-Bīrūnī, *Fī taḥqīq*, 95,8–16; trans. Edward C. Sachau, *Alberuni's India*, vol. 1, 194.

both are warm and dry in the fourth degree, representing the greatest extreme on his pharmacological scale.[14] Another typical aspect of this story is that the Arab physician is a Christian who feels naturally integrated into Islamic culture; his only comment on the foreign barbarians is the dry remark that now he has learned something he did not know before.[15]

The practice of medicine was often still in the hands of Christians; in particular, they set the tone in their elevated positions at court. Greek medicine met with resentment from those who objected to its foreign origins. One is reminded of the resistance in ancient Rome, led by Cato the Elder.[16] Al-Bīrūnī knew people who were horrified by the mere names of the Greek experts, ending as they did in an "s."[17] With visible malice, in a programmatic text titled "The Key to Medicine," the Muslim and avid philhellene Ibn Hindū describes the case of a theologian who suffered from severe diarrhea and had a physician prescribe a laxative in an attempt to prove that the medicine was ineffectual—with deadly results.[18] The spirit of this rejection developed into a kind of "prophetic medicine," which was based on the model of Mohammed and recommended the household remedies of popular medicine; over time, however, it also added Galenic elements.[19] We can see the natural conclusion of this development in the book by Muhammad Salim Khan that was mentioned at the beginning. To justify the use of elements from foreign medicine, people referred to the Prophet himself, who had also seen Christian and Jewish physicians for treatment according to the pious tradition of the ḥadīth.[20] People who wanted to hew more closely to pure Greek medicine tried to integrate it into earlier divine prophetic revelations, where the Asclepius myth offered a point of contact.[21] Asclepius was also the only one of the ancient gods whose name remained in the

---

14. Galen, *De simplicium medicamentorum temperamentis ac facultatibus* VIII: s.v. νᾶπυ and σκόροδον, 85 and 126.

15. Preissler, *Die Erlebnisse des syrischen Ritters Usāma ibn Munqid*, 148–50.

16. Vgl. Nutton, "The Perils of Patriotism," 30–58.

17. Al-Bīrūnī, *Kitāb taḥdīd*, 28; German translation in Strohmaier, "Al-Bīrūnī. In den Gärten," No. 5.

18. Ibn Hindū, 16,3–9; more on the polemics of Ibn Hindū in Rosenthal, "The Defense of Medicine."

19. Perho, *The Prophet's Medicine*, 49, 58, 62–64, 84–90, 100–110, 126–27.

20. Evidence compiled by Youssef, *Eine kritische Untersuchung*, 33–36.

21. Strohmaier, "Gedenken," 79–84; Strohmaier, "Asklepios und seine Sippe."

wording of the Hippocratic oath[22] that prospective physicians were required to take, according to the requirements of a manual for the market overseer.[23]

The Prophet Mohammed's preaching on the omnipotence of almighty God produced natural philosophical consequences for theologians, who assumed that the world was created anew in each atom of time, thus making the continuity of earthly things and their effects on one another a mere illusion. However, it is an exaggeration when Felix Klein-Franke concludes, "Naturally, this had unpredictable effects for the field of medicine."[24] The physicians who were trained according to Galen applied the *dynamis* of their medicines without worrying about the theologians' subtleties, even if they were pious Muslims—not to mention Christians, Jews and notorious heretics such as the great Persian clinician Rhazes, who believed the prophets of the book religions were swindlers, and instead chose to follow Socrates as his imam.[25]

Only especially ascetic individuals were able to reject medicine in its entirety, whether Galenic or "prophetic," when it came to understanding illness as a punishment or a special test. Abū l-Dardā', a contemporary of the Prophet, for instance, when he was sick, is said to have been asked, "What is your complaint?" "I complain of my sins," was the answer. "What do you desire?" he was then asked. "Forgiveness from my Lord." They asked, "Should we not call a doctor for you?" He responded, "The doctor is the one who ordained my suffering."[26] There was no shortage of mockery from enlightened parties; for instance, the above-cited Ibn Hindū states, "For those who fear that accepting the existence of medicine will interfere with what God, who is mighty and powerful, wills for His servant—they also should not eat when they are hungry or drink when they are thirsty, for perhaps God has condemned them to die of hunger or thirst. And if they ate or drank, they would be ignoring God's decision and their will would no longer correspond to His will."[27]

Al-Ġazālī (1058–1111), the reformer of Sunni orthodoxy in the eleventh century, addresses this objection in a positive sense. He divides

---

22. Strohmaier, "Ḥunayn ibn Isḥāq," 321–23 (reprinted in: Strohmaier, *Von Demokrit bis Dante*, 219–21).

23. Meyerhof, "La surveillance," 129, 131 (reprinted in: Meyerhof, *Studies*, XI).

24. Klein-Franke, *Vorlesungen über die Medizin im Islam*, 111–13; cf. the critical comments by Perho, *The Prophet's Medicine*, 67–69.

25. Urvoy, *Les penseurs libres*, 142–52; Stroumsa, *Freethinkers of Medieval Islam*, 87–120.

26. Wehr, *Al-Gazzali's Buch vom Gottvertrauen*, 94; cf. Perho, *The Prophet's Medicine*, 65–67.

27. Ibn Hindū, *Miftāḥ al-ṭibb wa-minhāj al-ṭullāb*, 14.

medicines into three groups; the first includes very obvious and natural things like water for thirst and bread for hunger. The second group includes cold medicines for warm illnesses and all the other remedies, which once again shows how deeply Galenic humoral pathology had infiltrated the general consciousness of Islamic culture. Pious persons are only warned to stay away from a third group, which includes incantations and magical cauterization, since the effects are only presumed and therefore trusting in them is a form of idolatry.[28] Nonetheless, this demonization may in fact have been seen as a recommendation by despairing patients, as shown by the frequent use of cauterization in Arabic popular medicine.

According to some reports, the Prophet had a more instinctual distaste for magic, or at least for things he considered to be magical. In Medina, he once saw some colleagues working to artificially pollinate palm trees. He found this to be a pointless and superstitious procedure, and he advised them not to do it. However, when the next year came and the trees did not bear fruit, Mohammed saw that he had been mistaken. As Johann Fück rightly emphasized, this story is plausible because the Prophet's authority is shown in a dubious light here, which contradicts the general tendency of the ḥadīth.[29] At the same time, it reveals his pragmatism, which often resulted in unclear compromises but at the same time allowed him to build his community. In this regard, other parts of the ḥadīth that describe his acceptance of the effectiveness of incantations are not implausible.

What was fatal for the further development of medicine, however, was the fact that he rejected the possibility of contagion.[30] The ḥadīth contains a striking statement that is found in several formulations: Lā ʿadwā wa-lā hāma wa-lā ṣafar ("There is no contagion, there is no owl; in other words, its reputation as an evil omen does not mean anything, and there is no animal that chews on the intestines when a person is hungry.")[31] The idea that an illness could be invisibly transmitted from one individual to another is thus equated with other superstitions. A Bedouin had countered the Prophet's statement with an example from his own experience, saying that his camels had been healthy as gazelles until a mangy camel joined them and infected

---

28. Wehr, *Al-Gazzalis Buch vom Gottvertrauen*, 91–94.

29. Fück, "Rolle," 21; reprinted in Fück, *Arabische Kultur*, 227.

30. A great deal of material available from Stearns, *Infectious Ideas*, and idem, *Contagion*, unfortunately not addressing the motifs of the prophet and their disastrous harmony with Greek humoral pathology, which lasted through the modern era and offered no way of handling the problem of contagion; for more detail, see also Strohmaier, "Ansteckung," 631–45.

31. Van Ess, *Der Fehltritt des Gelehrten*, 296–97.

them. The Prophet countered, "And who infected the first one?"[32] God was supposed to be the acting force behind all things, and if He was the originator of one illness, why not all of the following cases? In seeing the Creator at work everywhere, either helping or punishing, he did not want to allow that illness or its demonic sources could have independent powers—not even the power of attacking a living being on their own or moving to another individual. This principle is clearly formulated in the large *Lisān al-ʿarab* dictionary: "for instance, when a camel comes down with the mange, and people are careful not to keep it with the other camels for fear the mange could spread from one to the others, that they might suffer what the first one did. But Islam rendered this invalid. It had been assumed that illness could spread of its own accord, in response to which the Prophet, may peace be upon him, taught that this was not the case and it was God alone who causes illness and sends down the illness."[33] This even had military consequences, for instance during the first expansion into Syrian cultural lands when troops were faced with the question of whether they should capture a plague-infested city.[34]

In support of the Prophet's statement that they should not go in but also should not flee, al-Ġazālī also draws on the technical knowledge of physicians. Like them, he assumes that the plague is caused by the air. He adds that the contaminated air must not only come in contact with the body from the outside, but must also be breathed into the body for a longer period of time. Once this has happened, the illness is already lodged within you, and flight would be as useless and presumptive a remedy as incantations and the like. In order to emphasize the uselessness of fleeing, al-Ġazālī also draws on the idea of charity, asking who will care for the sick and possibly give them a chance of survival.[35] Here, Islam continues a Christian tradition that is not found in heathenism.[36] Al-Ġazālī was right to refer to the physicians. In humoral pathology, illness had been robbed of all individualism. The concept of the imbalance of the humors allowed for countless variations that could differ for each patient, and if an illness broke out among many people at once, even the Hippocratic author believed that it necessarily had to do with the air that they were all breathing in at the same time.[37]

32. Ullmann, *Medizin im Islam*, 243.

33. Ibn Manẓūr, 39, s.v. *iʿdāʾ*, translated in Fähndrich, *Abhandlung über die Ansteckung*, 31.

34. Van Ess, *Der Fehltritt des Gelehrten*, 228–311.

35. Wehr, *Al-Gazzali's Buch vom Gottvertrauen*, 98–100.

36. Lançon, "Attention au malade," 217–30.

37. Gourevitch, *La medicina ippocratica*, 425–33; see also Hippokrates, *De natura hominis* 9,3.5: 188,12–15; 190,12—192,7.

Only one voice has been recorded in literature, breaking through the alliance of medicine and theology in a special short monograph; not coincidentally, it belongs to a Christian, for whom Mohammed did not represent an ultimate authority. The physician and translator Qusṭā ibn Lūqā (who died in 912/913) was a Melkite, a Greek Orthodox Christian; we could also call him a Catholic, since he lived before the time of the schism. He begins his brief treatise "On Contagion (*Fī l-iʿdāʾ*)" with a subtle joke about Muslims (*ahl al-islām*) who think that illness can be transmitted purely by the mind despite their belief in the divine authority of their Prophet. His own argument is theological too; mentioning the Church father Gregory of Nazianzus, he argues that, if this were true, a mere idea would then become material reality, which would be like the omnipotence of the Creator and is thus absurd. There are purely mental transmissions, he says, such as "contagious" laughter, yawning, sleepiness, sexual excitement or the need to urinate, but they remain within this sphere and do not materialize. The transmission of illness from one person to another must therefore have a material substrate, and he describes it as a "spark" that jumps from a sick body to a healthy one.[38]

There is one other point where individual physicians in Arab-Islamic culture went beyond the materialist statements of ancient medicine, taking a more psychosomatic approach. Galen had been very undecided when it came to the question of the immortality of the human soul.[39] However, the New Platonism also taught by the Alexandrian school, which corresponded to Christian ideas in its teaching of the soul as an indestructible core of personality, was decisively picked up by Muslim philosophers, such as Avicenna, who is said to have used it in his medical practice as well.[40] Even in the receptive phase of the ninth century, the Nestorian court physician Yūḥannā ibn Māsawaih announced, in an inversion of Galen's thesis that the soul follows the makeup of the body, that the makeup of the body also depends on the constitution of the soul—and that a physician should therefore always encourage the patient even if he is not entirely sure about the effect of his treatment.[41]

---

38. Fähndrich, *Abhandlung über die Ansteckung*, §§3–6 and 21.

39. Galen, *De propriis placitis* 3:58–63.

40. Strohmaier, *Avicenna*, 68–71 and 120–23; other examples of Muslim physicians in Bürgel, "Psychosomatic Methods," 157–72.

41. Yūḥannā ibn Māsawaih, *Le livre des axiomes médicaux*, no. 39.

BIBLIOGRAPHY

Beck, Hans-Georg. *Byzantinisches Lesebuch*. Munich: Beck, 1982.
al-Bīrūnī, Muhammad ibn Ahmad. *Fī taḥqīq mā li-l-Hind*. Edited by Eduard Sachau. Leipzig: Harrassowitz 1925. ET = *Alberuni's India*. Translated by Eduard Sachau. London: Routledge & Kegan Paul, 1888.
———. *Kitāb taḥdīd nihāyāt al-amākin li-taṣḥīḥ masāfāt al-masākin*. Edited by P. G. Bulgakov. *Revue de l'Institut des Manuscrits Arabes* 8 (1962) 3–328.
Bürgel, J. C. "Psychosomatic Methods of Cures in the Islamic Middle Ages." *Humaniora Islamica* 1 (1973) 157–72.
Ess, Josef van. *Der Fehltritt des Gelehrten: Die "Pest von Emmaus" und ihre theologischen Nachspiele*. Supplemente zu den Schriften der Heidelberger Akademie der Wissenschaften. Philosophisch-historische Klasse 13. Heidelberg: Winter, 2001.
Fähndrich, Hartmut. *Abhandlung über die Ansteckung von Qusṭā ibn Lūqā*. Abhandlungen für die Kunde des Morgenlandes 48,2. Stuttgart: Steiner, 1987.
Fück, Johann. *Arabische Kultur und Islam im Mittelalter: Ausgewählte Schriften*. Edited by Manfred Fleischhammer. Weimar: Böhlaus, 1981.
———. "Die Rolle des Traditionalismus im Islam." *Zeitschrift der deutschen Morgenländischen Gesellschaft* 93 (1939) 1–32.
Galen: De simplicium medicamentorum temperamentis ac facultatibus VIII: Claudii Galeni Opera omnia. Edited by Karl Gottlob Kühn. Vol. 12. Leipzig: Cnobloch, 1826.
Galen: De propriis placitis 3: On My Own Opinions. Edited and translated by Vivian Nutton. Corpus Medicorum Graecorum V 3,2. Berlin: Akademie, 1999.
Gourevitch, D. "La medicina ippocratica e l'opera delle Arie, Acque, Luoghi: Breve storia della nascita e del potere di un inganno scientifico." *Medicina nei Secoli: Arte e Scienza* 7 (1995) 425–33.
Hippocrates. *De morbo sacro. Die hippokratische Schrift "Über die heilige Krankheit."* Edited and translated by Hermann Grensemann. Ars Medica II.1. Berlin: de Gruyter, 1968.
———. *Über die Umwelt (De aere aquis locis)*. Edited and translated by Hans Diller. 2nd ed. Corpus Medicorum Graecorum I 1,2. Berlin: Akademie, 1970.
———. *De aere aquis locis*. Edited and translated by Jacques Jouanna. 2nd ed. *Hippocrate, tome II*, 2e partie. Paris: Les Belles Lettres, 1996.
———. *De natura hominis*. Edited and translated by Jacques Jouanna. Corpus Medicorum Graecorum I 1,3. Berlin: Akademie, 1975.
Ibn Hindū, 'Ali ibn al-Husayn. *Miftāḥ al-ṭibb wa-minhāj al-ṭullāb*. Edited by Mahdi Mohaghegh and Muhammad Taqi Daneshpajuh. Teheran: McGill University Press, 1989.
Ibn Manẓūr, Muhammad ibn Mukarram. *Lisān al-'arab*. Vol. 15. Beirut: Dar Sadir, 1956.
Ibn Māsawaih, Yūḥannā. *Le livre des axiomes médicaux (Aphorismi)*. Edited by Danielle Jacquart and Gérard Troupeau. Hautes études orientales 14. Geneva: Droz, 1980.
Khan, Muhammad Salim. *Islamic Medicine*. 1986. New ed. London: Routledge & Kegan Paul, 2008.
Klein-Franke, Felix. *Vorlesungen über die Medizin im Islam*. Sudhoffs Archiv 23. Wiesbaden: Steiner, 1982.

Lançon, Bertrand. "Attention au malade et téléologie de la maladie: le 'nosomonde' chrétien de l'antiquité tardive (IVe–VIe siècles)." In *Les pères de l'église face à la science médicale de leur temps*. Edited by Véronique Boudon-Millot and Bernard Pouderon, 217–30. Théologie historique 117. Paris: Beauchesne, 2005.

Leipoldt, Johannes. *Von Epidauros bis Lourdes: Bilder aus der Geschichte volkstümlicher Frömmigkeit*. Leipzig: Koehler & Amelang, 1957.

Merkelbach, R. "Die Heroen als Geber des Guten und des Bösen." *Zeitschrift für Papyrologie und Epigraphik* 1 (1967) 97–99.

Meyerhof, Max. *Studies in Mediaeval Arabic Medicine*. Edited by Penelope Johnstone. Collected Studies 204. London: Variorum, 1984.

———. "La surveillance des professions médicales et para-médicales chez les arabes." *Bullletin de l'Instiut d'Egypte* 26 (1944) 119–34

Nutton, Vivian. "The Perils of Patriotism: Pliny and Roman Medicine." In *Science in the Early Roman Empire: Pliny the Elder, His Sources and Influence*, edited by Roger French and Frank Greenaway, 30–58. London: Croom Helm, 1986.

Perho, Irmeli. *The Prophet's Medicine: A Creation of the Muslim Traditionalist Scholars*. Studia Orientalia 74. Helsinki: Finnish Oriental Society, 1995.

Pormann, Peter E., and Emilie Savage-Smith. *Medieval Islamic Medicine*. New Edinburgh Islamic Surveys. Edinburgh: Edinburgh University Press, 2007.

Preissler, Holger. *Die Erlebnisse des syrischen Ritters Usāma ibn Munqid: Unterhaltsames und Belehrendes aus der Zeit der Kreuzzüge*. Orientalische Bibliothek. Munich: Beck, 1981.

Rosenthal, Franz. "The Defense of Medicine in the Medieval Muslim World." *Bulletin of the History of Medicine* 43 (1969) 519–32.

Stearns, Justin K. "Contagion." In *The Encyclopaedia of Islam* 3 (2010) 180–82.

———. *Infectious Ideas: Contagion in Premodern Islamic and Christian Thought in the Western Mediterranean*. Baltimore: Johns Hopkins University Press, 2011.

Strohmaier, Gotthard. *Al-Bīrūnī: In den Gärten der Wissenschaft: Ausgewählte Texte aus den Werken des muslimischen Universalgelehrten, übersetzt u. erläutert*. 3rd ed. Reclam-Bibliothek 20045. Leipzig: Reclam, 2002.

———. "Die Ansteckung als theologisches und als medizinisches Problem." In *Religion Versus Science in Islam: A Medieval and Modern Debate*, edited by Carmela Baffioni, 631–45. Oriente Moderno N.S. 19. Rome: Instituto per l'oriente, 2000. Reprinted in Strohmaier, *Hellas im Islam*, 118–27.

———. "Asklepios und das Ei: Zur Ikonographie in einem arabisch erhaltenen Kommentar zum hippokratischen Eid." In *Beiträge zur Alten Geschichte und deren Nachleben: Festschrift für Franz Altheim*, edited by Ruth Stiehl and Hans Erich Stier, 2:143–53, 448–54. Berlin: de Gruyter, 1970. Reprinted in Strohmaier, *Hellas im Islam*, 155–66.

———. "Asklepios und seine Sippe: Eine gräko-arabistische Nachlese." In *Words, Texts and Concepts Cruising the Mediterranean Sea: Studies on the Sources, Contents and Influences of Islamic Civilization and Arabic Philosophy and Science. Dedicated to Gerhard Endress on His Sixty-fifth Birthday*, edited by R. Arnzen and J. Thielmann, 151–58. Orientalia Lovaniensia Analecta 139. Leuven: Peeters, 2004.

———. *Avicenna*. 2nd ed. Munich: Beck, 2006.

———. "Das Gedenken an die Urheber der ärztlichen Kunst." In *Hellas im Islam: Interdisziplinäre Studien zur Ikonographie, Wissenschaft und Religionsgeschichte*, 79–84. Diskurse der Arabistik 6. Wiesbaden: Harrassowitz, 2003.

---. *Hellas im Islam: Interdisziplinäre Studien zur Ikonographie, Wissenschaft und Religionsgeschichte*. Diskurse der Arabistik 6. Wiesbaden: Harrassowitz, 2003.

---. "Ḥunayn ibn Isḥāq et le serment hippocratique." *Arabica* 21 (1974) 318–23. Reprinted in Strohmaier, *Von Demokrit bis Dante*, 216–21.

---. "La longévité de Galien et les deux places de son tombeau." In *La science médicale antique: Nouveaux regards. Études réunies en l'honneur de Jacques Jouanna*, edited by V. Boudon-Millot et al., 393–403. Bibliothèque historique et littéraire. Paris: Beauchesne, 2007.

---. "Medizin- und Wissenschaftsgeschichte der Islamisten." In *Parerga—Beiträge zur Wissenschaftsgeschichte: In Memoriam Horst Rudolf Abe*, edited by Jürgen Kiefer, 23–30. Akademie gemeinnütziger Wissenschaften zu Erfurt. Sonderschriften 37. Erfurt: Akademie gemeinnütziger Wissenschaften, 2007. Reprinted in Strohmaier, *Zwischen Islamismus und Eurozentrismus*, 60–66.

---. "Der syrische und der arabische Galen." In *ANRW* II,37,2 (1994) 1987–2017. Reprinted in Strohmaier, *Hellas im Islam*, 85–106.

---. *Von Demokrit bis Dante: Die Bewahrung antiken Erbes in der arabischen Kultur*. Olms Studien 43. Hildesheim: Olms, 1996.

---. "Zur Herkunft des Äskulapstabes." In *XXIIe Congrès International d'Histoire de la Médecine*, 503–4. Bucharest: Constantza, 1970. Reprinted in Strohmaier, *Von Demokrit bis Dante*, 65–66.

---. *Zwischen Islamismus und Eurozentrismus: Mosaiksteine zu einem Bild arabisch-islamischen Erbes*. Diskurse der Arabistik 18. Wiesbaden: Harrassowitz, 2012.

Stroumsa, Sarah. *Freethinkers of Medieval Islam: Ibn al-Rāwandī, Abū Bakr al-Rāzī, and Their Impact on Islamic Thought, Islamic Philosophy*. Theology and Science 35. Leiden: Brill, 1999.

Ullmann, Manfred. *Die Medizin im Islam*. Handbuch der Orientalistik. Erste Abt.: Der Nahe und der Mittlere Osten, Erg.-Bd. VI, 1. Abschnitt. Leiden: Brill, 1970.

Urvoy, Dominique. *Les penseurs libres dans l'Islam classique: L'interrogation sur la religion chez les penseurs arabes indépendants*. Paris: Flammarion, 1996.

Wehr, Hans. *Al-Ġazzālī's Buch vom Gottvertrauen. Das 35. Buch des Iḥyā' 'ulūm ad-dīn, Islamische Ethik*. Edited by H. Bauer. Islamische Ethik 4. Halle/Saale: Niemeyer, 1940.

Youssef, Farid. *Eine kritische Untersuchung der irrtümlich dem 'Abd al-Laṭīf zugeschriebenen Schrift "Medizinisches. Aus dem Koran und der Sunna."* Med. diss., Berlin, 2008.

3

Medicine in Islam
Contested Autonomy[1]

—Lutz Richter-Bernburg

AFTER THE RAPID MUSLIM-ARABIC conquests of the seventh century which encompassed the entire Fertile Crescent, the Iranian highlands, Egypt and North Africa, the following two to three centuries of Muslim religio-political leadership—as embodied by the caliphate—saw the development of a multi-ethnic, multi-religious culture whose dynamicism is evidenced by the permeability of its internal borders—even preceding the qualitatively and quantitatively ample witness of its materialized products.[2] The hegemony of Arabic Islam not only did not prevent the omnipresent exchange between conqueror and conquered in terms of languages, skills, traditions and religions, but actually may have promoted it. Creative potential was manifested in a wide range of areas, including religion, theology, philosophy, science, architecture, arts and crafts, technology, agriculture and horticulture.[3] The

---

1. Grateful acknowledgment is due István Ormos for generous sharing of views and contribution of references.

2. For obvious reasons, only a few titles can be mentioned here for an overview: Haarmann et al., *Geschichte*; Endreß, *Islam*; for general reference in Islamic studies, see *Encyclopaedia of Islam* [*EI*], and as a follow-up: Krämer et al., *Encyclopaedia of Islam Three* [*EI3*].—Despite the distortion involved, only the Christian calendar (now long since "globalized") will be used here.

3. Gutas, *Greek thought, Arabic Culture*; Rudolph, *Islamische Philosophie*; Watson, *Agricultural Innovation*; Bloom, *Islamic Art*; Ettinghausen, *Islamic Art*; Grabar, *The*

pragmatism and willingness to learn shown by the conquerors, who later became the ruling Muslim Arabs, have often been cited; and regardless of the role that religion and religious motivation played in their acculturation, overall it can be said that religious identity did not prevent Muslims during the early Islamic centuries, either in the area of religion in the broadest sense or in other areas, from adopting and appropriating their subjects' competencies.[4] Islam's initial Arabic monolingualism had been relativized by the Persian language since the tenth century,[5] and by Turkish since the thirteenth century,[6] although—for religious reasons—it did not disappear entirely; like the Latin of the Western Middle Ages, Arabic was able to establish a leading position as an educational and scientific language.

For medicine, as well as *mutatis mutandis* for other disciplines, the complex dynamics of these interactions within the caliphate meant that the appropriated late Hellenistic/Near Eastern practice was not simply perpetuated; instead, over the course of a few generations, a wide-ranging, sometimes downright scientific curiosity led to the (re)discovery and naturalization (through Arabic translations) of the respective "classical" authorities. In medicine, that primarily meant the teachings of Galen and Hippocrates, among many others.[7] In a secondary position, but particularly important for *materia medica*, translations of medical classics from Sanskrit—in come cases via intermediary Iranian versions—accompanied the

---

Formation of Islamic Art; Al-Hassan/Hill, *Islamic Technology*; Schacht and Bosworth, *The Legacy of Islam*. Readers should be warned about allegedly serious popularizing representations that are in reality full of factual errors, at their worst even misrepresenting history, such as Al-Hassani, *1000 Inventions*. Conversely this also applies to Gouguenheim, *Aristote au Mont-St.-Michel*.

4. Given some current tendencies toward ahistorical essentialization, to engage for a moment in the Arabic equivalent of "carrying coals to Newcastle" by "carrying dates to Hadjar" (an oasis proverbially known for its date palms, surrounding the modern city of Hofuf in the—officially thus called—Eastern Province of Saudi Arabia) may not be too harshly judged; with diachronic and diatopic fluidity, orthodoxies as well as heterodoxies are subject to historical change and thus to fluctuations in their sphere of influence (and perception), both as dogmatic systems and as real historical actors, mediated through their adherents.

5. Cf. Fragner, *Persophony*.

6. Cf. *EI*, ^{2}X [2000] 715b–16b, s. v. Turks, III 2 [Ambros et al.]; Doerfer, "Chaghatay Language;" Turan, "Anatolia;" Cahen, *Pre-Ottoman Turkey*; Bombaci, *Histoire de la littérature turque*.

7. See here and in the following (even without special references) Pormann and Savage-Smith, *Medieval Islamic medicine* (Bibliography); cf. *EI*, ^{2}X [1999] 451b–61a [Savage-Smith et al.]; Endreß, *Literatur*, 116–52; Ullmann, *Die Medizin im Islam*; Sezgin, *Geschichte des Arabischen Schrifttums*.

Greek works.⁸ Even if the effects of such Islamic Galenism on the care for and treatment of, patients cannot unreservedly be called positive, its fundamental naturalism does it credit; the natural causes of illness corresponded to a natural treatment, which could include certain occult or sympathetic-based elements. At the same time, medicine in Islam cannot simply be reclaimed for Galenism; aside from academic medicine, many demotic and often superstitious practices remained, enjoying a high level of popularity that was also often perpetuated by material constraints.

Beyond the previously mentioned (linguistically and technically outstanding) Graeco-Arabic translations,⁹ the flowering of Islamic Galenism is documented by a whole series of illustrious authors, by no means limited to the names discussed later on in Medieval Latin. In addition to their resonance in the Occident, their credentials are certainly irreproachable, but they should be considered *primi inter pares* within their own cultural context; it was simply by coincidence that other members of their group were never translated and thus failed to be included in the Western canon.¹⁰

One area where the religiously colored creative adaptation of "inherited" practices clearly benefited potential patients was in hospitals. Care facilities for patients needing treatment and healing had been familiar to the Nestorian Christians of Mesopotamia since the pre-Islamic era, and regardless of how plausible later Arabic reports on the founding of the earliest hospital in the caliphal capital of Baghdad—under the first Abbasids, in the late eighth century—may have been, there is no doubt about its Nestorian origins. This is illustrated by its Arabicized name *bīmāristān* ("place for the sick"), a loan from the regional Persian vernacular.¹¹ Beginning with the "charity tax" as the religious duty of every Muslim,¹² beneficence was considered one of the most noble proofs of piety in Islam, and it had its own legal status in the form of foundations (Arabic *waqf*, plural *awqāf*).¹³ As a result, correspondingly organized foundations benefiting hospitals and other

---

8. Ullmann, *Die Medizin im Islam*, 103–7; Sezgin, *Geschichte des Arabischen Schrifttums*, 187–202.

9. Cf. Ullmann, *Wörterbuch*.

10. In addition to the titles mentioned in n. 7 above, see Abattouy, "Intercultural transmission;" Speer and Wegener, *Wissen über Grenzen*; Richter-Bernburg, "Oranges, Quiddities and Algorisms;" Richter-Bernburg, "Iran's Contribution to Medicine;" Jacquart, *La science médicale occidentale*; Weisser, "The Influence of Avicenna on Medical Studies in the West," *Encyclopaedia Iranica*, s.v. "Avicenna xiii."

11. The Syriac-Aramaic written language of these same Christians used a transliteration of the Greek ξενοδόχειον instead; see Pormann and Savage-Smith, *Medieval Islamic Medicine*, 21.

12. Nagel, *Koran*, translated the Arabic *zakāh* as "cleansing tribute."

13. See *EI*, ²IX [1995] 59b–99b, esp. 59a–63a [Behrens-Abouseif].

medical facilities can be found throughout history, up to the present day. Of course, before discussing the rightfully famous examples, a caveat should be raised—one that is always relevant for the premodern period—that until the responsibility for supervising foundations passed to modern governmental administrations in the nineteenth century, only rudimentary tools existed to ensure the foundation's proper and sustainable functioning.[14] Thus a foundation's ability to function was strongly dependent on favorable or unfavorable circumstances. There were fundamental differences between town and country as well as among regions. From the capital Baghdad, where members of the political elite had founded several hospitals by the tenth century, the institution spread throughout the Fertile Crescent (e.g., Jerusalem) and to Iran (e.g., Shiraz and ar-Rayy [near today's Tehran]). Starting with the era of the Seljuks, their satellites and successor dynasties, Syria and Egypt as well as Anatolia were the focal points; here, an architectural ambition was at times displayed that went well beyond mere functionality.[15] Depending on the founder's vision and according to the amount of money that had been donated, a hospital could feature a large number of specialized medical and care personnel, wards for various illnesses and separated by patient gender, a pharmacy with specialized staff, and a medicine budget for inpatient treatments.[16] Both in the ninth and tenth centuries—the first, "classical" culmination of medical scholarship—and later in twelfth-thirteenth-century Syria, for which we have a particular wealth of sources, the best-equipped hospitals were distinguished by the possibility of offering clinical lessons, in other words combining patient care with medical instruction and training. One example of such a combination of practice and theory, of in- and

---

14. According to Islamic law, charitable foundations could only be established by private individuals using their personal assets, even if such persons happened to be rulers over large dominions; although the validity of such deeds was on principle unlimited, there were no effective control mechanisms beyond the founder's lifetime. In reality, foundation assets were often alienated, which meant that the dependent institutions literally fell apart. In addition, "normal" depreciations of the original assets could not be balanced out institutionally.

15. Cf. *EI*, ^{2}I [1960] 1222b–26a [Dunlop et al.]; Hillenbrand, *Islamic Architecture*, 617 (index of individual monuments), s.vv. Divriği, Edirne: külliye, madrasa, mosque; 639 (subject index), s.v. Hospitals; *EI*, ^{2}VIII 964a–b, s. v. Saldjūkids, VI 2: *Art and architecture in Anatolia* [Rogers]; Mayer, "Feldstudien"; Jacobi, *Pascal Coste*, esp. 103, 125–27 (the same hospital, established by Sultan al-Manṣūr Qalāʾūn, from 1284–85); Behrens-Abouseif, *Cairo of the Mamluks*, 244–46, no. 36 (hospital of Sultan al-Muʾayyad from 1420).

16. Cf. Issa Bey, *Histoire des Bimâristans (Hôpitaux)*, esp. 61–69 (excerpted translation of the founding deed).

out-patient care in hospitals and private practice and academic writing, is Abū Bakr ar-Rāzī (d. 925), the Rhazes of the Latin Middle Ages.[17]

One special feature of inpatient treatment was care for mentally ill people, though this was often limited to keeping them calm by tying them down;[18] an oft-cited exception is the music therapy program in the hospital founded by the Ottoman sultan Bayazid II in Edirne,[19] even if this was ultimately based on ancient speculations about the psychotropic effects of music.[20]

The social reality of hospitals as facilities for those who had fewer resources and no other access to medical care—and particularly the mentally ill—is reflected by a shift in meaning of the abovementioned Arabic word for "hospital," which gradually came to mean "mental institution." Those who were better positioned in society either visited physicians in their own practices or requested home visits.

Another example of the religiously motivated Islamic appropriation of (late) antique antecedents were thermal baths (Arabic *ḥammām*), which were essential in order to fulfill the duty of ritual purity. There was a certain similarity to hospitals here, in that the wealthy had baths in their own homes, but the privately funded public baths provided, beyond their religious purpose, cosmetic and health care and served as social venues.[21]

If thus far the immediate or coincidentally mediated effects of religious attitudes and behaviors in traditional Islam have been described as fundamentally positive for both medical education and practice, yet it is important to go back to the abovementioned truism about the historical changeability of religion. At the very time when Islamic Galenism was flowering in the tenth century, and increasingly since then, openness and

17. See "al-Rāzī," *EI*, ^{2}VIII [1994] 474a–477b [Goodman]; Richter-Bernburg, "Al-Razi;" Richter-Bernburg, "Abu Bakr Muhammad al-Razi's (Rhazes) Medical Works;" Richter-Bernburg, "Abū Bakr al-Rāzī and al-Fārābī."

18. Since the fixtures for chaining inmates already existed, hospitals could also be used as prisons for people who incurred the authorities' anger and were not slated for immediate execution; for an example from Baghdad of the late twelfth century, see Richter-Bernburg, "Ibn al-Māristānīya."

19. Goodwin, *History of Ottoman Architecture*, 143–51, 472–73.

20. Horden, *Music*; esp. Shiloah, "Jewish and Muslim Traditions of Music Therapy," 142, no. 56. For an example of an Arabic reflection on the tradition of ancient music therapy practice and its contemporary application, see Ibn Hindū [d. 1029], "Key to medicine," 17:4–16, 56:12–57:9.

21. Cf. *EI*, ^{2}III [1966] 139b–46a [Sourdel-Thomine et al.]; Grotzfeld, *Das Bad*; Warner, "Taking the Plunge;" Goodwin, *History of Ottoman Architecture*, 204, 248–49, 281; Hillenbrand, *Islamic Architecture*, 626 (index of terms), *ḥammām*; 635 (subject index), bath; Jacobi, *Pascal Coste*, 119, 157, 198–201.

tolerance of diversity—for instance toward sciences and philosophies that were "non-Arabic" in origin—were challenged by religious tendencies; while these were often contradictory, they had in common a criticism or even rejection of Galenism. These tendencies included magical understandings of the protective power of the divine word of the Koran; xenophobic bigotry; and an increasingly narrow self-declared Sunni orthodoxy that mirrored real sociopolitical crises beginning in the early tenth century. Often, the theologumenon of divine justice that paralleled human justice was replaced by that of an arbitrary omnipotence that consequently denied the efficacy of secondary causes.[22]

However, even where this conclusion was not drawn, "orthodox" views of the scientific scope of the message from God's envoy Mohammed—a message that was based on divine revelation—shifted away from an acknowledgement of autonomous reason. In the field of medicine, and increasingly since the fourteenth century, the result was "prophetic medicine."[23] Its claim of categorical superiority over merely human and forever fragmentary knowledge in Galenism immediately ran up against the medical inadequacy of the religious sources, the Koran, and Mohammed's divinely inspired exemplary conduct in word and deed, so that Galenic doctrine largely had to be incorporated after all.[24] The internal contradiction that characterizes the entire spectrum of medical writing based on the prophetic model can be seen quite clearly in the discussion of contagion, about which the corpus of "authentic prophetic words" provided contradictory evidence. The refusal to recognize such contradictions also had a centuries-long tradition within the relevant discipline of "prophetic tradition," one that was unaffected by the obvious hermeneutic inconsistency. Even the experience of the "Black Death" beginning in 1347 did not change anything for most proponents of "prophetic medicine;" most of the plague writings continued to insist that the plague was not communicable, based on the authority of an alleged

---

22. Not without sarcasm, Ibn Hindū criticizes all three approaches in his above-mentioned *Protrepticus* "Key," 14:13—16:13; on Islamic theology, cf. Nagel, *Geschichte der islamischen Theologie*; Nagel, *Die Festung des Glaubens*, esp. 148–56; Perler and Rudolph, *Occasionalismus*.

23. Cf. Perho, *The Prophet's Medicine*; Ullmann, *Medizin*, 185–89; Justin Stearns, *Infectious Ideas* (to be read with caution).

24. Here, see Perho, *The Prophet's Medicine*, though with a more positive emphasis; for one sample reference, see Ibn Qayyim al-Jauzīya, *Zād al-Maʿād fī hady khayr al-ʿibād*, esp. IV 70–338. The author, despite his unrestrained use of scholarly medicine, goes so far as to depict the chasm between "academic" and prophetic medicine as wider than that between the quackery of itinerant vendors and scholarly medicine (ibid., 183:3–5); for the most part, though, he considers the respective proportions as equal.

prophetic word.²⁵ Objections were raised only by a minority of people, well-considered though their arguments might have been.²⁶

The religiously motivated attack on medicine, whether underhanded or open, as what could without anachronism be described as a secular science and art (τέχνη),²⁷ led to the development of various argumentative defense strategies. The most common of these, repeated for centuries, followed the opponents' precedent in drawing on a presumed saying by Mohammed; according to this dictum, all scholarship and science can ultimately be divided into two categories: a category relating to "religious actions" and a category relating to "bodies" (in other words, human beings); fittingly, the two terms rhyme in Arabic.²⁸ Consequently religious studies are associated with a knowledge of norms and commandments without which orthodoxy and orthopraxy would not be possible; conversely, medicine—as the study of the human organism—is said to provide the physical requirements for fulfilling religious duties. In this function, as an *ancilla fidei*, it thus becomes legitimate, even required, according to Islamic law. The argument often uses another "prophetic word" here, according to which God has created a cure

25. Cf. van Ess, *Der Fehltritt des Gelehrten*.

26. Ullmann, *Die Medizin im Islam*, 242–50, esp. 246ff; the Hispano-Arabic vizier and intellectual Ibn al-Khaṭīb (d. 1375) stands out because of his critical sobriety; unflinching historical criticism of so-called prophetic medicine is also articulated by Ibn Khaldūn, the renowned historical theorist (d. 1406; see Rosenthal, trans., *Ibn Khaldûn*, esp. III 150); cf. EI ²XI [2000], pp. 2b–4b [Shoshan/Panzac].

27. Here, too, Ibn Hindū is an eloquent, if by no means unique witness (esp. Ch. 2, pp. 7–8); his authorities are the Greeks: Hippocrates, Aristotle, Galen. He has a prominent predecessor in ʿAlī b. al-ʿAbbās al-Majūsī [writing within the years 974–977; in Latin "Haly Abbass"], the author of the compendium *al-Kāmil fī ṣ-ṣināʿa aṭ-ṭibbīya*, later known in Latin as the *Pantegni* or the *Regalis dispositio* (ed. Būlāq 1877, I 3:12–14); using terms that echo Galen, he praises the rank of medicine and says it is universally indispensable. On al-Majūsī cf. Micheau, "ʿAlī ibn al-ʿAbbās al-Maǧūsī." Ar-Rāzī and Ibn Sīnā ("Avicenna") do not find it at all necessary to "justify" medicine explicitly.

28. In the present context too, debaters frequently availed themselves of a device which had originated early on in Islamic tradition; purportedly "prophetic" utterances were quoted—or produced ad hoc—in order to buttress one's own argument. In mid-tenth century, approaching the full florescence of Islamic Galenism, the adage was attributed to the jurist ash-Shāfiʿī (d. 820), much revered as an authority of religious law; such attribution might be accepted as a reflex of the religious-philosophical debates which took place at the time of composition of the pertinent bio-hagiographical works; s. Jalāl ad-Dīn as-Suyūṭī, *al-Manhaǧ as-sawī wa-l-manhal ar-rawī fī ṭ-ṭibb an-nabawī*, 90:3–7 with n. 2. At any rate, possibly the first medical author to use the formulation about the "duality of sciences," Abū Sahl Bishr b. Yaʿqūb as-Sijzī, still felt free to ascribe it with panegyric intention to the dedicatee of his work, the amir Abū Aḥmad Khalaf b. Aḥmad (r. 963–1003; it has not yet been possible to narrow the author's dates any further unless a dependence on al-Majūsī were assumed and thus c. 980 as *terminus a quo*); see Dietrich, *Medicinalia Arabica*, 66–69, no. 22, esp. 66.

for every illness except old age. However, it should be kept in mind that apologists of "prophetic medicine" sometimes also considered the ink with which the healing verses of the Koran were transcribed to be such a cure; the water in which it was dissolved was treated as an elixir.[29] When it came to pure scholarly medicine in the Middle Ages, a religious explanation was generally added to the secular, philosophical explanation that would earlier on have been sufficient by itself.

The above-mentioned, centuries-old authorial convention of justifying, in the prologue to medical writings, the subject *sub specie fidei islamicae* clearly shows the persistence of literary patterns on the one hand; on the other, it just as clearly shows a real or anticipated pressure to produce such justification. After all, the purely secular justifications also provided by tradition were often ignored even by those later authors who were not proponents of "prophetic medicine."[30] Even if this observation cannot be based on a quantitative evaluation of relevant writings, on the basis of a selection of Arabic and Persian *medicinalia* it would seem to be well-founded qualitatively.[31] A few examples should serve as an adequate illustration here. The fact that the dedication to a caliph of a medical treatise in the late eleventh century, the time of the Sunni Restoration, is undergirt with a religious justification of medical science is only unsurprising if the Sunni Restoration is quasi-automatically distanced from "non-Arabic" science.[32] Approximately a century later, the Baghdad-based, equally strict Sunni religious scholar Ibn al-Jauzī (d. 1200) undertook at least a rhetorical harmonization of the religious and rational justifications, of written documents—from the Koran and the Mohammedan model—on the one hand and technical medical

---

29. Even Ibn Qayyim al-Jauzīya could only produce companions of the prophet Mohammed as authorities, but without the technically required chain of transmitters; see *Zād al-Maʿād* IV 181:-6, etc. Despite his noticeable reticence on these practices, he leaves no doubt about his conviction that charms are effective against the evil eye (ibid., 176–84).

30. In a fifteenth-century commentary on symptomatology and etiology that has been studied for centuries, the healing power of Mohammed's dispensation is cited before embarking on the subject with a quotation from Galen a few lines later; see Dietrich, *Medicinalia Arabica*, 122–24, no. 52.

31. The Arabic materials are provided by Albert Dietrich in his abovementioned *Medicinalia Arabica*, based on manuscript studies in Turkey and Syria. The Persian materials are not individually cited here because they simply, through the eighteenth century, rehearse the earlier arguments; see Richter-Bernburg, *Persian medical manuscripts*.

32. This is a reference to Abū ʿAlī Yaḥyā Ibn Jazla ("Byngezla;" d. 1100) in the prologue to *Taqwīm al-abdān* ("Tabulated information on bodies;" in Latin *Tacuini aegritudinum*) for the Abbasid al-Muqtadī (r. 1075–94); see Dietrich, *Medicinalia Arabica*, 101–2, no. 40.

knowledge on the other;³³ despite all his programmatic reverence for the religious—and medically unproductive—canon, even Ibn al-Jauzī succumbs to the urge to draw on medical literature in a concrete context.³⁴ As already noted, regardless of how certain theoretical religious reservations about Galenism affected everyday life,³⁵ there was also a certain diversity of normative convictions among devout Sunnis, as documented by Ibn al-Jauzī's younger Iranian contemporary Fakhr ad-Dīn ar-Rāzī (d. 1209), a religious scholar with a solid education in philosophy. After a brief, almost ritualized reference to the Prophet's concept of "duality," he bases his apology of medicine entirely on traditional rational and philosophical arguments.³⁶ These were time and again deployed in Mesopotamia, Iran and Anatolia until the late fifteenth century.³⁷

As a result, in analyzing the diverse, even at times contemporaneous pronouncements, possible regional differences as well as the given author's personal interests must be taken into account; "orthodoxy" did not wear the same garb everywhere—nor did it have the same impact everywhere. Another example from around 1200, but this time from Ayyubid-era Egypt,³⁸ can be found in a compilation of medical examination knowledge dedicated to the incumbent vizier, in other words not a man of religion. The volume expresses the hope—to be read as an appeal—for future generous support of medicine in keeping with the richly endowed religious disciplines; in any case, according to the author's hard-to-verify claim, the distribution of resources put medicine at a clear disadvantage.³⁹

33. Dietrich, *Medicinalia Arabica*, 110–12, no. 46.

34. See above, n. 24; for a sharp criticism of Ibn al-Jauzī, see Ullmann, *Medizin im Islam*, 186.

35. E.g., the rejection of religiously proscribed substances such as wine as a medicine, as reported by "medical historian" Ibn abī Uṣaybiʿa (d. 1270); see also Ullmann, *Medicine in Islam*, 10, 231–32. Leclerc used him extensively in his *Histoire de la médecine arabe*.

36. Dietrich, *Medicinalia Arabica*, 77–79, no. 28, in a commentary on Avicenna's al-Qānūn ("Canon"), Book I; on Fakhr ad-Dīn s. Arnaldez, *Fakhr al-Dîn al-Râzî*.

37. Dietrich, *Medicinalia Arabica*—here in chronological order: 112–13, no. 47 (Ibn Hubal, d. 1213); 80–83, no. 29 (Quṭb ad-Dīn ash-Shīrāzī, d. 1311); 115–17, no. 49 (Najm ad-Dīn ash-Shīrāzī, d. 1330); 91f, no. 34 (Muḥammad al-Aqsarāʾī, d. 1378); 125–28, no. 53 (Masʿūd al-Ḥasanī, fl. 1472); 128f, no. 54 (Muẓaffar ad-Dīn al-Amshāṭī, d. 1496).

38. I.e. the dynasty of Saladin; see *EI3*, 2007–2, pp. 191a–204a.

39. Dietrich, *Medicinalia Arabica*, 195–98, no. 91; written in the decade before 1207 (the year when the author ʿAbd al-ʿAzīz as-Sulamī died) for Ṣafī ad-Dīn Ibn Shukr, the vizier of Saladin's brother and true successor al-Malik al-ʿĀdil Saif ad-Dīn ("Saphadin").

Perhaps the most lasting effect of this need to provide a religious, and thus backward-looking, justification for medicine can be seen in the closing off of a future as once hinted at by "Rhazes."[40] Even if Galenic medicine by no means disappeared, it was robbed of any prospect of positive change by its being tethered to the Mohammedan ideal, in other words the ever-receding ostensible highpoint of creation and history. Through an ironic quirk of history, "prophetic medicine" at present enjoys unebbing popularity alongside contemporary scientific medicine.[41]

BIBLIOGRAPHY

Abattouy, Mohammed, Jürgen Renn, and Paul Weinig, eds. "Intercultural Transmission of Scientific Knowledge in the Middle Ages: Graeco-Arabic-Latin." *Science in Context* 14:1/2 (2001).

Abusharaf, Rogaia Mustafa. *Female Circumcision: Multicultural Perspectives.* Pennsylvania Studies in Human Rights. Philadelphia: University of Pennsylvania Press, 2006.

Afary, Janet. *Sexual Politics in Modern Iran.* Cambridge: Cambridge University Press, 2009.

Aldeeb Abu-Sahlieh, Sami A. *Male and Female Circumcision among Jews, Christians and Muslims: Religious, Medical, Social and Legal Debate.* Warren Center, PA: Shangri-La, 2001.

Arnaldez, Roger. *Fakhr al-Dîn al-Râzî: Commentateur du Coran et philosophe.* Études musulmanes 37. Paris: Vrin, 2002.

Behrens-Abouseif, Doris. *Cairo of the Mamluks: A History of the Architecture and Its Culture.* London: Tauris, 2007.

Bloom, Jonathan M., ed. *Early Islamic Art and Architecture.* The Formation of the Classical Islamic World 23. Aldershot, UK: Ashgate, 2002.

Bombaci, Alessio. *Histoire de la littérature turque.* Paris: Klincksieck, 1968. Original: *Storia della letteratura turca.* Thesaurus litterarum: Sez. 1, Storia delle letterature di tutto il mondo. Milan: Nuova Accademia, 1956.

---

40. S. Richter-Bernburg, "Al-Razi."

41. The analysis of today's scientific medicine takes up a great deal of attention in Islami(ci)st discourse, as well as in the practical policies of so-called Islamic states like Iran, as can be seen from many recent websites. The following are just a few highlights chosen at random: Abusharaf, *Female circumcision*; Aldeeb Abu-Sahlieh, *Male and Female Circumcision*; Eich, *Moderne Medizin und islamische Ethik*; Darby/Svoboda, "A Rose;" Rispler-Chaim, "Artificial insemination;" ead., *Islamic medical ethics*. Also relevant to medical ethics—in other words, questionable—are the high number of sex change surgeries in Iran, especially for MTF (male-to-female) procedures (e.g., http://archive.radiozamaneh.com/english/category/write-ups/transexual; on this discussion, cf. Bucar, "Bodies;" Shakerifar, "Visual" [includes a discussion of *Be like others*, a documentary by Tanaz Eshaghian, 2008 (cf. http://en.wikipedia.org/wiki/Be_Like_Others)]; Gherovici, *Please select*; Kugle, *Homosexuality*; Janet Afary, *Sexual politics*.

Bucar, Elizabeth M. "Bodies at the Margins: The Comparative Case of Transsexuality." In *Religious Ethics in a Time of Globalism: Shaping a Third Wave of Comparative Analysis*, edited by Elizabeth M. Bucar and Aaron Stalnaker, 49–64. Palgrave Macmillan's Content and Context in Theological Ethics. New York: Palgrave Macmillan, 2012.

Cahen, Claude. *Pre-Ottoman Turkey: A General Survey of the Material and Spiritual Culture and History c. 1071–1330*. Translated by J. Jones-Williams. London: Sidgwick & Jackson, 1968.

Darby, Robert, and J. Steven Svoboda. "A Rose by Any Other Name? Rethinking the Similarities and Differences between Male and Female Genital Cutting." *Medical Anthropology Quarterly* 21 (2007) 301–23.

Dietrich, Albert. *Medicinalia Arabica: Studien über arabische medizinische Handschriften in türkischen und syrischen Bibliotheken*, 65–69. Abhandlungen der Akademie der Wissenschaften in Göttingen, Philologisch-Historische Klasse 3, 66. Göttingen: Vandenhoeck & Ruprecht, 1966.

Doerfer, Gerhard. "Chaghatay Language and Literature." In *Encyclopaedia Iranica*, edited by Ehsan Yarshater, 5:339a–43b. Costa Mesa, CA: Mazda, 1992.

Eich, Thomas. *Moderne Medizin und islamische Ethik: Biowissenschaften in der muslimischen Rechtstradition*. Religion und Gesellschaft 2. Freiburg: Herder, 2008.

Encyclopaedia of Islam [EI]. 12 vols. 2nd ed. Leiden: Brill, 1960–2005.

Endreß, Gerhard. *Der Islam: Eine Einführung in seine Geschichte*. 3rd ed. Munich: Beck, 1997.

———. "Die wissenschaftliche Literatur." In *Grundriß der arabischen Philologie II. Literaturwissenschaft*. Edited by H. Gätje and W. Fischer. Wiesbaden: Reichert, 1987.

———. "Die wissenschaftliche Literatur." In *Grundriß der arabischen Philologie III: Supplement*. Edited by H. Gätje and W. Fischer. Wiesbaden: Reichert, 1992.

Ess, Josef van. *Der Fehltritt des Gelehrten: Die 'Pest von Emmaus' und ihre theologischen Nachspiele*. Heidelberg: Winter, 2001.

Ettinghausen, Richard, Oleg Grabar, and Marilyn Jenkins-Madina. *Islamic Art and Architecture 650–1250*. 2nd ed. New Haven: Yale University Press, 2001.

Fragner, Bert G. *Die "Persophonie": Regionalität, Identität und Sprachkontakt in der Geschichte Asiens*. ANOR 5. Berlin: Das Arabische Buch, 1999.

Gherovici, Patricia. *Please Select Your Gender: From the Invention of Hysteria to the Democratizing of Transgenderism*. New York: Routledge, 2010.

Goodman, Lenn E. "al-Rāzī." *Encyclopaedia of Islam*, 8:474a–77b. 2nd ed. Leiden: Brill, 1994.

Goodwin, Godfrey. *A History of Ottoman Architecture*. Baltimore: Johns Hopkins Press, 1971.

Grabar, Oleg. *The Formation of Islamic Art*. Rev. ed. New Haven: Yale University Press, 1987.

Grotzfeld, Heinz. *Das Bad im arabisch-islamischen Mittelalter: Eine kulturgeschichtliche Studie*. Wiesbaden: Harrassowitz, 1970.

Gouguenheim, Sylvain. *Aristote au Mont-St.-Michel: les racines grecques de l'Europe chrétienne*. Paris: Seuil, 2008. German ed.: *Aristoteles auf dem Mont Saint-Michel: die griechischen Wurzeln des christlichen Abendlandes*. Commentary by Martin Kintzinger. Darmstadt: WBG, 2011.

Gutas, Dimitri. *Greek Thought, Arabic Culture—the Graeco-Arabic Translation Movement in Baghdad and Early 'Abbasid society (2nd–4th/8th–10th centuries)*. London: Routledge, 1998.
Haarmann, Ulrich, Heinz Halm, and Monika Gronke, eds. *Geschichte der Arabischen Welt*. 5th ed. Munich: Beck, 2004.
Al-Hassan, Ahmad Y., and Donald R. Hill. *Islamic Technology: An Illustrated History*. Cambridge University Press, 1986.
Al-Hassani, Salim T. S., gen. ed. *1000 Inventions: The Enduring Legacy of Muslim Civilization*. 3rd ed. Washington, DC: National Geographic, 2012.
Hillenbrand, Robert. *Islamic Architecture: Form, Function and Meaning*. Edinburgh: Edinburgh University Press, 1994; reprinted with amendments, 2000.
Horden, Peregrine, ed. *Music as Medicine: The History of Music Therapy since Antiquity*. Aldershot, UK: Ashgate, 2000.
Humphreys, R. Stephen. *Islamic History: A Framework for Inquiry*. Rev. ed. Princeton: Princeton University Press, 1991. 1st ed., Minneapolis: Bibliotheca Islamica, 1988.
Abū l-Faraj Ibn Hindū [d. 1029], *Miftāḥ aṭ-ṭibb wa-minhāj aṭ-ṭullāb* ["Key to medicine and students' curriculum"]. History of Science in Islam I. Mahdī Mohaqqeq and Mohammad-Taqī Dānešpažūh eds.; Tehrān: McGill University Institute of Islamic Studies, Tehran Branch, in collaboration with Tehran University, 1989/1368.
Ibn Qayyim al-Jauzīya. *Zād al-Maʿād fī hady khayr al-ʿibād*. Edited by Muṣṭafā ʿAbd al-Qādir ʿAṭā. 6 vols. Beirut: Dār al-kutub al-ʿilmīya, 1419/1998.
Issa Bey, Ahmed. *Histoire des Bimâristans (Hôpitaux) à l'époque islamique*. Cairo: Barbey 1928.
Jacobi, Dominique, Thierry Conti et al., eds. *Pascal Coste—toutes les Égypte*. Marseille: Bibliothèque municipale & Éditions Parenthèses, 1998.
Jacquart, Danielle. *La science médicale occidentale entre deux renaissances (XIIe s.—XVe s.)*. Variorum Collected Studies Series 567. Aldershot, UK: Ashgate, 1997.
Krämer, G. et al., eds. *Encyclopaedia of Islam Three [EI3]*. Leiden: Brill, 2007–2015.
Kugle, Scott Siraj al-Haqq. *Homosexuality in Islam: Critical Reflections on Gay, Lesbian and Transgender Muslims*. Oxford: Oneworld, 2010.
Leclerc, Lucien. *Histoire de la médecine arabe*. 2 vols. Paris: Leroux, 1876. Reprinted, Burt Franklin Research & Source Works Series 18,1–2; Science classics 6,1–2. New York: Franklin, 1971.
Mayer, Wolfgang. "Feldstudien am Maristan des Sultans al-Mansur Qalaʿun [sic for Qalaʾun] in Kairo." *Mitteilungen des Deutschen Archäologischen Instituts, Abteilung Kairo* 59 (2003) 289–304 (Ill. 49–51).
Micheau, Françoise. "ʿAlī ibn al-ʿAbbās al-Maǧūsī et son milieu." In *Constantine the African and ʿAlī ibn al-ʿAbbās al-Maǧūsī: The Pantegni and Related Texts*, edited by Charles Burnett and Danielle Jacquart, 1–15. Studies in Ancient Medicine 10. Leiden: Brill, 1994.
Nagel, Tilman. *Die Festung des Glaubens: Triumph und Scheitern des islamischen Rationalismus im 11. Jahrhundert*. Munich: Beck, 1988.
———. *Geschichte der islamischen Theologie*. Munich: Beck, 1994.
———. *Der Koran: Einführung, Texte, Erläuterungen*. Munich: Beck, 1983.
Perho, Irmeli. *The Prophet's Medicine: A Creation of the Muslim Traditionalist Scholars*. Studia Orientalia 74. Helsinki, 1995.
Perler, Dominik, and Ulrich Rudolph, eds. *Occasionalismus: Theorien der Kausalität im arabisch-islamischen und im europäischen Denken*. Abhandlungen der Akademie

der Wissenschaften zu Göttingen, Philologisch-historische Klasse. Folge 3, 235. Göttingen: Vandenhoeck & Ruprecht, 2000.

Pormann, Peter E., and Emilie Savage-Smith. *Medieval Islamic Medicine*. New Edinburgh Islamic Surveys. Edinburgh: Edinburgh University Press, 2007.

Richter-Bernburg, Lutz. "Abū Bakr al-Rāzī and al-Fārābī on Medicine and Authority." In *In the Age of al-Fārābī: Arabic Philosophy in the Fourth/Tenth Century*, edited by Peter Adamson, 119–30. Warburg Institute Colloquia 12. London: Warburg Institute/Turin: Nino Aragno Editore, 2008.

———. "Abu Bakr Muhammad al-Razi's (Rhazes) Medical Works." *Medicina nei Secoli—arte e scienza* 6 (1994) 377–92.

———. "Al-Razi [sic]." In *Arabic Literary Culture 500–925*, edited by M. Cooperson and S. M. Toorwa, 299–308. Dictionary of Literary Biography 311. Detroit: Thomson Gale, 2005.

———. "Ibn al-Māristānīya: The Career of a Hanbalite Intellectual in Sixth/Twelfth Century Baghdad." *Journal of the American Oriental Society* 102 (1982) 265–83.

———. "Iran's Contribution to Medicine and Veterinary Science in Islam AH 100–900/ AD 700–1500." In *The Diffusion of Greco-Roman Medicine into the Middle East and the Caucasus*, edited by John A. C. Greppin, Emilie Savage-Smith and John L. Geriguian, 139–67. Anatolian and Caucasian Studies. Delmar, NY: Caravan, 1999.

———. *Persian Medical Manuscripts at the University of California, Los Angeles—A Descriptive Catalogue*. Humana Civilitas 4. Malibu, CA: Undena, 1978.

———. "Oranges, quiddities and algorisms." In *The Rise of Islam*, edited by V. S. Curtis and S. Stewart, 61–70. The Idea of Iran 4. London: Tauris, 2009.

Rispler-Chaim, Vardit. "Artificial Insemination." In *EI3* (2007) 158b–60a.

———. *Islamic Medical Ethics in the Twentieth Century*. Social, Economic and Political Studies of the Middle East 46. Leiden: Brill, 1993.

Rosenthal, Franz, trans. *Ibn Khaldûn—The Muqaddimah: An Introduction to History*. 3 vols. Bollingen Series 43. New York: Pantheon, 1958.

Rudolph, Ulrich. *Islamische Philosophie: Von den Anfängen bis zur Gegenwart*. Beck'sche Reihe 2352. Munich: Beck, 2004.

Schacht, Joseph, and Clifford Edmund Bosworth, eds. *The Legacy of Islam*. 2nd ed. Oxford: Clarendon, 1974. German trans: *Das Vermächtnis des Islams*. Zurich: Artemis, 1983.

Sezgin, Fuat. *Geschichte des Arabischen Schrifttums [GAS] III: Medizin, Pharmazie, Zoologie, Tierheilkunde bis ca. 430*. Veröffentlichungen des Institutes für Geschichte der Arabisch-Islamischen Wissenschaften. Leiden: Brill, 1970.

Shiloah, Amnon. "Jewish and Muslim Traditions of Music Therapy." In Horden, *Music*, 69–83.

Shakerifar, Elhum. "Visual Representations of Iranian Transgenders." *Iranian Studies* 44 (2011) 327–39.

Speer, Andreas, and Lydia Wegener, eds. *Wissen über Grenzen: Arabisches Wissen und lateinisches Mittelalter*. Miscellanea Mediaevalia 33. Berlin: de Gruyter, 2006.

Stearns, Justin K. *Infectious Ideas: Contagion in Premodern Islamic and Christian Thought in the Western Mediterranean*. Baltimore: Johns Hopkins University Press, 2011.

Jalāl ad-Dīn as-Suyūṭī. *al-Manhağ as-sawī wa-l-manhal ar-rawī fī ṭ-ṭibb an-nabawī*, ed. Ḥasan Muḥammad Maqbūlī al-Ahdal. Beirut: Mu'assasat al-kutub ath-thaqāfīya; and Sanaa: Maktabat al-jīl al-jadīd, 1406/1986.

Turan, Osman. "Anatolia in the Period of the Seljuks and the Beyliks." In *Cambridge History of Islam*, edited by P. M. Holt et al., 1:231–50. 1st ed. Cambridge: Cambridge University Press, 1970.
Ullmann, Manfred. *Die Medizin im Islam*. Handbuch der Orientalistik. Abt. I, Erg-Bd VI 1. Leiden: Brill, 1970.
———. *Wörterbuch zu den griechisch-arabischen Übersetzungen des neunten Jahrhunderts*. Wiesbaden: Harrassowitz, 2002.
———. *Wörterbuch zu den griechisch-arabischen Übersetzungen des neunten Jahrhunderts, Supplement I–II*. Wiesbaden: Harrassowitz, 2006, 2007.
Warner, Nicholas. "Taking the Plunge: The Development and Use of the Cairene Bathhouse." In *Historians in Cairo: Essays in Honor of George Scanlon*, edited by Jill Edwards, 49–79. Cairo: The American University in Cairo Press, 2002.
Watson, Andrew M. *Agricultural Innovation in the Early Islamic World: The Diffusion of Crops and Farming Techniques, 700–1100*. Cambridge Studies in Islamic Civilization. Cambridge: Cambridge University Press, 1983.
Weisser, Ursula. "The Influence of Avicenna on Medical Studies in the West." In *Encyclopaedia Iranica*, edited by Ehsan Yarshater, 3:107a–10a. London: Routledge & Kegan Paul, 1989.

4

Medical Concepts and Therapeutic Networks among Tamasheq Nomads in Mali

—Anna K. Münch

INTRODUCTION

SCARRED BY YEARS OF intense drought that decimated their herds and turned large areas of the Azawad into inhospitable desert, marginalized by foreign occupation forces, and isolated by violent uprisings from their own ranks, the Tamasheq in North Mali are once again forced to survive by adapting to the limited resources within their environment. Sparse rainfall obliges them to be highly mobile and often places them far from urban centers and public services such as schools and health care facilities. In particular, nomadic women and children, whose lives are largely restricted to the protective shadows of the tent and encampment, have difficulties in accessing external health services. They hardly ever go into villages or towns and don't have the economic means to reach health resources outside of their own networks. Very little is known about their internal networks, their conceptions of illness, their understanding of the human organism, their ideas about the etiology of diseases and their concomitant responses and behavior.

The Kel Alhafra (Arabic *al-ḥufra*) of the Republic of Mali are a Tamasheq group comprising 194 families of about 950 individuals, who migrate as nomadic pastoralists with mainly camels, goats and sheep from the Algerian border to the shores of the river Niger.[1] Unlike other Tamasheq fractions, the Kel Alhafra have no families of traditional healers who pass on their knowledge from generation to generation and serve as contact persons in case of illness. The Kel Alhafra form a subgroup of the Kel Ānṣar,[2] located east of Timbuktu, all of whom belong to the class of the *inəsləmān (Sg. anəsləm)*,[3] the Islamic scholars, who devoted themselves from the eleventh/twelfth century to the study of the Qur'an and Arabic sciences. Although there are respected marabouts[4] who can apply the Qur'anic text to treat sickness, in the female milieu there are no explicitly designated women with traditional healing knowledge. At birth, the umbilical cord is always cut by a relative or neighbor, and when a woman or her child are sick, interventions depend on the type and quality of her own healing knowledge, her social support system and the opportunities she has to use these effectively.

How, in general, the Kel Alhafra understand health and sickness, what the dominant ideas about the human body are, how a norm-defining value system operates and in what ways it determines the scope available to or the restrictions placed on them, are issues that will be addressed in the following.

---

1. The primary nomadic space for the Kel Alhafra is Azawad, which stretches from 17°N northwards of Timbuktu deep into the Saharan desert. This semi-arid area is divided into two administrative districts, Timbuktu and, further north Kidal; the Kel Alhafra live in the former, and more precisely in the commune of Ber.

2. As Muslims and promoters of Islam, the Kel Anṣār take their name from the Arabic *al-anṣār*, the medical followers of the prophet Muhammad who took him up among their number and supported him after his *ḥiǧra* to Mecca.

3. The *inəsləmān* in Mali comprise not only the Kel Anṣar (in the districts of Niafunké, Goundam, Timbuktu, Rharous), but also the Kel Ǝssuk (in the Niger Bend, particularly the districts of Rharous, Bourem, Gao, Ansongo, Ménaka and Kidal) as well as the Ijəllad (in the district of Bourem). On the Kel Anṣār, see Marty, "Etudes sur l'islam et les tribus du Soudan"; Norris, *The Tuaregs*.

4. Typologically, the *inəsləmān* have a similar function as the Arabic *murābitīn* groups that were disparaged by the French colonial administration as "marabout" (see *Encyclopedia of Islam* (2), (Leiden: Brill, 2000) X, 379). The *murābitīn* featured in some ways an "elite education," insofar as the privilege of reading and writing (religious texts) was officially acknowledged. Whether the Kel Alhafra—as were often the Arabic *murābitīn*—belonged to a Sufi community, remains undetermined.

LIFEWORLDS AS SYMBOLIC CONSTRUCTIONS

At first sight, the world of the Kel Alhafra appears to be a dualistic one, divided into seemingly oppositional pairs that constitute the entire universe: day and night *ašāl d-ehāḍ*, sun and moon *tāfukk d-iyor*, heaven and earth *išənnawān d-ākall*, fire and water *efew d-aman*, heat and cold *tākusse d-təssəmḍe*, rainy season and dry season *akāsa d-ewelān*, light and darkness *ənnor d-tihāy*, north and south *afālla d-ajuss*, feminine and masculine *eyy d-tunte*, body and spirit *tayəssa d-unfas*, life and death *tāmudre d-tamətānt*, this life and the next life *āddunya d-ālaxirāt*, paradise and hell *ālžānnāt d-ālžāhannām*. Together, however, these pairs form a mythical living space, *āddunya*,[5] in which all directions and positions are directed toward an affective focus, namely Mecca, *mākkāt*, the center of the Islamic world.

In this way, the mythical[6] comprehension of the Islamic world fulfills an identificatory purpose, because it constitutes an explanation of the world in which every element stands in meaningful relationship to every other element. Potential oppositions are tempered by a holistic world view,[7] and emphasis is placed on the complementarity of all phenomena: day can only be classified as such if I know what night is; I can only comprehend life when I am able to conceive its end and thus death—*wār təzzayād tāmudre a-fāl wār təssanād ā-wa aqqālān taməttant*, the Kel Alhafra say, "you do not know life if you are not aware of the significance of death." Every conceivable being is essentially monistic, and anything that one tries to place outside this mythological space must, ultimately, be situated in reference to it and thus encompassed by it.

For the Kel Alhafra, the condition or status of things in their world is first made possible by the Islamic creation myth. This constructs a clearly demarcated basis for perception, determining the position of things and the activities of daily life while also establishing a coexistence between the human body and its surroundings, one in which the human is always

---

5. The Kel Alhafra apply the term *āddunya* not only as the opposite of *ālaxirāt* but also, in their cosmological understanding, as a designation for the entire universe. This illustrates that the bipolar world construed by the Kel Alhafra is not an absolute, self-contained system but one that reflects the occasional incoherence of the lifeworld.

6. Myth is to be understood here in the original sense given to it by the Greeks and not as the purely material explanation of the world envisaged by Auguste Comte. For Plato, mythos (μῦθος) is a creation of humans that unlike logos (λόγος) is transmitted not by constructive education but in suggestive narration. Aristotle describes mythos as a symbolic emulation of action, a construction of the elements of the act, the soul of a drama, always subjective, a projection and expression of human skills. (On the Greek use of the term myth, see Nesselrath, "Mythos-Logos—Mytho-Logos," 1–26.

7. On the holistic worldview of Islam, see Jachimowicz, "Islamic Cosmology."

understood as dominant over nature. God created existence by naming it, and he taught Adam[8] and no other living being (the angels included) the names of things.[9] Humans were accorded certain cognitive faculties that place them above all other living beings: they have the "knowledge of the visible" *tāmusne ta ti-tənhəy*, but its complementary pole, "the knowledge of the invisible" *tāmusne ta wār ti-tənhəy*, remains withheld.

Instead of the Arabic term *āddunya*, older people among the Kel Alhafra often use a Tamasheq word-image: *tesāyt n-ākall fuk*. In Tamasheq, *tesāyt* is a woven dish used in preparing millet to separate the grain from the chaff. Viewed metaphorically, the world in this sense comprises "the sieve of the entire earth," whereby the millet stands for everything that exists. The conceptual meaning of this term is constituted in a gesture, that of tossing the pounded millet. In this act, grain and its complementary coat are separated. The naturally visible things of the world remain in the *tesāyt*, while the chaff falls through it, disappears and from that moment on is understood as the invisible and inapprehensible under the *tesāyt*. On the *tesāyt n-ākall* as lifeworld, the Kel Alhafra are engaged with the physical space of the here and now with its concrete, variably characterized regions that are always directed toward the *qiblāt*, the sanctified direction of prayer, eastward, toward Mecca. Nevertheless, aware of the invisible above and beneath the earth, the lifespace with its interchangeable dimensions always forms a homogenous and indivisible whole for the Kel Alhafra.

In analogy to the macrocosm, the tent for the Kel Alhafra, forms a microcosm, constructed according to the same oppositions and homologies that regulate the entire universe. The tent *ihānan* (sing. *ehān*) is oriented by Mecca toward the east *s-emāināj*, such that its entrance is always on the western, *s-ātārām*, side. In this way, anyone entering the tent does so with his or her face toward the east, thus bringing the divine auspiciousness, *ālbarāka*,[10] of the holy city into the microcosm. At the same time, because

---

8. In Tamasheq the human is also called *āwadəm*: *āw*, descended from, *adəm*, Adam.

9. In Qur'anic teaching, the human is "created with My own hands" *halaqtu biyadayya* (38/75), "and [I] breathed My spirit in him," *wa nafaḥtu fīhi min rūḥī* (38/72), and God created Adam after his image, *lataqabbahu-l-waǧh fa'inna-llāhu ḥalaqa ādam 'ala ṣūratihi*, as expressed by a *ḥadīṯ* from the Ṣaḥīḥ al-Buḫārī (see Buḫārī: *istiḏān* 1; and Muslim: *birr* 115, Ǧannah: 28, Ḥanbal, Ibn: *musnād* Vol. II, 244, 251, 315, 323). Adam was characterized by the special gift of knowledge because God taught him the name of all things: *wa 'allama Adama –l-asmā'a kullahā* . . . (2/31).

10. *ālbarāka* derives from the Arabic root *baraka* and literally means, "to kneel down." Chelhod writes that in the Semitic, this "kneeling down" is always associated with sexual union, with the fertilizing power of the man, and that it was only later, after Islamization, that this male "vital force" acquired its signification as the divine

the tents are low structures, it is necessary to bend down to enter the tent, and thus one bows symbolically in the cardinal direction that is connoted as holy. The east, *emāināj*, is symbolic for Mecca, for the shared origin and genealogical linking of each individual believer with this center. As the sacred cardinal direction, the east is always positively connoted. The believer prays in the direction of the *qiblāt*, and the Kel Alhafra take care that no impurities are found in the eastern part of the tent and that no unclean acts take place there. Defecation and urination toward the east are frowned upon, as is throwing any form of refuse in this direction.

The east-west opposition that represents holy and profane, sunrise and sunset, light and dark, day and night, pure and impure, is mirrored by an analogous contrast between the north, *afālla*, and the south, *ajuss*.

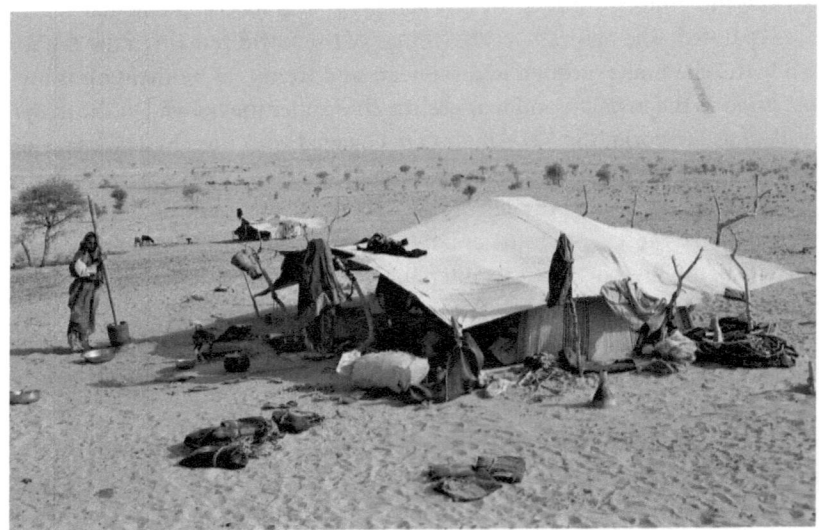

Figure 1:
Tent (*ehān*) aligned toward the east, with its opening toward the west.
(In Killa, November 2006)

"benediction."

For the Kel Alhafra today, *ālbarāka*, embodies in its Islamic sense the divine power of blessing, an arbitrary gift of God that manifests itself in the world when it adheres to objects and people. It is still associated with fertility, with generative, procreative, creative, and especially healing powers. Not only marabouts and healers possess *ālbarāka*, but also medicinal plants, valuable food sources such as camel's milk or fertile pastures have also internalized this divine power. On *ālbarāka* see: Chelhod, "La baraka chez les Arabes ou l'influence bienfaisante du sacré," 68–88; Westermarck, *Ritual and Belief in Morocco*, vol. 1, 35–261; Geertz, *Observer l'Islam*, 58–59; Rasmussen, "Accounting for Belief"; Nicolaisen, "Essais sur la religion et la magie touarègues," 118–19; Kriss and Kriss-Heinrich, *Volksglaube im Bereich des Islam*, vol. 1, 4pp.

Among the Kel Alhafra, the north of the tent is the woman's side; the south is assigned to the man. But again, the "mythical-ritual system," in which the tent and everyday life of the Kel Alhafra are integrated, cannot function contrastively without simultaneously unifying. Everything is subsumed into an order, and if the north stands for the feminine, damp, cold, impure, weak, left, and tempting spirits, the south as masculine, warm, pure, right, strong and steadfast is not conceivable without its opposite.

The Kel Alhafra represent the human body according to the same structural principles that apply to the spatial partition of the world as macrocosm and the tent as microcosm.[11] The body is described with such oppositions as inner and outer, *āmmās d-afālla*, upper part and and lower part, *s-afālla n-tāsa d-ider n-tāsa*, front and back, *s-dat d-s-ḍarāt*, right and left, *ayəl d-tasālje*, contributing to an overall design homologous to that of the tent or the world. God created the human in his image, *'ala ṣūratihi*, the Kel Alhafra say, citing an Islamic tradition,[12] and it is assumed that in essence the human body is complete and pure and that impurity is to be ascribed merely to each human's personal comportment with his or her body.

LOCAL FRAMEWORKS FOR HEALTH, SICKNESS, AND HEALING

"Tāylassed?" "Are you saved and redeemed?" is the opening question of every Tamasheq greeting; *"ma tāxlaqād?"*—"How are you?" or, literally, "How are you created (by God)?" In the Qur'anic perspective, only one answer is possible: *"ālxer yās, təbarāk allah!"*—"Only the good, the best, the most excellent, God be praised!" To respond to the question negatively would be to attribute defectiveness to God the creator who is responsible for all human life. At the same time, the expression *təbarāk allah* embodies a person's gratitude for the grace, *ālbarāka*, and the benevolence of God.

Not only their greeting but all of creation and this lifeworld in the sense of nature are essentially teleologically determined. The Kel Alhafra believe that in nature nothing happens as a result of its own innate force. For them, there is no causal link, no laws of nature in the sense of a physical connection between cause and effect. Reality is the creator alone, and is

---

11. See Bourdieu: "On observe à peu près universellement que la plupart des distinctions spatiales sont établies par analogie avec le corps humain qui constitue le schème de référence par rapport auquel le monde peut s'ordonner ..." *Trois études d'ethnologie Kabyle*, 289.

12. *lataqabbahu-l-wağh fa'inna-llāhu ḥalaqa ādam 'ala ṣūratihi*, as a *hadīṭ* from the *ṣaḥīḥ al-buḥārī* says. See Buḥārī, M.I.I., *istiḏān*, 1; see also: Muslim, I., *birr*, 115, Ğannah: 28, Ibn Ḥanbal, A.I.M., *musnād*, vol. II, 244, 251, 315, 323.

responsible for everything that happens and is. In this theistic understanding, the creator alone is responsible for all diseases.[13] There may indeed be bacteria, *mikrobtān*, poisons, *āssāmān*, the cold, *təssəmḍe*, the heat, *tākusse*, and other things that elicit diseases, but nothing happens independently of the will of God, *derhan n-Māssināy*. He endows these causal factors with their disease potential and characteristics, while also granting healing powers to a therapeutic method. For the Kel Alhafra, disease represents a manifest form of the supernatural power of God, *temātert n-Māssināy*, and thus cannot be simply perceived as bad or evil, because God is merciful and does not meaninglessly impose a burden on humans. Disease, rather, reflects *tāmusne ta wār ti tənhəy*, "the knowledge of the invisible," which encompasses a hidden divine wisdom that is not always comprehensible or obvious to humans.[14] Through suffering, *ayāna*, the individual comes closer to God, must submit him- or herself to God's will and recognizes in his or her weakness the boundlessness of divine power.

A human can have no influence on the appearance and causes of diseases, except in so much as he or she sins, earning as a result God's punishment, *ālyazzāb*, in the form of an illness for which the individual is then responsible. The Kel Alhafra believe that everyone must look after and preserve their health as a part of God's creation and that a sick person must do everything in her or his power to achieve a cure. At the same time, however, everyone has a day predetermined by God on which he or she will die, *ašāl wa n-tāyrəst təmda*. Like disease, the event of death is never arbitrary but is rooted in divine providence and cannot be influenced by human beings. Nevertheless, every sick person contemplating the divine power is expected to appeal to God for a cure. Since God alone is responsible for life and death, the Kel Alhafra are deeply suspicious about the effectiveness of both traditional and modern medication. God's knowledge encompasses everything and when a life has reached its appointed end, nothing can delay the predestined death.[15] A therapy can never counteract divine providence and may only be effective if the disease has been sent as a test and purification or as

---

13. See also here the Qur'anic understanding 6:17: *wa 'in yasaska –llahu bi-durrin fa-la kāšifa lahu 'illa huwa wa 'in yasaska bi-ḫaīrin fa-huwa ʿalā kulli šay'in qadīrun*—"and if He visits thee with good, He is powerful over everything, He is omnipotent over His servants."

14. "'*innama-l-ġaybu li-llāhi*" (10:21) but also surah 6:59: "With him are the keys of the Unseen; none knows them but He. He knows what is in land and sea; not a leaf falls, but He knows it. Not a grain in the earth's shadows, not a thing, fresh or withered, but it is in a Book Manifest."

15. See surah 63:11: *wa lan yuʾaḫḫira-llahu nafsan 'iḏan ğāʾa ʾağaluhā wa-llahu ḫabīru bi-mā taʿmalūna*—"But God will never defer any soul when its term comes, And God is aware of the things you do."

a punishment,[16] to bring the suffering individual closer to God and to lead him or her back to the righteous path. Only God's mercy in the form of a cure for the disease can release one from one's torments.

Disease as Test and Purification

On one hand, the Kel Alhafra understand diseases as trial and purification. Diseases are elicited by natural elements and the stars, by natural catastrophes, poisonous animals, infection, accidents and hereditary factors. Therefore humans beings bear no responsibility; such causal events have been scheduled by the divine power long before their appearance in this lifeworld, *fāll tesāyt n-ākall fuk*,[17] and are sent to believers as a trial and purification, to test their patience, *tāẓidert*, and piety, *āliman*.

Infection, *emāls*, is viewed first and foremost by the Kel Alhafra as the creation of a condition of sickness in a formerly healthy person. Since God alone can create, once again he alone is the origin of the illness. While the Kel Alhafra have empirical experience of the mechanical transmission of a disease, they can provide no concrete explanations for such transmission and cannot construct a theoretical picture for the process of an infection. In the absence of such conceptions, infectious diseases are often misrecognized as hereditary diseases, as is the case for tuberculosis, *tāsut talābasāt*, and skin mycosis, *ākorkor*. Because entire families may be afflicted by these diseases, the Kel Alhafra conclude that God has marked the family with the disease and that it is passed on from generation to generation, although such a "hereditary line," *etāri dāy imārawān*, may be broken or modified by the creator's will. The wind, *aḍu*, can also spread diseases, against which the infected individual is defenseless, just as he or she carries no guilt for afflictions and suffering passed on by the parents.

Disease as Divine Punishment

On the other hand, diseases can be sent as divine punishment. In this case, the individual concerned shares the responsibility for his or her condition.

---

16. In this context, certain Kel Alhafra sometimes cite the following saying of the Prophet from *Ṣaḥīḥ al-Buḥārī*: "Neither tiredness nor sickness, neither care nor grief, neither pain nor sorrow afflicts a Muslim, not even a single miniscule thorn can prick him that is not God's punishment for his errors."

17. See surah 57:22: *"mā 'aṣāba min muṣībatin fī-l-'arḍi wa la fī 'anfusikum 'illā fī kitābin min qabli 'an nabra'ahā 'inna ḏālika 'alā-llahi yasīrun"*—"No affliction befalls in the earth or in yourselves, but it is in a Book, before We create; that is easy for God."

A debt, *ābākkaḍ*, has been imposed, such that through suffering, one may reflect on and recognize one's weakness, helplessness and subjection to the all-encompassing divine power.[18] *a-fal osās āwadəm har iksuḍ Māssināy*, "if a human has difficulties, he is reminded of God," the Kel Alhafra say. Through suffering, the sick person comes closer to God and appeals to Him for forgiveness for all sinful behavior and inattention to the divine creation.

Healing

The Kel Alhafra not only associate illness directly with the divine creative power; they also believe in the miraculous nature of healing, which they do not believe can be explained in any way by physiological factors alone. They do not attribute the effect of a drug to the medicine itself or to the skill of the doctor, but solely to the wisdom of God. Doctors and drugs are simply instruments, they are never the actual reason someone is healed. For the Kel Alhafra, religious attitudes to illness and healing are more important than choosing the right treatment.

For this reason, they will accept a divinely and religiously inspired healer such as a marabout much more readily than a medically trained doctor. This is because the healer acts as an intermediary between divine power and the sick person, with the devout declaration of God's word playing a major role in healing.

CONCEPTIONS OF THE HUMAN BODY

The Kel Alhafra conceive of the human body as a mixture of the various forces that comprise the entire universe. Every single organ exists in relation to all other organs, and should even the tiniest part of the balanced wholeness of the body change, the entire organism responds.[19]

---

18. See here surah 4:123: *"man ya'mal su'a yuǧzabihi wa la yaǧid lahu min dūn-i-llahi walīyan wa la naṣīran."* "Whosoever does evil shall be recompensed for it, and will not find for him, apart from God, a friend or helper."

19. Concepts of a cosmological balance reflected in the microcosm of the body are also found in other cultures, as described, for example, by the following authors: Basso, *Western Apache Witchcraft*; Bastien, "Qollahuaya-Andean Body Concepts"; Bourdieu, *Esquisse d'une theorie de la pratique*; Cunningham, "Order in the Atoni House"; Ebin, "Interpretations of Infertility"; Ferro-Luzzi, G., "Women's Pollution Periods"; Griaule, *Conversations with Ogotemmeli*; Harwood, "The Hot-Cold Theory of Disease"; Hugh-Jones, C., *From the Milk River*; Leslie, ed., *Asian Medical Systems*; McGilvray, *Symbolic Heat*; Reichel-Dolmatoff, *Amazonian Cosmos*; Vogt, *The Zinancantecos of Mexico*; Zahan, *The Religion*.

Components of the oppositional partners in the universe are assigned by the Kel Alhafra to the categories "hot," *wa n-tākusse*, and "cold," *wa n-təssəmḍe*:[20]

Universe—*āddunya*	
wa n-tākusse	**wa n-təssəmḍe**
Day—*ašāl*	Night—*ehāḍ*
Sun—*tāfukk*	Moon—*iyor*
Life—*tāmudre*	Death—*taməttant*
Fire—*efew*	Water—*aman*
Heat—*tākusse*	Cold—*təssəmḍe*
This world—*āddunya*	The next world—*ālaxirāt*
Light—*ənnor*	Darkness—*tihāy*
South—*ājuss*	North—*afālla*
Masculine—*eyy*	Feminine—*tunte*
Dry—*əquur*	Wet—*immihād*
Visible—*āẓẓahir*	Concealed—*ider*

Figure 2: Composition of the universe from oppositional pairs

In an analogy to these categorized energies that govern the universe, the human body is also comprised of a cold and a hot life principle, *tākusse d-təssəmḍe*, whose equilibrium is dependent on its balance in the natural world. The natural environment, foods and illnesses are classified into hot and cold categories and they can influence the corporeal balance between *tākusse* and *təssəmḍe*. In a healthy individual, *tākusse* and *təssəmḍe* are well adjusted, but if this equilibrium is disturbed and a large discrepancy develops between the two categories, the organism is weakened and will fall sick. In the understanding of the Kel Alhafra, heat, *tākusse*, is a living heat, a driving force based in the heart from where it stimulates the living processes

---

20. The polarized assignment of elements into "hot" and "cold" categories that are responsible for certain events through the immanent tension between their opposing forces was a popular explanatory model among the pre-Socratic natural philosophers. Anaxagoras, for example, opposed a cold, wet, dense and dark category (earth) to a hot, dry and tenuous one (ether). Parmenides associated hot and light with the element fire, cold, dark and heavy with night/darkness. See Lloyd, G., *Polarity and Analogy*, 57.

Such classificatory systems whose corresponding pairs are bound to one another by an inner correlation that often reflects a deeper-lying one can also be found, however, in earlier cultures. See here Guthrie, *A History of Greek Philosophy*, Vol. 1, 251–56; Hertz, "La prééminence de la main droite," 553–80; Byl, "Le dualisme ou les couples d'opposées," 210–37.

in the body via the blood.[21] As will be seen, the inner workings of the body are perceived as a kind of "cooking," and attention must always be paid to ensuring that an optimal temperature is maintained so that the body neither overheats nor cools down too much.

Humans can, however, develop an affinity—a temperament—for one or other direction that may shift according to context and that he or she will spend a lifetime trying to counterbalance. The Kel Alhafra divide these individuals into *kel tākusse*, people of the warmth/heat, and *kel təssəmde*, people of the cold. People of the warmth/heat, *kel tākusse*, have a tendency to retain too much heat in their bodies. This renders them nervous, impatient and irascible. They sweat easily and heavily, try to avoid the sun and hot places, and suffer from frequent headaches and nosebleeds, when the internal heat begins to accumulate in the head. The *kel tākusse* have a tendency to eat too much and to drink too little, which means that they do not urinate very often, and their excreta are hot and have a bad smell. In contrast, the people of the cold, *kel təssəmde*, tend toward too little heat in their bodies because the "cooking processes" in their organs are functioning on a low flame. Individuals in this category demonstrate a passive, if not apathetic, character, always have cold hands and feet, and generally suffer from a poor digestion, with the result that their excreta are odorless because they do not absorb nutrients adequately and food often passes undigested through their gut. *kel təssəmde* tend to drink a lot, but suffer from a lack of appetite, and they prefer warm and sunny to cold and damp places.

Kel tākusse among the Kel Alhafra compensate for their hot temperament through a diet rich in foods of the "cold" category, while the *kel təssəmde* attempt to counteract their overcool temperament with foods that are classified as "hot." At the same time, both *kel tākusse* and *kel təssəmde* have a low tolerance for foods and illnesses of their own category. Depending on their affinity to one or other character, "cold" or "hot," individuals can react totally differently to the same foodstuffs or illnesses. In the traditional medicine, therefore, it is crucial to first identify the patient's temperament and the character of the illness in order to prescribe a therapy that will be effective. In general it is said of the *kel tākusse* that they often have a shorter lifespan than the *kel təssəmde* but that they are also less susceptible

---

21. The idea of an "implanted heat" is well attested in antiquity and in the medieval Arabic-Islamic literature as *al-ḥarāra al-ġarīziya*, and is responsible for the organism's entire metabolism. According to both Aristotle and the author of the hippocratic texts this "inborn" heat has a particularly important function during reproduction. See Deichgräber ed., *Hippokrates*; see chapter "Die Entstehung der Körperteile und Organe nach 'De carnibus' und Aristoteles," 28–30; Roussel, "Ether et chaleur dans l'embryologie aristotélicienne," 157–80.

to disease. If they fall sick, the illness is usually severe and serious, but in general they respond rapidly to appropriate treatment. With their cold bodies, the *kel təssəmḍe*, on the other hand, are susceptible to chronic diseases that are difficult to cure and, though they do not necessarily shorten the life of the *kel təssəmḍe*, may condemn them to a life of permanent suffering. The Tamasheq say, "*wa n-tākusse enematin, wa n-təssəmḍe āmarhin,*" "those of a hot character are the ones who die, those of a cold character are the invalids."

DISEASE CATEGORIES

According to the symptoms, the Kel Alhafra assign disease to the category of hot or cold. "Hot" diseases, *torhənnawen n-tākusse*, are always acute: the signs appear suddenly and the course of the disease is brief and severe. In the case of diseases that are potentially fatal, death can occur rapidly in the absence of therapeutic intervention. Diseases of a "hot" character are usually visible on the surface of the body and manifest as inflammations, flatulence, congestion, secretions or bloody excreta from within the body. Fever, *tenāde*, that can be felt on the overheated body, is always an indication of a disease in the "hot" category. All externally visible skin diseases and diseases that originate from the river or water pools, for example intestinal parasites, *imijlān*, or the Guinea worm, *atləb*, are classified as "hot." However, the end stage of certain diseases, such as *idmārān wi lābasnen* (pneumonia) for example, whose onset was not necessarily due to "hot" causes, can also in serious cases turn into an acute, life-threatening "hot" condition. In general, "hot" diseases may cause a great deal of suffering for a fairly short period of time, but with the appropriate therapy they can disappear as quickly as they emerged.

"Cold" diseases, *torhənnawen n-təssəmḍe*, on the other hand are chronic. They hide in the body over a period of time before they become apparent and when they do, the disease may already have reached a well-advanced stage. Because someone with a "cold" disease often ignores or does not notice it for a long time, the disease settles within the body, is difficult to cure, and the disease course is described by the Kel Alhafra as sluggish and protracted.[22] The Kel Alhafra identify, in general, things (e.g., food, nature etc.) that have a "warming" effect on the body as the cause of

---

22. The traditional healer Walett Faqqi in the text "isefran" defines "cold" and "hot" much as they are characterized by the Kel Alhafra: "In general, 'hot' diseases develop quickly, in one direction or the other; 'cold' maladies develop so slowly that they are not perceptible until an advanced and dangerous stage." Walett Faqqi, F., *Isefran*, 12.

"hot" diseases, while things that have a "cooling" impact on the organism are answerable for "cold" diseases. Diseases of a "hot" character, *torhənnawen ti n-tākusse*, are always treated with therapies that have a cooling effect on the overheated organism. Likewise, following this theory of opposite curing opposite (*contraria contrariis*[23]), "cold" diseases are given a warming treatment. Some diseases though have, according to the Kel Alhafra, a hybrid temperament: they can be provoked by either hot or cold things, or during the course of the disease its thermal character can switch; in both cases, the treatment must be appropriate to the disease character.

Considering the classification of the Kel Alhafra's disease repertoire, there is quite clearly a preponderance of diseases classified as "hot" over those of a "cold" or hybrid character. When asked for the reasons behind this imbalance, the Kel Alhafra replied that many of the "hot" diseases have only appeared in recent years, along with the major droughts and the changes in their habits.

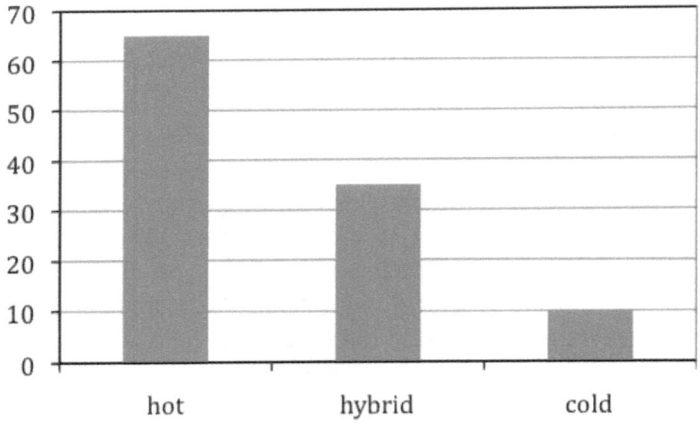

Figure 3: Frequency of the diseases characterized as "hot," "hybrid," and "cold."

"Today there are many diseases that we do not recognize," *"ašāl-i təhee torhənnawen tājotnen wār nəzzej,"* said Ninde, a woman aged about 70 in an encampment at Inkomen.[24] The dietary changes have brought with them *amāyrəs*, a condition of general debilitation, she continued, and the new foods, mainly classified as "hot," together with the shortage of milk, and malnutrition, also encourage the development of "hot" diseases, especially

---

23. The theory that every dyscrasis can be treated with its opposite is found in Galen: *"yanbaġī an tuʿāliġa kulla mizāġin bi-diddihi"*—"you must treat every temperament with its opposite." Ḥunain ibn Isḥāq, ed. M. Meyerhof, 179, 15.

24. Discussion at In Komen, November 2005.

skin diseases. In addition, the failure of the rains has forced families to move further south in the direction of the river, to the cities, and to temporary jobs. Many decide to become sedentary, either totally or in part.

Growing desertification and changes to lifestyles and dietary traditions have severely disturbed the delicate balance by which the Kel Alhafra understand health. It is expressed not only in the frequency of "hot" illnesses, but also in the emergence of "new" diseases that are unfamiliar to the Kel Alhafra and cannot be cured by their traditional therapies. These include a "new fever," which may occasionally be thought to be meningitis, malaria or even the "fever from Abidjan," which is carried in particular by immigrant workers returning home from Ivory Coast. It can be understood not only as malaria, but also as "a new fever" in the sense of AIDS.

THERAPEUTIC NETWORKS BETWEEEN THE SACRED AND THE SECULAR

The Kel Alhafra are exceedingly mistrustful of the state health care services whose employees, the nomads believe, exploit their situation for their own benefit. A physical suffering is kept hidden for as long as possible and confided, if at all, only to familiar peers. Demonstrating a high degree of self-control, a sick Kel Alhafra will only break out of his/her networks when the disease is well advanced. When a healer from outside is consulted, he or she is almost invariably a practitioner from the folk sector who shares the cultural background of the Kel Alhafra. Because a marabout or a traditional healer is endowed with *ālbarāka*, the divinely inspired power of blessing, and practices a holistic treatment which takes into account all aspects of the patient's circumstances, the Kel Alhafra feel much closer to such healers than to biomedically trained doctors or state-trained health personnel.

Although the Kel Alhafra acknowledge the immediate effects of modern pharmaceuticals, in particular those that are given as injections of infusions, they nevertheless think that modern drugs only fight the symptoms, and thereby superficially relieve the patient from his or her complaint, but do not remove the disease out of the body. After treatment with modern medicines, the disease will reappear later in a different form or another part of the body. There is in every disease an element of divine wisdom, not always comprehensible to humans, and thus a total cure requires and comprises not only a physical healing but also an inner spiritual cleansing—both aspects are important in regaining inner equilibrium and good health.

In this contemporary situation where the Kel Alhafra are torn between rebellion and capitulation, between an idealized past and an uncertain future, between a nomadic lifestyle and settlement in villages or cities, and not least between traditional and modern medicine, religious values are being reassessed as a source of greater stability in such precarious times. A general return to and reinterpretation of religious values is apparent, in which coreligionists are forming a social network set within the context of a shared Islamic origin, history and culture. Because virtues such as piety and godliness now win both recognition and respect, the role of the marabout within the nomadic society is gaining in significance and influence. This revived piety has two important consequences for health concepts and behavior among the Kel Alhafra. On one hand, it brings with it a religious fatalism in certain circles that smothers any personal responsibility and action; children in particular suffer in such cases, because they are absolutely dependent on their parents. The second effect is the rejection of secular influences, including modern medicine. The effectiveness of modern medicine is placed in doubt, not only because it does not offer a holistic approach to the patient's suffering and treatment, but also because it is perceived as the product of profit- and power-greedy western industrialized nations and their sidekicks in the local health care sector. "āṣ ṣexāt ašəkrəš n-alxer," they say in Tamasheq, "health is a garden of good fortune." "mušan torhənna tojarāt āṣ ṣahāt-nanāy," the Kel Alhafra add, "however, sickness surpasses our means," because they are subject to the divine power, and recovery is decided by God alone.

BIBLIOGRAPHY

Arberry, Arthur J., trans. *The Koran Interpreted: A Translation*. London: Oxford University Press, 1964.
Basso, Keith H. *Western Apache Witchcraft*. Anthropological Papers of the University of Arizona 15. Tucson: University of Arizona Press, 1969.
Bastien, Joseph W. "Qollahuaya-Andean Body Concepts: A Topographical-Hydraulic Model of Physiology." *American Anthropologist* 87 (1985) 595–611.
Bourdieu, Pierre. *Esquisse d'une théorie de la pratique: Précédé de trois études d'ethnologie kabyle*. Travaux de droit, d'économie, de sociologie et de sciences politiques 92. Paris: Seuil, 2000. English trans.: *Outline of a Theory of Practice*. Translated by Richard Nice. Cambridge: Cambridge University Press, 1977.
al-Buhārī, Muḥammad Ibn Ismaʿīl. *ṣaḥīḥ al-buḥārī. al-ṣāmiʿ aṢ-ṣaḥīḥ*. Liechtenstein: Thesaurus Islamicus Foundation, 2000.
Byl, Simon. "Le dualisme ou les couples d'opposées." In *Recherches sur les grands traités biologiques d'Aristote: Sources écrites et préjuges*. Mémoires de la classe des lettres ser. 2, 64. Brusselles: Académie royale de Belgique, 1980.
Chelhod, J. "La baraka chez les Arabes ou l'influence bienfaisante du sacré." *Revue de l'Histoire des Religions* 148 (1955) 68–88.

Part 2

Religion, Illness, and Care of the Sick in Asiatic Health Care

5

A Focus on the Law or on the Individual?

The Uncoupling of Religion and Health Care and the Emergence of Medical Science in Ancient China[1]

—Paul U. Unschuld

The WHO's definition of "health" as a "state of complete physical, mental and social well-being" met with a great deal of critical commentary, not least from theologians. A more recent example of these critical voices is Prof. Ulrich Körtner, a professor of Systematic Theology at the Evangelisch-Theologische Fakultät (Faculty of Protestant Theology) at the University of Vienna. He writes:

> The WHO's definition reinforces a sense of entitlement according to which health in an overarching sense is not due to grace or good luck, but is a right. The religious longing for healing is transformed into a right to happiness, to freedom from suffering and to children who are free from any illness. To the extent that the WHO sees health not as an ability but a state, humans' opportunity and ability to suffer is completely overlooked.

---

1. See also Unschuld, "When Health Was Freed from Fate."

Suffering is seen only as that which should not exist, rather than being accepted as an aspect of life that complements happiness.[2]

There are several phrases in this statement that are worth discussing. Medical historians will primarily be interested in the repeated emphasis on what, from a theological perspective, is a recent and undesirable development in how humanity deals with sickness. Körtner and others imply that things were different in the pre-modern era—and this is precisely the idea that I want to investigate more closely today. In fact, historical sources show that in Chinese antiquity, there was apparently a much more striking emphasis on the natural-science-based idea of uncoupling religion from medical science than was the case in European antiquity. To be sure, there remained a close connection between medical science and religion in China in subsequent centuries—as continues to be the case today—but the cultural construct that we call medical science meant drawing a conscious boundary between the age-old idea of a near-total dependency on numinous powers on the one hand and a new world view on the other that promised to reward every individual with good health and longevity if they complied with laws and morals as allegedly asked for by certain natural laws.

I would like to argue that the implicit idea of a right to health, which Körtner and other theologians criticize in the WHO's definition of health, is by no means a recent development. The right to health is the basis for uncoupling religion and medical science. The idea of health as a right—and this is true of ancient China as well as Europe—is the basis for creating the field of medical science as we know it today.

Medical science is the fairly easily definable result of a clearly defined cultural revolution, and can be placed with relative ease on a chronological timeline. I would claim that, in the cultural history of humanity, no other change in world view has been as deep-seated or as long-lasting. What makes it particularly fascinating is that this revolution first took place in the eastern Mediterranean region, what we normally refer to as ancient Greece, and then a few centuries later on the eastern edge of the Eurasian continent, in China. In both cultural areas, a completely new type of medical science emerged: a type of medicine that we still foster and further develop today, that we continue to teach in our medical schools as the only acceptable way to respond to illness.

What was different about this new medical science was its three-part creed. I consciously use the term creed here because the underlying idea used to guide the medical science then and ever since was and is nothing other than a profession of faith. The three parts are easy to list:

2. Körtner, *Unverfügbarkeit des Lebens?*, 41–43.

1. All natural occurrences are based on laws. These laws apply regardless of time, space or persons—be they humans or numinous.
2. We human beings are able to recognize these laws. Persistent searching will lead to deeper and deeper insights; no limit is in sight.
3. If we are aware of the laws of nature, that is sufficient in order to understand human existence as well as the entire universe in which this existence takes place.

None of these creeds can be scientifically proven in opposition to alternative ideas, and yet even today they remain the basis for our work in the fields of natural science and medical science.

No evidence of these laws of nature had been discovered yet, either in Greece or in China, and yet some of the intelligentsia began to believe that such laws were behind all forms of creation, existence and decay. In this context, a medical science arose in which people saw themselves as part of a system of natural laws that would punish them if they violated the laws. At the same time, in addition to fulfilling a moral obligation, it gave them the chance of enjoying a long life without illness. The new medicine came with a promise of freedom from suffering and sickness as long as people followed the rules, the natural laws.

Based on Harald Holz' comparative legal philosophical investigations of China and Europe, we can conclude that in both Chinese and Greek antiquity, the idea developed—whether consciously or unconsciously—that there was a kind of justice in mankind's interactions with the universe in which they lived.[3]

This counterpart to mankind was never given a specific name. And yet the counterpart became a contractual partner. This represents the true cultural understanding of medical science.

People enter into a contract with their counterpart. The identity of the counterpart remains unclear. What is clear, however, is that the parties have a relationship based on mutual claims against one another. As Harald Holz puts it, this can also be described as justice. The relationship allows each side to claim its rights (justified claims against the other party) and obligations (justified claims by the other party against oneself).

The contract, once again citing Harald Holz, is determined by the principle of doing right and being right, in other words a claim for justice that awards "each his own" in terms of both rights and obligations.[4]

---

3. Holz, "Rom und China," 16ff.
4. Ibid., 6.

A person who shared this sense of existential justice acknowledged his obligations and demanded his rights in exchange. To the same extent, he was also aware of his unknown counterpart's claims. This counterpart had the right to bring people to life, as men or as women, perhaps with a beautiful body, perhaps as a cripple, and ultimately to remove its creations from life as well. Between these starting and ending points, the unknown counterpart was obligated to give people the opportunity to enjoy a life without suffering. In order to enjoy this, people also had to do what was right and fulfill their obligations. The people's obligation was to act in accordance with the laws of nature. In exchange, they were given the right to a life free from suffering, or rather a life of good health.

Medical science represents the effort to help people claim their rights from this unknown counterpart. Another way of putting it is that medical science has spent the last two millennia searching for the details of the conditions established in the contract, so that it can give humanity the chance to fulfill its own part of the contract.

Medical science's role is to tell people what they must do and what they must avoid in order to claim their rights. Illness, then—it is almost unnecessary to add—is the consequence of humankind's violation of an obligation. Just as health is not a gift or an act of mercy, but a right that comes from complying with obligations, illness in the age of this new medicine is no longer the result of the unfathomable whims of more or less clearly visible numinous forces, for instance many gods or the one God; instead, it is a clearly defined exercise of power by the unknown counterpart when people grossly fail to fulfill their obligations. This exercising of power is associated with pain, physical deformity and premature death.

In its role as an attorney, capable of reducing the sentence and leading the way back to health even if there is no way to prevent the breach of the law, medical science can take two fundamentally different paths. Since we see medical science as the product of an idea about the right to good health, based on natural laws, it makes sense for us to stay at the level of legal philosophical comparisons for a while as we weigh the diagnostic and therapeutic alternatives.

In the history of law, from antiquity to the present, and particularly in the comparison of continental European legislation with Anglo-Saxon legislation, we can see a dichotomy of approaches. In brief, these involve abstract law on the one side, and cases of precedence as the basis for making decisions on the other. A nearly identical dichotomy of approaches has also distinguished medical science in its efforts to find the appropriate treatments for illnesses.

In Chinese history, medical science is comparable to the continental European approach of finding justice. The basis for diagnosing illnesses is an understanding of abstract laws and principles. The new form of Chinese health care knowledge created at the beginning of the Han Dynasty, in other words since the 2nd century BCE, placed the collective norm above the individual patient; individual cases of illness always had to be traced back to the general norm.

Thus numerous individual cases came together to form an abstract collective. Of course, this perspective was not entirely new. Historically, there were already collective concepts in use, such as malaria. Each individual malaria patient differs from every other malaria patient in terms of his or her own experience of the illness. Nonetheless, even in prehistoric times, the view had clearly already become established that all of these individually differing cases could be assigned a shared label, namely *nüe*, which today is translated as "malaria." The new medical science inherited many such historical labels, and set itself the task of redefining them on the basis of a violation of the yin-yang and five-phase norms, according to the newly discovered laws of nature.

But what specifically was taking place? We are in the fortunate position, thanks to written sources, of being able to follow the emergence of this new medicine out of the pre-medical, non-medical healing arts—much more clearly than in ancient Greece. In fact, the sources even allow us to identify a watershed moment in intellectual history, approximately in the middle of the 2nd century BCE. This watershed was nothing other than the uncoupling mentioned in the title, of religious healing arts on the one side and health care approaches on the other.[5]

If we define the concept of religion very broadly as a construct that places people in an existential relationship with numinous powers, whether these be ancestors, the spirits of the dead, a pantheon or perhaps only a single god, then we can describe a form of religious healing in China that begins around the eleventh century BCE. This was the idea that either the ancestors or evil spirits, in other words demons, were able to harm the health of living people. We know that the Chinese subscribed to this idea because of reliable written sources from the first millennium BCE. Of course, the specifics of the practices associated with this idea are known only from the second century on, and in much greater detail beginning in the fourth century.

In particular, Daoism played an important role here. As Michel Strickman so knowledgeably showed in his book *Chinese Magical Medicine*, local cults for dealing with illness and misfortune were common in Chinese

---

5. Unschuld, *What Is Medicine?*, 44ff.

antiquity.[6] These cults believed in local deities who needed to be consulted and asked for help in healing illnesses. The Daoist religion attempted to dethrone these local gods and to unmask them as spirits from the underworld of the dead, saying that they in fact had caused the illnesses that they were called by the exorcist cults to heal. Thus the model of Daoism did not question the impact of the spirits of the dead. However, it did set a goal of limiting the evil deeds of these spirits and lessening the effects of their actions. It developed what one might call a typical Chinese image of heaven and hell as giant bureaucratic structures. The authorities of heaven were called upon to rectify the damages caused by those in the world of the dead. The underworld, too, had its own authorities and military, its own writing and even its own flora. It was a world of evil, of intrigue, of battles and of long, painful trials. New arrivals in the underworld were evaluated by three high judges and condemned to endless torment according to the severity of their guilt. However—and this is decisive—the punishment did not apply merely to the criminal, but could also extend to many generations of his patrilinear descendants.

In this view, the details of which cannot all be explained here, a living person who contracted an illness was very rarely responsible for his own suffering. Most of the time, he was experiencing the collective curse of his clan from the world of the dead. For very serious crimes, a new arrival in the world of the dead could have all of his descendants wiped out, to the ninth degree of kinship. The living and the dead thus ormed a chain of mutual responsibility across many generations. The good deeds of the living could ease the existence of the dead who were in hell. Conversely, the living were often forced to pay for the deeds of their departed forebears. If one spirit brought a claim against another, the torture could begin immediately, and could also involve the living descendants. The symptoms of an illness were thus an indication that an ancestor in the world of the dead was involved in criminal proceedings. Here, too, I will keep my remarks brief. Daoism offered its priests as attorneys for the dead. Priests were trained to infiltrate the world of the dead and to act as defendants or prosecutors in order to lessen the suffering of their clients.[7]

From the sources dating to the middle of the first millennium, it can be seen that this idea of an interaction between the living and those who were long dead was gradually supplemented or even replaced by the idea that the happiness and well-being of the living was due to the good deeds of their distant ancestors, while suffering and illness were due to the failures of

---

6. Faure and Strickmann, *Chinese Magical Medicine*, 40.
7. Ibid., 3 et passim.

the more recent dead. Fundamentally, however, the idea remained that only part of an illness is the patient's own fault. The individual's moral dependency on his living or dead relatives made it very likely that a patient was paying for failures that were not his own. Ultimately, the view was strengthened that arbitrary demons took possession of the living, without bringing any ancestors into play.

Here we have described one of the religious models that has persisted in China until the present day. It forces people to follow a certain set of morals so that they, and perhaps their descendants many years from now, can benefit from their good deeds. In an essay as brief as this one, these observations will have to suffice; for the many different ways in which the basic principles of Daoism were implemented by the population can hardly be listed in just a few pages. In short, the individual was not responsible for his own existence. Fate could befall him because others had sinned and because their punishment applied to him as well. Medical science, on the other hand, offered liberation. Medical science is the basis for individual existential self-determination. Medical science is the alternative to religion and religious healing. There is no middle ground that connects the two. Medical science takes away the power that the gods, the spirits of the dead or the one God hold over living people—in Europe as well as in China.

For now, let us remain in China. In order to understand the development of the medical healing arts, or simply medicine, in the initially defined sense of an alternative to religious healing, it makes sense to take a look at the Mawangdui manuscripts and other writings from the early second century BCE. Here we read, for instance, about a "compulsion to belch," an "inability to lift the head toward heaven," as well as "retention of urine" and "cramps in children."[8] What we fail to find in these texts is a conceptual distinction between the state of being ill and the underlying disease itself—in other words, between the more or less visible and palpable signs of suffering on the one hand and the disturbances deep within the organism that cause these signs of suffering, as symptoms, on the other.

Precisely this step beyond the conceptual watershed was taken sometime in the second century BCE. For the first time in Chinese history, the new medicine drew a clear distinction between outward signs of suffering and the concept of a disease that was responsible for these symptoms. From this point on, therapy was, ideally, focused on the disease rather than on the individual case.[9]

---

8. Harper, *Early Chinese Medical Literature*, 208, 209, 233.
9. Unschuld, *Huang Di Neijing Suwen, Nature, Knowledge*, 205 ff.

After this time, disease meant a deviation from norms set by natural law, deep within the human organism. The deviation from the norm was in turn the result of a violation by the owner of this organism, in other words the person. The laws of nature from which the norms for health-promoting behavior were derived can be found in the yin-yang and five-phases doctrines that originated in the third and second centuries BCE. The plausibility of these natural-law doctrines came from centuries of experiencing and observing the ongoing forces of nature as well as human social behavior; the three-hundred-year phase of the "Warring States," from the sixth to the third century BCE, left a lasting impression that still shapes Chinese culture and mentality today. The core concept of the yin-yang teaching can be found in the classic text of Chinese medical science, written in the centuries either just before or just after the birth of Christ. It reads: "Mutual domination—this is harmony. If there is no mutual domination, this is disease."[10] In another place, the message reads: "To be familiar with domination and revenge—this is a model valid for all mankind. There is nothing else to the Way of heaven."[11]

The natural laws of yin-yang and the five phases offer the knowledge that people need in order to survive in an environment where defeat and retribution dominate. They clearly explained, in detail, how people should behave—in terms of the ratio of waking and sleeping, what to eat, what clothing to wear in different seasons and different temperatures, in terms of sexual behaviors and many other aspects. Fidelity to the law, in other words behavior that followed the teachings of the systematic correspondence of all things, guaranteed good health. Violating the law meant punishment. By defining the illness that caused the state of being ill, it could be determined where the violation had taken place and how it should be appropriately treated.

Being ill, then, is a punishment. This idea can also be found in the realm of religious healing. However, medical science clearly states that it is always the offender himself who receives the punishment. In other words, if someone is sick, it is his own fault. Herein lies the key cultural historical significance of the development of medical science. Medical science is a sign that the individual has been liberated from his linkage with his ancestors. It is also a sign of liberation from the arbitrary will of one god or many numinous beings. Medical science is based on the realization that understanding natural laws shows us the path to self-determined health. It may not

---

10. Unschuld with Tessenow, *Huang Di Nei Jing Su Wen. Huang Di's Inner Classic.* Vol. 2, 282.

11. Ibid., 617.

be possible for everyone to achieve this health through self-determination right at this moment. However, the exploration of the laws of nature opens up larger and larger freedoms. Thus it is not surprising that, in the history of European medical science, whenever a significant breakthrough appeared at the horizon, theology attempted to prevent its realization—this is true until today, for example, in terms of the potential of stem-cell research. Every new step toward the self-determination of health reduces humanity's need to follow the strict moral codes of a religion. Above all, compliance with strict moral codes is guaranteed by a fear of illness or other suffering as punishment for violating these codes. By defining the laws of nature, which are responsible for sickness and health regardless of whether or not religious morals are followed, medical science gives people the freedom to disregard these morals and thus the associated faith in spirits, gods or the one God.

The physiological and pathological basis for the new Chinese medicine's view of disease and the state of being ill came from a completely new idea: that all of the organism's functions were connected with one another and with the individual body parts and tissues through primary, secondary and tertiary vessels. Transporting blood and vapors through these channels was the pivotal point of life. An undisrupted transport was essential to health; a disrupted transport caused illness. Inserting a needle into these vessels, in varying combinations of a limited number of insertion points—known as acupuncture—is the method of choice for reversing a violation of the norms.

The theory of vessels that underlies acupuncture is, in fact, a projection: a projection of the new road and transport network of the recently unified empire onto the individual human organism. Before the unification of the empire in 221 BCE, the last remaining states from the time of the Warring States existed largely in isolation from one another. Like the organs of the human body, they were not seen as parts of a great exchange, but as individual pieces existing alongside one another. This now changed with the unification of the empire. In the new empire, the former individual states created an organic whole. The well-being and woes of this organic whole depended on a harmonious give and take between its individual parts. This new reality of the state order was soon reflected in medical texts, as the new reality of the physiological order.[12]

The Chinese elite of that time, however, was divided in how they responded to the deep-reaching structural change that is only hinted at here. Right from the start, some Chinese social philosophers preferred a completely different system of order than the one represented by the newly

12. Unschuld, "What is Medicine?," 50 ff.

formed empire. These were the intellectuals who rejected the large, bureaucratically governed, multi-centric social organism, which was based on exchange, trade and change, because they believed it to be ungovernable and detrimental to the harmony of human coexistence. For simplicity's sake, let us call these opponents Daoists, because it is in Daoist writings that we find explicit proof of this opposition.

In fact, the writings of the Daoists describe a system of healing arts that reflects their prejudices against manmade morals and laws as well as their rejection of the unified empire. This dichotomy of political views was now also expressed by differing degrees of willingness to look for abstract deviations from the norm as an underlying disease that caused individual cases of being ill. Daoist healing did not agree with this tendency in the new medical science. Thus we find two opposing approaches in the history of Chinese healing, whose only legitimization consisted of an order-oriented, in other words social-philosophy-based, opposition.

Since some of the health care experts refused to accept the vessel theory as the key to understanding physiology and pathology, and thus rejected acupuncture as well, since it was only legitimized through this theory of vessels; and since the same thinkers refused to interpret the reality of life on the basis of natural laws, there was no basis or incentive for them to recognize a fundamental deviation from the norm in the individual cases of illness. The ideological alternative to the new medicine expressed itself in a continuation of pharmaceutical therapy as a persistent form of individualism. For one thousand years to come it failed to integrate the natural science of the yin-yang and five-phases doctrines into the application of pharmaceutical recipes.

Every new case of an illness is slightly different than the ones before it, and stands alone. Each individual recipe that had proven effective in the past was taken seriously. However, each individual recipe was effective only in a limited number of cases at best, so it seemed inevitable to believe in the individuality of the cases and to offer as many recipes as possible for as many forms of the illness as possible.

The difference from the theoretical principles of acupuncture is abundantly clear at the height of this development, between the twelfth and sixteenth centuries. As before, acupuncture continued to get by with a limited number of insertion points. The various combinations of these points made it possible to effectively treat the limited number of deviations from the norm. The pharmaceutical tradition, on the other hand, was forced to constantly expand its initially small number of drugs and recipes, since it was unable to recognize each concrete case of suffering as a variation on a limited number of deviations from the norm.

As early as the eighth century, the official material medica compendium of the Tang Dynasty described 850 individual drugs. In the twelfth and thirteenth centuries, this number increased to 1700 substances. Finally, in the sixteenth century, the ultimate peak was reached with the publication of the *Bencao gangmu*. Li Shizhen, the author of this encyclopedic survey of all known pharmaceutically used herbal, animal, mineral and man-made substances, described just under 1900 individual drugs in his life's work.[13]

The dynamic nature of material medica corresponded to the increasing wealth of literature on recipes. Where the Mawangdui manuscripts described about 200 recipes, the work of Tang-era physician Sun Simiao (581–682?) featured 5300 recipes, a number that was soon exceeded by Wang Tao's *Waitai biyao* with 6000 recipes—not to mention the *Shengji zonglu* with 20,000 recipes and the *Pujifang* in the early fifteenth century, with no fewer than 61,000 recipes.

In the eleventh and twelfth centuries, though, before this development reached its height, several pharmaceutical authors more or less stepped on the brakes. Kou Zongshi (around 1116) wrote a book on *material medica*, the *Bencao yanyi*, that included just 500 drug descriptions; Wang Haogu (thirteenth century) believed 224 medications were sufficient, and Zhu Zhenheng (1281–1358) kept the number to just 153 substances. However, this was not the only change in the pharmaceutical tradition.[14]

The abovementioned authors linked the effects of pharmaceutical substances in the human body with the deviations from norms that had already been in use in acupuncture medicine for a thousand years already, in other words with the limited number of concepts for disease that were behind the unlimited number of individual symptoms of illness.[15] This rendered the large number of drugs unnecessary.

The point was no longer the effectiveness of the individual drugs, but rather their value within the normative context of yin-yang and the five phases. The authors created the first Chinese system of pharmacology; at the same time, however, they brought to an end—at least for some users of pharmaceutical medicine—the trend toward unlimited individuality in diagnosis and therapy, which had become an increasingly impracticable expansion of both individual substances and the number of recipes.

When we look at the situation near the end of the imperial era, in other words during the Qing Dynasty in the eighteenth and nineteenth centuries, we thus see not just the parallel existence of the natural-law and

13. Unschuld, *Medicine in China*, passim.
14. Ibid., 85–127.
15. Ibid., 154ff.

individualistic approaches to Chinese healing, but also the efforts to create what today would be known as a crossover—combining the collective approach with the individualistic approach.

As an example, let us look at the instructions for "black gold pills." This recipe was recommended for treating a large number of gynecological ailments. It was thus a recipe for a disease collective that was assumed to manifest itself as numerous individual symptoms. The crossover came from the possibility of adapting the basic collective recipe to the individual case by adding and omitting individual components. The texts that recommend "black gold pills" name more than a hundred such modifications to account for the individual experiences of gynecological ailments.

To conclude: Approximately two thousand years ago, a remarkable initiative was launched in China with the aim of liberating people from their entrapment by the moral failures of others and their dependency on the arbitrary whims of numinous powers. The new medicine of the era put its adherents in a position of self-determination. This condition of self-determination was, and still is today, an ideal. Even today, the health of passive smokers depends on the behavior of others; many people's health depends on pathogenic environmental conditions, and even today, children are born with deformities that are inherited or caused by their mothers' grossly negligent behavior during pregnancy. Still, there is a clear distinction between these circumstances and a religious non-medical attitude. Medical science is legitimized by its faith in the eternal progress of knowledge in the natural sciences, which increasingly give people the power to determine whether nonsmokers will continue to be endangered by smokers, whether the masses will be harmed by environmental damages and whether children will be born with abnormalities. Man, or rather mankind—according to the ideal of medical science—can decide how much health to allow itself, and is no longer dependent on any other instance when it comes to making this decision.

BIBLIOGRAPHY

Harper, Donald. *Early Chinese Medical Literature: The Mawangdui Medical Manuscripts.* Sir Henry Wellcome Asian Series 2. London: Kegan Paul, 1998.

Holz, Harald. "Rom und China: Zwei Weltreiche im Vergleich unter rechtsphilosophischen Aspekten." In *Rechtsdenken: Schnittpunkte West und Ost,* edited by Harald Holz and Konrad Wegmann, 1–36. Strukturen der Macht 13. Münster: Lit, 2005.

Körtner, Ulrich H. J., *Unverfügbarkeit des Lebens? Grundfrage der Bioethik und der medizinischen Ethik.* Neukirchen-Vluyn: Neukirchener, 2001.

Strickmann, Michael. *Chinese Magical Medicine*. Edited by Bernard Faure. Stanford University Press, Stanford, 2002.

Unschuld, Paul U. "When Health Was Freed from Fate: Some Thoughts on the Liberating Potential of Early Chinese Medicine: East Asian Science." *Technology and Medicine* 31 (2010) 9–22.

———. *Huang Di Neijing Suwen: Nature, Knowledge, Imagery in an Ancient Chinese Medical Text*. Berkeley: University of California Press, 2003.

———. *Medicine in China: A History of Ideas*. 25th anniversary ed. Comparative Studies of Health Systems and Medical Care. Berkeley: University of California Press, 2010.

———. *Medicine in China: A History of Pharmaceutics*. Comparative Studies of Health Systems and Medical Care. Berkeley: University of California Press, 1976.

———. *What Is Medicine? Western and Eastern Approaches to Healing*. Translated by Karen Reimers. Berkeley: University of California Press, 2009.

Unschuld, Paul U., with H. Tessenow. *Huang Di Nei Jing Su Wen. Huang Di's Inner Classic. Basic Questions. An Annotated Translation*. Vol. 2. (in collaboration with Zheng Jinsheng.) Berkeley: University of California Press, 2011.

6

Buddhist Principles of Tibetan Medicine?

The Buddhist Understanding of Illness and Healing and the Medical Ethics of the *rGyud-bzhi*

—Jens Schlieter

INTRODUCTION

TIBETAN MEDICINE (Tibetan: *gso ba rig pa*), like Chinese, Indian and Greek systems of medicine, is a well-developed model, rooted in an independent tradition, of etiology (causes of illness), diagnosis, therapy and medicinal arts. By analyzing types of constitutions and their specific dispositions toward illness, Tibetan doctors attempt to determine which illness is present. Ideally, the therapy consists of restoring the balance of the three "bodily humors": wind, bile and phlegm.

Even if an important root of Tibetan medicine goes back to the non-Buddhist Indian medical teachings of the *Āyurveda*, it is nonetheless clear that by the time the fundamental work of classical Tibetan medicine—the twelfth-century "four-root Tantra" (*rGyud bzhi*)—was composed, there was a strong connection between Tibetan medicine and Buddhist teachings and ideas. Based on the guiding question about the relationship between religion and the treatment of illnesses, I would first like to explore the central Buddhist concepts that helped shape Tibetan medicine's ideas about ailments, suffering, illness and healing. Using selected examples, I will investigate the extent to which there are differences between pre-modern Tibetan medical texts and today's Western therapeutic ideals. These examples have to do with the approach that physicians should take with incurable patients (hopeless prognosis) according to the *rGyud bzhi*, and the form of ethics that should guide physicians in dealing with patients overall.

If the normative presentation of medical ethics among Tibetan doctors is found to have a certain Buddhist ethos, we might assume that—in keeping with the karmic idea of "perpetrator ethics"—the actions of the physician, rather than the sufferings of the potential victim ("victim ethics") are the main focus. If, on the other hand, medical ethics are shown to have been "buddhicised" at a later stage, it is also possible that the medical ethics were only partially harmonized with the more strongly Buddhist, soteriological ethics; in this case, any remaining tensions in the concept would need to be described.

ILLNESS AND SUFFERING

The concept of illness currently in use today can be differentiated into three main meanings: (a) a case of illness that affects one person, (b) a type of illness (within the classification of pathologies), and (c) an abstract concept in opposition to the state of health.[1] In Buddhist source texts, too, illness and healing can be categorized into these three levels: as healing of a specific illness through medicine; as a teaching about the fundamental causes of illness; and on an overarching level, where the Buddhist teachings or the Buddha himself (or another healing figure) are used as medicine to heal suffering. Depending on the level, the categories represent the cycle of mortality, desire,[2] or rebirth itself.[3] For the various schools of Buddhism, one of the central teachings of the historical Buddha Śākyamuni is schematized as the "four noble truths." The first begins in the style of a standard passage: "Birth is suffering, illness is suffering, death is suffering."[4] The suffering caused by illness is thus a fact of human existence. Since one of the stated goals of

1. Cf. Meyer, "Introduction," 11.
2. On the concept of suffering desire, see Pruett, *The Meaning and End of Suffering.*
3. Cf. Birnbaum, *Der heilende Buddha,* 19 f. Cf. also Butzenberger and Fedorowa, "Wechselbeziehungen," 89.
4. E.g., *Mahāsatipaṭṭhāna-Sutta,* D II.290–315.

Buddhist healing practice is to overcome the conditions of suffering, overcoming "illness" is also part of the Buddhist "therapy."[5]

The first truth, suffering, is followed by truths about the causes and/or the "formation of suffering," about the "relief of suffering" and the "path toward relief." The structure of this schema, as has often been noted, resembles a schema used in traditional Indian medicine.[6] In the words of the Buddhist commentator *Buddhaghosa* (5th cent.): "The truth of suffering must be considered an illness; the truth of how suffering comes about must be considered the cause of the illness; the elimination of suffering . . . must be considered healing; the truth of the path must be considered medicine."[7]

According to an investigation of the sources by Albrecht Wezler,[8] however, it seems unlikely that the Buddha (or the sources containing his teachings), as claimed, was guided by an existing medical schema. This schema includes 1.) the diagnosis of "illness" (Sanskrit *roga*), 2.) its etiology (Sanskrit *rohagetu*), 3.) the medicine (*bhaiṣajya*) and 4.) the elimination of the suffering (*ārogya*). Instead, it seems much more plausible that the Buddha was the first to design such a schema.[9] In any case, a clear parallel can be seen between the attitudes of a physician and the Buddha, who explicitly believes suffering to include pain, worry, depression, the fading of the senses, etc., and who also explains the genesis of this suffering in an empirical, physiological, psychological and karmic sense. In this regard, when speaking of Buddhist "existential diagnostics," it is better to refer to *the sufferings* rather than *the ailment* of a person.[10] According to this approach, the suffering and pain that accompany handicaps are not seen as necessary impositions by a higher power or fate; at the same time, the existential intensity of the

---

5. Cf. Schlieter, "Endure, Adapt, or Overcome?" 309–36.

6. This observation can be found, for instance, in Butzenberger and Fedorowa, "Wechselbeziehungen," 95–96.

7. Buddhaghosa and Ñāṇatiloka, *Visuddhi-magga* (512,7–9)/and *Der Weg zur Reinheit*, 596.

8 Wezler, "On the Quadruple Division of the Yogaśāstra, the Caturvyūhatva of the Cikitsaśāstra and the 'Four Noble Truths' of the Buddha," 290–337.

9. Wezler's conclusion: "the quadruple division was discovered by the Buddha; it was thereafter taken over by the author of the relevant sūtras" (Wezler, "On the Quadruple Division of the Yogaśāstra, the Caturvyūhatva of the Cikitsaśāstra and the 'Four Noble Truths' of the Buddha," 336.)

10. According to Geertz, "Religion als kulturelles System," 68, the question from a religious perspective is less about how suffering "is to be avoided, but rather how to suffer." Early Buddhism, by contrast, actually advises eliminating suffering. On the differentiation between ailment and suffering, see also the article "Heil/Leid" by the same author, 203–5; see also Edwards, "Three Concepts of Suffering," 59–66.

dimension of suffering (which is more strongly emphasized in the concept of an ailment) should be noted.[11]

Suffering can have physical as well as mental causes. What is important here is to what extent the Buddhist teachings (or the teaching as such) make sense as a universal treatment for all kinds of suffering, in other words also as a way to relieve illnesses.[12] Some of the passages suggest that it is possible for people to achieve freedom from suffering even during their lifetimes. However, in the passages that tend to describe human life itself through the metaphor of an ongoing "illness," such as the observations on the disgust and decay of the body, there is no mention of relieving illnesses. There are various depictions in the Mahāyāna literature suggesting that certain healing figures like the medicine Buddha, as the "King of Healers" (Sanskrit *Baiṣajyagururāja*, Tibetan *'od kyi rgyal po* or *sangs rgyas sman la*), are able to relieve all suffering, but this is more an expression of wishful and petitioning prayers than faith in a concrete medical and therapeutic effect. Instead, there are indications that skepticism dominated when it came to the potential for healing specific illnesses. Both the Vinaya rule, stating that people suffering from certain illnesses should not be accepted into the order, and the chapters defining "untreatable illnesses" in Indian and Tibetan medical texts, which I will discuss in further detail below, seem to confirm this.

Nonetheless, it must be noted that when suffering is defined from a Buddhist perspective, there are no other overarching interpretations regarding the higher meaning of the suffering. Suffering is clearly not an anthropological constant caused by the will of a creator. A fundamental Buddhist theorem that is also significant in the ethical debate is that all beings strive to achieve "happiness" (*sukha*) and to avoid "suffering" (*duḥkha*): "If we mentally explore the world in every direction of the compass, we [nonetheless] will not find anyone whom we value more than ourselves. In the same way, the others also value themselves the most highly; thus those who value themselves should not injure others."[13] The fundamental texts of Mahāyāna Buddhism, which is predominantly practiced in Tibet, also assume a fundamental, universally shared preference for avoiding suffering in all sensi-

---

11. "Suffering" is thus also the better term in the sense that it defines the chronological extension of the experience of an ailment, which is clearly just as much a part of the Buddhist conception as in the definitions of "suffering" in English; cf. Cassell, *The Nature of Suffering and the Goals of Medicine*, 33: "suffering can be defined as the state of severe distress associated with events that threaten the intactness of person."

12. It is clear that the *Vinaya* discusses this; the monks were to go out into the world "for the benefit and joy of many" (*bahujanahitāya bahujanasukhāya*, Vin I.21) and spread the word. Promoting "well-being" (*hita*) is thus part of their professional 'mission'; see also Promta, "Law and Morality: The Buddhist Perspective," 13.

13. P. I.75 = *Udāna* 5.1 (*Piyatarasutta*).

tive beings, which simultaneously represents the basic axiom of Buddhist ethics.[14] For instance, the famous exercise on the "equality of the other and of oneself" (Sanskrit *parātmasamatā*) in Śāntideva's *Bodhicaryāvatāra* states: "Since everyone experiences suffering and happiness in the same way, I must protect them as I do myself. Just as the one body, consisting of various body parts like the hand, etc., must be protected, so too must this whole diverse world, whose beings experience the same happiness and the same suffering."[15]

Based on the definition of "suffering," then, there should not be any fundamental difficulties in integrating the types of medical treatments that aim to reduce suffering due to illness—at least at a general level, since the specific treatment of ailments is still influenced by other complex conditions that at best are generally based on religious statements about suffering.

ILLNESS AND HEALING

According to the above schema, health is defined in Buddhist sources as the absence or relief of illness (Sanskrit *ārogya*).[16] What is interesting about this understanding is that it is also expressed linguistically by the terms used: "without being ill" (*ārogya*), or "non-sickness" (*ārogyatā*).[17] By contrast, the term "medicine" is interpreted in Indo-Tibetan Buddhist teachings as an "antidote" that must be excreted when the patient recovers. In the famous canonical allegory of the poisoned arrow, the physician who pulls the arrow from the wound is acting like the Buddha, who also provides his teachings for the sake of "recovery."[18] Medicine helps maintain the health of one's own body and spirit.[19] In general, the Buddhist perspective argues that, in order to gain acceptance for medical treatments, adequate karmic healing actions can only be carried out on the condition of a "long life." This view is also set forth in the *Dīghanikāya*: "Their lives are useful to ascetic beggars and brahmans because the longer such virtuous and well-behaved ascetic beg-

---

14. Cf.. M I.341; see also Harvey, *An Introduction to Buddhist Ethics*, 33ff.

15. Bca VIII. 91–92, quoting the translation by Steinkellner, *Śāntideva*, 102ff.

16. For more on the Theravāda Buddhist concept of illness, see Nanayakkara, "Disease," 633.

17. Bhikkhu Pāsādika, "Health and Its Significance in Buddhism," 149.

18. *Cūḷamāluṅkya-Sutta*, M I.426–432, cf. Demiéville, *Buddhism and Healing*, 14ff.; cf. also Soni, "Buddhism in Relation to the Profession of Medicine," 135–51.

19. In addition, certain illnesses prevent acceptance into the cloister according to the rules of the order (cf. Haldar, *Development of Public Health in Buddhism*). The usefulness of medicine thus also affects the achievement of the goal of healing in a different way.

gars and brahmans remain alive, the greater the [karmic] service that they provide" (D II.332). This is also one of the reasons that the Vinaya says, "Those who are sick and wish to die despite the availability of medicine and helpers, refusing food, are committing an error" (Vin III.82).

In general, it can be said that health is interpreted in Indian, Tibetan and Chinese medicine as the restoration of balance (e.g., between the bodily humors of wind, bile and phlegm), in other words a homeostasis. Mental as well as physical illnesses—according to some texts—are always more or less present; thus from a Buddhist perspective, even embryos and fetuses suffer. This stands in opposition to the modern Western perspective that the mother's womb is an idyllic paradise free from suffering, to which some long to return later in life.

Interestingly, in the texts of the Pāli canon bodily illnesses are defined as those that cannot be intentionally influenced. Passages discussing the teaching of the five components of the personality state, for instance: "If this body, o you monks, were the self, the body would not bring forth any illness [P. ābādha], and one would have the ability to decide for the body, 'This is how my body shall be; this is how it shall not be.' Because namely, o you monks, the body is not the self, and that is why the body brings forth illness, and one does not have the ability to decide, 'This is how my body shall be; this is how it shall not be.'"[20] By contrast, "inner hygiene" can be influenced by following the "path toward purification,"[21] which culminates in the purification of one's own spirit.

The next question is which causes can more specifically be held responsible for human illnesses. One particularly noteworthy idea is that they are caused by "(continuing) actions" (Sanskrit *karma*), in other words linking illnesses back to the impulses for negative action that come from unwholesome behavior or thoughts of earlier lives.[22] It should be observed, however, that even what is probably the earliest source to discuss the idea of "karmically caused" illness rejects the idea that all suffering, and thus all illness, is caused by karma.[23]

---

20. Vin I, *Mahāvagga* 1,6,38 ff., cf. Butzenberger and Fedorowa, "Wechselbeziehungen," 94.

21. Dhp 279, see Norman and von Hinüber, *Dhammapada*, 78.

22. On the diversity of ideas about karma in Theravāda and Tibetan Buddhism, see also Matthews, "Post-Classical Developments in the Concepts of Karma and Rebirth in Theravāda Buddhism," 123–144; also Schmithausen, "Critical Response," 203–30.

23. The text (*Sīvaka-Sutta*) names eight causes of worldly suffering: dysfunctions in wind, bile and phlegm, and in their combination; changes in climate; detrimental behavior (P. *visamaparihāraja*); sudden events not influenced by karma (*opakkamika*); and maturing karma, cf. Schmithausen, "Critical Response," 209.

Other texts add to this schema the basic mental "poisons" of greed, hatred and willful blindness as further causes of bodily illness.[24] The latter are also considered to be important causes of illness in Tibetan Buddhist medicine, since these poisons lead to an improper, unhealthy and ultimately destabilizing lifestyle. As a result, from an even broader perspective, eliminating the "blinding of the spirit" creates an existence that is free from suffering.[25] The *rGyud bzhi*, the standard work of Tibetan medicine, mentions—as a valid opinion—that uncertainty should be seen as the actual, overarching cause of illness; because as long as creatures are equipped with a lack of knowledge (Tib. *ma rig*), they will be unable to free themselves from illness (*nad*),[26] because "the cause of all illnesses is one thing only: a lack of knowledge, due to a failure to understand the meaning of the loss of self."[27]

The model of health inculturated through Buddhism is thus "perpetrator-centered," since the patient's healing process is at least partially driven by the patient himself and must begin with the patient. Thus illness is interpreted morally, to a certain degree. Some modern Buddhist ethicists assert that while karma can be used to explain the current status quo, it cannot be extended into the future as a determinant;[28] however, they say, any medical treatment is a wasted effort if the karma of the past is still in effect. Still, because it is not possible to determine the extent to which a certain illness is directly caused by karma, and because the relationship between deeds and illnesses is conditional rather than deterministic, it is in turn the physicians' duty to make every effort to heal the patient. Karma is thus only one of the causes, and it is not surprising that medical texts in particular indicate other factors; after all, a karma-based determinism would undermine the entire basis of practical medical treatment.[29] In addition, according to the teachings of Tibetan medicine, illnesses are only partially caused by negative karma.[30]

---

24. Cf. Demiéville, *Buddhism and Healing*, 24.

25. Cf. the statements by the 14th Dalai Lama, "Gesundheit und Krankheit," 21–22.

26. "Four-Root Treatise" (*rGyud bzhi*, hereinafter: Gzh), *Bdud rtsi snying po yan lag brgyad pa gsang ba man ngag gi rgyud*. Lhasa: Bod ljongs mi dmangs dpe skrun khang [1982], II.8; 34,17.

27. Gzh II.8; 34,15 f.: *nad rnams kun gyi rgyu ni gcig pu ste / bdag med don ma rtogs pas ma rig ces/.*

28. Ratanakul, "Buddhism, Health, Disease and Thai Culture," 18.

29. Cf. Zysk, *Asceticism and Healing in Ancient India*, 30.

30. Cf. *rGyud bzhi* II.12, translated, e.g., in Clark, *The Quintessence Tantras of Tibetan Medicine*, 88–98.

Furthermore, the view is often expressed that the emphasis on the temporary nature of "primary" suffering, as well as the belief that this life is not the only one, creates a greater sense of peace for Buddhists at the end of life.[31] In the West, this view is influenced by Jon Kabat-Zinn, for instance, who developed a therapeutic program for pain and stress management based on elements of modernized Burmese awareness meditation (*vipassanā*). Obviously, pain is still physically experienced by those who are experienced in concentrative meditative practices, but they are said to be less prone to self-abandonment and despair because the exercises can be used to positively influence the pain. Paradoxically, however, these practices are much more commonly learned and exercised by Western lay Buddhists than by cradle Buddhists in Southeast and Central Asia; in fact, they were, up to the modern revival, for centuries hardly practiced at all by monks and nuns in the cloisters.[32]

The Buddhist paradigms regarding illness and healing certainly affect the personal interaction with illness to some extent, although a decontextualized perspective hardly seems possible. The differences in beliefs, practices and life contexts between the urban middle class of a city population and the farming families living in villages, not to mention nomads, are simply too great (something that could be said of pre-modern Tibet as well). Finally, the competing supply of regional healers must not be forgotten. At the same time, it is clear that while the concept of karma plays a role in ultimately clarifying suffering, it does not limit medical practice to simply diagnosing the karmic relevance of an illness—despite the karma constraint, therapeutic freedom can be exploited if, as in many cases, the effects of karma as a contingency formula are not interpretatively applied precisely in those places where medical therapy is no longer helping.

BUDDHIST TEACHINGS AS MEDICINE

For contemporary discourse, particularly by the monastic experts on biomedicine, the competing relationship between their own soteriological practice and medicine is also important. The Vinaya rules prohibit monks and nuns from practicing any kind of medical profession and only permit a few medicines for general use,[33] but—according to Kenneth Zysk's thesis—it is precisely in these early Buddhist contexts, without the hindrances of

---

31. Bhikku Mettānando, "Buddhist Ethics in the Practice of Medicine," 203.
32. Cf. Sharf, "Buddhist Modernism and the Rhetoric of Meditative Experience."
33. Cf. D I.12, D I.69; Vin I.199–252; Dh 244; see also Mahinda, "Medical Practice of Buddhist Monks: A Historical Analysis of Attitudes and Problems."

brahmanic purity laws and professional limitations, that causal treatments and proto-scientific medicine experienced an upswing. Without a doubt, teachings on medical treatments as well as medical centers were able to develop in cloisters, both in the Theravāda Buddhist tradition and in the Mahāyāna tradition.[34]

Another push toward the liberalization of medical practices took place in Mahāyāna Buddhism through the Bodhisattva ideal. The Bodhisattva, a religious role model, acts as a "Bodhisattva healer" to relieve others' ailments and to show them the way out of suffering. This also affects the self-conception of the medical ethos. A fairly concrete description of the medical activities to be performed by a Bodhisattva can be found in Tsong kha pa's commentary on the chapter about the "Stages of the Bodhisattva" in the work *Yogacārabhūmi*, credited to Asaṅga. The text distinguishes between physical and mental suffering; it calls upon the Bodhisattva to give medicine to those with bodily illnesses, to lead the blind, to carry crippled people to their destinations, etc.[35]

In fact, it must be remembered that in addition to the ideas opposing causal medical therapy, the Mahāyāna also showed an early tendency to promote Buddhist teachings as such, or even the Buddha himself, as cures. An interesting line of argument compares the Buddha to an expert physician, since the Buddha, as the "best physician" (Sanskrit *bhiṣagvara*),[36] himself becomes the medicine in these pious traditions. The Mahāyāna philosopher Nāgārjuna also metaphorically describes the Buddha as the highest physician, who uses the medicine of good teachings to "treat all false opinions."[37] In the work *Yuktiṣaṣṭikā*, on the other hand, Nāgārjuna states that "false views" (Tibetan *log pa shes pa*) are those that produce the "faults of corruption" (Tibetan *non mongs skyon rnams*) that cause ailments.[38] Tracing illness back to uncertainty as the primary cause, which then produces the three poisons (greed, hatred, envy) that in turn are manifested at the fine-matter

---

34. The Vinaya commentary *Samantapāsādikā* contains detailed regulations about the practices that were permissible for Theravāda monks in the 5th century (II.469–72); cf. Mahinda, "Medical Practice of Buddhist Monks: A Historical Analysis of Attitudes and Problems," 459–62.

35. See Tsong kha pa, *Byang chub sems dpa'i tshul khrims kyi rnam bshad Byang chub gzhung lam*, fol. 17b (in: Collected Works [1975], Vol. 2, New Delhi: N.G. Demo); translated in Tatz, *Asanga's Chapter on Ethics with the Commentary of Tsong-Kha-Pa*, 122.

36. Cf. Butzenberger and Fedorowa, "Wechselbeziehungen," 98.

37. Nāgārjuna, *Catuḥstava* III.51; cf. also Butzenberger and Fedorowa, "Wechselbeziehungen," 98. Cf. also Mppś, k 1, 58c; trans. in Lamotte (1970), *Le Traité*, Vol. I., 17.

38. Cf. Butzenberger and Fedorowa, "Wechselbeziehungen," 98.

somatic level as the "faults" (Sanskrit *doṣa*) wind, bile and phlegm, is a theory that is also expounded in the Lotus Sūtra[39] and in the *rGyud bzhi*.[40]

Evidence of honoring the Buddha as the highest healer, in indirect opposition to the "profane" medical practice, can also be found in the sūtra literature, which is devoted to honoring the medicine Buddha, known as the *Bhaiṣajyaguru*. To give just one example: "If a woman who is in labor and experiencing great pain is able to honor this Tathāgata in complete faith, to praise his name and his being, she will be freed from her pain and her child will come into the world without deformities ... The child will have sharp senses, intelligence and a peaceful spirit. It will rarely be sick, and no inhuman being can steal its life force" [etc.].[41]

Signs of a medicine shaped by religion can also be found in the *rGyud bzhi*. For instance, Chapter 7 of the 2nd Tantra (on signs of death) states that it is a sign of pending healing if a monk appears to the patient.[42] However, the role of the Bodhisattva as a healer only begins to influence the general principle through the idea that the Bodhisattva himself can become a form of medicine. In the famous *Vimalakīrtinirdeśa*, when an epidemic begins to spread, a Bodhisattva takes on the role of distributing the medicine of "immortality" (Tibetan *bdudryud*) that heals the sick.[43]

And the Indian Mahāyāna scholar Śāntideva states, using specifically medical terms, "May I be a healing herb for the sick, and may I be a doctor and a caretaker for them until the sickness does not return"[44] (Bca III.7)—a passage that was clearly also used as a normative principle for the healing profession, since it is also cited in the hagiographic biography of a famous Tibetan doctor, among other places.[45] In summary, it can thus be said that a tradition of piety sees the Buddhist teachings themselves as the actual medicine.

---

39. Cf. Sharma, "Medicine in Buddhist and Jaina Traditions."

40. In the 2nd tantra, *bshad rgyud*, Ch. 8; cf. Clark, *The Quintessence Tantras of Tibetan Medicine*, 75–76.

41. According to the Chinese version of a lapis lazuli radiance sūtra, trans. in Birnbaum, *Der heilende Buddha*, 205–230, 221.

42. See Clark, *The Quintessence Tantras of Tibetan Medicine*, 68.

43. Cf. Demiéville, *Buddhism and Healing*, 47.

44. Cf. Steinkellner, *Śāntideva*, 38.

45. Cf. Dar mo Sman rams pa Blo bzang chos grags (*1638, died around 1697), "Biography of gYu thog the Elder," *gYu thog gsar rnying gi rnam thar*, translated by Rechung Rinpoche and Kunzang, *Tibetan Medicine*, 301, where this verse by Zhi ba lha (Śāntideva) is cited from the *Bodhicaryāvatāra*.

CASE STUDY: DOCTORS' ETHICS AND TREATMENT OF PATIENTS ACCORDING TO THE RGYUD BZHI

Medical ethics in the narrower sense may include the codices and declarations of behavioral rules of the professional medical ethos; in a broader sense, medical ethics also include "all of the rules and norms, convictions and attitudes, codifications and institutions that aim to coordinate actions in the medical field with ethical standards."[46] Thus physicians' behavior is subject to two different sets of criteria, namely a pragmatic set regarding the correct or incorrect treatment of patients and a moral set guided by the difference between good and evil. The two are "inextricably linked,"[47] in the sense that together they form the physicians' ethos.

In addition, it should not be ruled out altogether that the traditional medical ethical ideals as formulated in Buddhist texts may deviate in important ways from *general* Buddhist ethics. The ideals for physicians' behavior can create "special codes" in several senses: for instance in the question of whether patients must be told the truth in the event of a hopeless diagnosis, as general ethics would expect. Another example where a special code could apply is the case of active or passive suicide assisted by a doctor. Buddhist scholars could also be expected to criticize the physicians' ethos, or there could be secondary Buddhist shaping or framing of professional physicians' ethos.

One example of the religious shaping of the physicians' ethos is found in one of the three classic Indian medicine texts, the *Carakasaṃhitā*.[48] This text contains the oldest known (brahmanically embedded) physician's oath in Indian tradition.[49] The *Carakasaṃhitā* states, "Everyone admires a twice-born (i.e. *brahmin*) doctor who has self-discipline, is polite, wise and a master of his field ... For someone who is drawn into the spell of death due to a terrible sickness, there is no religious or worldly benefactor like the one who knows how to extend his life. No gift can compare to the gift of life."[50]

Finally, we must consider the descriptions that help generally explain the relationship between representatives of the Buddhist teachings on the one hand and the medical profession on the other, as well as between both

---

46. Honnefelder, "Medizinische Ethik: 2. Systematisch," 652.
47. Ibid.
48. See Sharma, ed. and trans., *Caraka-Saṃhitā: Agniveśa's Treatise Refined*.
49. See also Benner, "The Medical Ethics of Professionalised Ayurveda," 185–203; on the "physician's oath" (*Ātreya-Anuśāsana*) of the *Caraka Saṃhitā*, see also the translation by Menon and Haberman, "Oath of Initiation: from the Caraka Samhita," 130–32.
50. CaS VI.1., 4, 51 ff., translated by Wujastyk, "Medizin in Indien," 23.

of these and their clientele (patients and "laypeople"), since—in the sense of metaphorical-narrative behavioral orientations—they can also be bioethically "active" behind the scenes, even today. These orientations can have subtle effects, as can be seen from the religiously influenced history of the term "patient" (a noun formed in the sixteenth century from the Latin *patiens*, "to undergo, to bear, to suffer"; pres. particip. Lat. *pati*); the same root is used in "passive" and "passion," as in the "story of Christ's suffering").[51]

Another interesting question is whether Buddhist medical ethics also express a professionalization of the medical field, which, as can be seen from the Hippocratic oath,[52] is not only intended for the good of the patient, but also regulates access to the medical practice, in other words by keeping the number of competitors as small as possible.

Well-formulated, written professional ethics clearly fulfill multiple functions. On the one hand, these functions help form an autonomous professional community. Conflicts that arise during the treatment of the patients are not handled by arguing with the patient, who then feels mistreated, but are handled internally wherever possible. In other words, it is not that the doctor has made a mistake; instead, either the treatment was *lege artis* and the fault lies in the patient's perception of it, or else the doctor's incorrect treatment of the patient demonstrates that he is not (or no longer is) a doctor within the professional community. Naturally, this only applies if there is no certified medical training at corresponding institutions to standardize the access to the market. This does not seem to have been the case in the age of Hippocrates, nor in twelfth-century Tibet, when the *rGyud bzhi* was compiled.

Traditionally, medical ethics seem to have been formulated only to a limited extent by doctors who practiced on a Buddhist basis—for the reasons described above. However, this does not rule out the possibility that ethical teachings played a large role in the verbal instruction of student doctors.[53] In the medical texts of the Mahāyāna, on the other hand, elements of Bodhisattva ethics are applied to the suffering patient, for instance sympathy and loving care.[54] The decision as to how doctors should behave

---

51. Cf. Stolberg, *Homo patiens*.

52. Cf. here Neuhaus, "Ich schwöre bei Apollon dem Arzte," 37–40.

53. The paucity of sources for early discussions of medical ethics is probably due to the verdict of the canonical sources, which prohibit monks and nuns from performing medical work. This verdict may have contributed to the fact that medical ethics in later Mahāyāna traditions do not represent a regionalized type of ethics, but instead merge with the general ethics of the Bodhisattva, for instance in the *Vimalakīrtinirdeśa*.

54. For instance in Tibetan sources like the *rGyud-bźi* and the *Vaiḍūrya sṅon-po*, etc. Cf. Rechung Rinpoche and Kunzang, *Tibetan Medicine*, 91 f., 282 ff.

toward patients and their relatives when they see a low chance of recovery or survival for the patient is primarily determined by an ethical recommendation: explaining everything to the patient,[55] on the one hand because of the ethos of truthfulness and on the other so that, as mentioned earlier, the dying person can prepare to have the right spiritual attitude at the moment of death.[56]

For heuristic reasons, let us give a schematic model of the relationship between doctor and patient here.[57] This will allow us to more precisely classify the aspects of the ethos given below, based on a case study of Tibetan Buddhist medical texts.

Relationship model:	Convictions of the patient:	Obligations of the doctor:	Concept of patient responsibility:	Role of the doctor:
a) informational	established and defined; known to the patient	provide information	patient has control and the ability to choose	competent technical expert
b) interpretative (supportive / advisory)	vague, conflicting, requires interpretation	clarify the patient's convictions; suggest measures	patient needs to be convinced of the desired values / goals; patient's choice of treatment is implemented	advisor and supporter
c) deliberative	open to development and revision during the conversation	same as (b), but more committed and more leading	patient develops own moral attitude	friend or teacher
d) paternalistic	'objective'; shared by the patient and doctor	promote the well-being of the patient without taking patient's wishes into account	patient agrees to "objective values"	custodian

In this overall model, however, the autonomy of the patient, in other words the desire and the need to make his own decisions, is assumed as a given.

55. This is also true in Tibetan medicine; cf. Rechung Rinpoche and Kunzang, *Tibetan Medicine*, 88.

56. Cf. Bhikkhu Pāsādika, "Health and its Significance in Buddhism," 155–56.

57. From Emanuel and Emanuel, "Four Models of the Physician-Patient Relationship." Their preferred model is the deliberative relationship, which in my opinion mainly involves a pedagogical component.

This need is certainly more strongly manifested in very individualized societies than in societies with close family relationships. Still, even in the context of Western societies, it has been shown that many patients feel the need to discuss their medical decision-making options primarily with family members, friends or acquaintances whom they consider to be competent.[58]

The above paternalistic model, on the other hand, assumes an understanding on the part of the doctor that was probably common in premodern contexts. According to this model, the doctor knows what is best for the patients. Modern Buddhist medical ethicists have noted that, based on the Buddhist behavioral codices, doctors should primarily act as a "noble friend" or "spiritual advisor" (Sanskrit *kalyāṇamitra*). "If all doctors were to see themselves as good friends to the patient and cultivate the qualities of a good friend, many problems of legislation that surround neo-Christian medical ethics would disappear. Legislation serves only to fill the gap of uncertainty created by a doctor's approach to practice."[59] Also worth noting here is the increasingly clear fundamental attitude of many Buddhists that a legal system is unnecessary thanks to the perpetrator-centered idea of self-fulfillment and personal practice.

PHYSICIANS' ETHOS IN THE *RGYUD BZHI*

Butzenberger and Fedorowa, Bhikkhu Pāsādika, and others supported the thesis that the rigorous rejection of patients with incurable diseases, as found in the two major classical works of brahmanic Hindu medicine, the *Carakasaṃhitā* (approx. second–first century BCE) and the *Suśrutasaṃhitā* (approx. fourth century), had been replaced by a Buddhist ethos of compassion, for instance as seen in the Buddhist-influenced medical text of the Vāgbhaṭa, *Aṣṭāṅgahṛdayasaṃhitā* (seventh century):[60] "The theoretical conception of suffering is no longer absolute and unconditional in Buddhism; instead, this role falls to the recommended behavior toward suffering... Ultimately, this unconditional, categorical ethics of compassion wins out over the pragmatically motivated... partial ethos of medicine. Suffering as a challenge sets its own standards."[61]

---

58. Cf. Clarke and Hall, et al., "Physician-Patient Relations: No More Models," 16–19.

59. Mettānando, "Buddhist Ethics in the Practice of Medicine," 201.

60. Cf. Butzenberger and Fedorowa, "Wechselbeziehungen," 105–6. For more on the Buddhist influences, see also Meulenbeld, *History*, 603ff.

61. Cf. Butzenberger and Fedorowa, "Wechselbeziehungen," 107.

A clear sign of this is that the medical texts *Carakasaṃhitā* and *Suśrutasaṃhitā* include instructions for performing an abortion[62]—which after all violates the general Buddhist ethics of non-injury—while these are missing from Vāgbhaṭa's *Aṣṭāṅgahṛdayasaṃhitā*.[63]

In fact, in general, Vāgbhaṭa's work embeds physicians' activities within Mahāyānic ethics. This can be seen, for instance, in the introductory verses to the text, which is the only classical work in Indian medicine to have been included in the Tibetan Buddhist canon:[64] "Honor be to him, the unmatched doctor who destroys passions and the like as well as the illnesses that constantly adhere and spread throughout the entire body by creating greed, blindness and dissatisfaction."[65] In the Tibetan version, the physician's ethos is tied even more explicitly to the Buddhist ethics of compassion.[66] Given the background of the Buddhist "perpetrator ethics," it should not be surprising that here, as in the *rGyud bzhi*, the benefits of medicine are also—and perhaps especially—laid out for the doctor.

In the *rGyud bzhi*, as in the classical Āyurveda texts, there is a separate chapter dealing with doctors' professional ethos. It is the last chapter (no. 31) of the "Explanatory Treatise" (*bshad rgyud*), and bears the title "The doctor who is also a healer" (*gso ba sman pa po*).[67] It not only describes the ethos of the physician; in addition—again like the larger Āyurvedic treatises—the formulation of industry ethics here (with a clear structural similarity to the contents of the Hippocratic oath) particularly serves to distinguish the medical profession from presumptive doctors, quacks and autodidacts.

In contrast to the Hippocratic oath, however, the *rGyud bzhi* does not contain any principle with the same scope as the *nil nocere*. This is not surprising, since the commandment to do no harm is already at the core of Buddhist ethics. The same is true of abortion, which is also not discussed in the *rGyud bzhi*. Even the issue of a stillborn fetus does not seem to be mentioned in the *rGyud bzhi*. An entire chapter is devoted to this case in

---

62. Cf. Lipner, "The Classical Hindu View on Abortion," 41–69.

63. Cf. Kumar, *Ayurvedic Concepts of Human Embryology*, 59–60.

64. E.g., in *Derge* (D) bsTan 'gyur, he (119), 44b1–335a7 (D Nr. 4310); Sanskrit edition: Emmerick and Das, *Vāgbhaṭa's Aṣṭāṅgahṛdayasaṃhitā*.

65. Ah I.1, 1; using the translation by Butzenberger and Fedorowa, "Wechselbeziehungen," 104.

66. Cf. Vogel, *Vāgbhaṭa's Aṣṭāṅgahṛdayasaṃhitā*, 44 ff. The Tibetan translation includes, for instance, an additional opening verse that honors the Buddha as the highest physician (also known as the medicine Buddha). In addition, the first Sanskrit verse includes references to the Buddhist theory of the three poisons.

67. Gzh 95–101.

the *Aṣṭāṅgahṛdayasaṃhitā*,⁶⁸ and the work recommends and describes the medically indicated uterine abrasion. It is certainly conceivable that Tibetan doctors passed down possible abortion practices in addition to the revised Buddhist medicine presented in the *rGyud bzhi*. However, this does not seem to be very likely, since such practices are not even mentioned in the harsh criticisms of false medical practice, which is also covered in the work. From this it may be concluded that abortions were not very common. Or were they so taboo that those who performed them agreed to maintain strict silence on the matter? Given the fact that pre-modern abortion practices were often associated with significant risks for the mother, this would not be unlikely.

The chapter on medical ethics begins by listing six prerequisites that a doctor must fulfill: (1) he should have an intelligent mind (Tibetan *blo ldan*), should (2) pursue a purely caring intention (Tib. *bsam pa dkar ba*), (3) fulfill certain (Tantric) "oaths" (*dam [bca'i] tshig*, skt. *samaya*), (4) have practical skills, (5) be industrious and conscientious, and (6) be familiar with the common practices in the world (*mi chos mkhas*). These six prerequisites are then further explained. Here, we will primarily look at the ethically and institutionally significant descriptions.

On the creation of pure intention, the text continues, "Caring intention is associated with the thought of awakening (Tib. *byang chub*, San. *bodhicitta*). From preparation to complete execution, the primary goal is to see the [suffering of the] *Saṃsāra* and to trust [in one's ability] to provide a benefit (well-being), and [to develop] a lack of bias due to hatred, love, good and evil, [which is associated with] the four [healing states of] compassion (Tib. *snying rje*), benevolent love (*byams pa*), sympathetic joy (*dga' ba*) and equanimity (*btang snyoms*). The desire to achieve the highest level of enlightenment is achieved when one practices without interruption after entering into the main practice. The practitioner should examine [the patients] as required, and should be without resentment [toward them]. One who masters this will easily provide healing; many of those who recover (literally "survivors") will become his friends." (Gzh 96,4–9).

The fruits born from the activities of the medical profession are clearly named at the end of the chapter: in addition to food and goods, there is also power, influence and wealth. However, the ultimate fruits of the medical profession always have to do with the doctor himself: obtaining healing karma for himself. It is amazing how little these ethics differ from the corresponding treatises on the general ethics of the Bodhisattva (for instance

68. On the treatment of dead or "misdirected" fetuses (Sanskrit *mūḍhagarbha*), see also the chapter Śarirasthāna (2) trans. in Hilgenberg and Kirfel, *Vāgbhaṭa's Aṣṭāṅgahṛdayasaṃhitā*, 171–78.

in the form developed in Sgam po pa and in Lam-rim literature). Does this mean that medical ethics are based entirely on ethico-religious ethics, or are there conflicts in the medical field where the recommended action diverges from the general Bodhisattva ethics?

Next come the "oaths" (Tib. *dam tshig*), similar in form to the medical oaths in the European tradition, which are in turn listed as 11 separate points. In Tantric Buddhism, the term *dam tshig* refers to the obligations that the pupil takes on from his teacher.

The first six obligations are those that doctors must always "keep in mind" (*blo bzhag*): to see (1) their "initial instructor" (*slob dpon*) as a Buddha (*sangs rgyas*) [in the sense that he is an embodiment or emanation of the Medicine Buddha Bhaiṣajyaguru], (2) his teachings as words of the wise (*drang srong*, San. *ṛṣi*), (3) the "medical (written) teachings" (*gso dpyad*) as the "flow of transmission" (*bka' rgyud*), (4) the other adepts (*mchen*), in other words medical students, as friends and brothers (*grogs spun*), (5) the "patients" (*nad pa*) as their own sons (*bu tsha*), and (6) blood and pus (*khrag rnam*) from the perspective of a "dog and pig" (*khyi phag*), in other words, not to be disgusted by them.

The next two oaths must be "taken" (*bzung bya*), namely recognizing (7) the bearer of medical knowledge (*rig 'dzin*) as the "(Dharma) protector" (*bka' srung*) and (8) his tools as protection. Finally, the last three oaths are to be "recognized" (*shes bya*): doctors must recognize medicines (9) as a valuable substance (*nor bu*) that works like a wish-granting jewel, (10) as a "divine nectar" (*bdud rtsi*, San. *amṛta*) that heals all sicknesses (*nad rnams sel ba'i bdud rtsi*), and finally (11) as the first sacrificial substance (*mchod rdzas*) from the bearer of knowledge. More specifically, the doctor must envision himself as Bai-ḍūrya-rgyal po, the king of medicine, and his medicines as the begging bowl filled with nectar that the Medicine Buddha holds in his right hand.[69] In order to complete this identification, he must recite a lengthy devotional formula that formally resembles the introduction to the Hippocratic oath, followed by the mantra of the Bhaiṣajyaguru.

These oaths describe a typical ideal for the behavior of a physician. The main aspect focuses on legitimizing the path of succession, but also on helping the practitioner identify with his role as a Bodhisattva.[70]

69. Accordingly, the introductory statement to the *rGyud bzhi* describes how doctors should identify with the medicine Buddha who radiates healing knowledge. Physician Khangkar, *Lectures on Tibetan Medicine*, 1) says, "the doctor should not take himself or herself as an ordinary living being but at this particular moment, meditate and visualise that he or she is a deity of the medicine Buddha and is imparting the medical teachings in such a form and spirit."

70. Is this a sign of a religious reformation of the physicians' ethos, or an indication

Another feature is what, from a contemporary Western perspective, would be called a paternalistic medical ideal: the doctor is called upon to treat patients like his own children; he is described as acting like a protector and a father (*pha*) for the creatures (wandering in the Saṃsāra). (Gzh 98,16) The main idea here is probably an emotional relationship, but it cannot be ruled out that this also affects his communication with patients. The next section explains "behavior in [medical] practice" (*rnam pa bzo ba*), which is enacted through physical, verbal and mental aspects (physical skill, intelligence). What is relevant for the doctor-patient relationship here is mainly the statement on the doctor's speaking, namely that "the doctor can provide joy to the patient through loving words." (Gzh 97) Next, the "efforts through action" (*bya ba la brtson*) are explained: "The industrious *efforts for others* should be directed toward the patient, for [promoting] his well-being (Tib. *don*) without delay or distraction." Finally, the sixth paragraph also includes a reference to the doctor's benevolent self-concept: "If the doctor is seized by compassion for normal needy persons [the poor], his leading intent is carried out by the highly praised ones [Buddhas]."[71] According to the exact meaning of the word, the doctor is "medicine" (*sman*), "because he treats illnesses and benefits the body ('does good')" (Gzh 98).

This is one of the very rare places where the *rGyud bzhi* refers to the altruistic virtues of the physician. However, even here it does not advise any concrete, individually motivated behavior; the doctor's benevolent *intent* is said to be implemented *by the Buddhas*. Nonetheless, it is still part of the modern self-concept of Tibetan physicians, as described by the most famous Tibetan doctor of the twentieth century, Lobsang Dolma Khangkar, that the needy and monks are treated for free, and their livelihood and practical needs are financed by payments from other patients.[72]

Part IV of the chapter on medical healers, where doctors and healers are classified according to their deeds, is amazingly extensive. This section not only includes descriptions of ideal models and behaviors for doctors, but also describes—in vignettes and metaphorical comparisons—deviations from the medical idea. The highest ideal is that of the "unmatched healer" (*sman pa bla na med pa*), who has overcome the "three poisons" that are responsible for creating illness—in other words, the Medicine Buddha himself (99,1). This is followed by the "excellent doctor" (*khyad par*

---

that the systematization of medical knowledge simultaneously represented an institutionalization of physician education in monastically dominated circles?

71. *thun mong phongs pa rnams la snying rjes bzung / mthon po rnams kyis rang gis mdo don sgrub* / 97,13f. See also *Baiḍūrya sngon po*, I.405.

72. Khangkar, *Lectures on Tibetan Medicine*, 68. On physicians' ethics, see also ibid., 66 ff.

can), who is upstanding and is gifted with love, transcendental perception (*mngon shes*) and understanding of others (consciousness, *gzhan rig*) (99,2), and who "sees benefits for others as a benefit to himself" (*gzhan gyi don la rang don sems*, 99,5f.). Even the "normal [doctor]" (*phal pa*) is a friend of the [wandering] creatures" (*'gro ba'i gnyen*) who can point to an authentic instructional lineage. Still, by far the largest section is devoted to those who only pretend to be doctors. They are all considered "destroyers of life" (*srog gi gshed*, 99,3).[73]

These types of "bad doctors," says the text in summary, are "demons in the form of doctors," because "when they cast the lasso of the god of death, they are in control of life." (Gzh 100,5).

The extent to which this self-concept of pre-modern Tibetan Buddhist doctors deviates from the contemporary physicians' codex,[74] for instance as seen in the abovementioned Geneva doctor's oath, will not be analyzed in detail here. However, as Dr. Dawa (director of the largest Tibetan medical school in exile, the Mentseekhang in Dharamsala) stated in a 2005 interview, the chapter in the *rGuyd bzhi* on healers and physicians is still memorized by medical students today, and thus provides a certain kind of orientation.

ON TREATING PATIENTS WITH A HOPELESS PROGNOSIS

What duties, then, have Buddhist scholars and physicians assigned to those who treat the dying?

The fact that, according to the pre-modern Tibetan Buddhist understanding, a "proper death" takes priority over living as long as possible, is shown by a text about treating the dying titled "Freedom Through Listening in the Transitional State" (*bar do'i thos grol*), also known as the "Tibetan Book of the Dead" in the West. The text appears to describe a type of assisted suicide for spiritual purposes. In the first lesson, devoted to the "Bardo of the moment of death" (*'chi kha'i bar do*), in other words to those who are about to die or who have just died, the spiritual helper is called to do the following: "When you notice that the breath has stopped, you should lay the patient on his right side in the lion position and press firmly on both arteries

---

73. On the false physicians and/or improper behavior, see also Thangka No. 37, illustrating the *Baiḍūrya sngon po*, in Parfionovitch and Gyurme Dorje, *Tibetan Medical Paintings*, 89.

74. Virtue-based ethical attempts to establish a contemporary ethics of medicine come somewhat closer to the Tibetan physicians' ideal, for instance when virtues like sympathy, intelligence, fairness, proportion, integrity and selflessness are suggested; see Zimmermann-Acklin, "Tugendethische Ansätze in der Bioethik," 205.

that bring about sleep until they have stopped pulsing."⁷⁵_ftn1#_ftn1 Could this in fact be seen as active assisted suicide (which is certainly not considered to be beneficial in general Buddhist ethics)? This question is difficult to answer because the definition of death varies by culture. In other words, the performance of this practice could itself indicate that the patient in question is considered to be irrevocably dead, even if the dying process is not yet entirely complete. In any case, the process of dying is described in different ways in Tibetan Buddhist texts, but generally states that the "wind that preserves life" (Tib. *srog*) withdraws from the two side channels or "arteries" in the "left channel" (Tib. *rkyang ma rtsa*) and the "right channel" (Tib. *ro ma rtsa*) into the main channel, and then ends in the heart.

However, the "Book of the Dead" clearly states that a "pulsing" can be felt in the abovementioned channels that are to be compressed. The medical anatomical Thangka illustrations of the *Baiḍūrya sngon po* use almost the same words to describe two channels running along the neck (Tib. *snying rtsa gnyid log*), which, when compressed, cause unconsciousness. Thus it is likely that from a Western medical point of view, both cases are referring to the carotid arteries (*carotis*), whose Greek description "numbed" (*karōdis*) also indicates the numbing effect of applying external pressure to them.[76]

The second example, which comes from the *rGyud bzhi*, clearly shows that according to this standard work of pre-modern Tibetan medical practice, there was by no means an overarching charitable obligation for doctors working in the Buddhist tradition to protect or extend the patient's life at any cost. Instead, the guiding principle was to recognize the definitive signs of death that made further treatment pointless from a medical standpoint—not to mention the cases where patients did not seem worthy of treatment from a moral perspective. This is explained more precisely in the 26th chapter of the "Explanatory Tantra" (*bshad rgyud*), which bears the title "Four parameters for accepting or rejecting patients for treatment." It defines four classes of patients: those who are easy to treat, those who are difficult to treat, those who are nearly impossible to treat (*sgo tsam*), and those who are to be "rejected" (*spang ba*) (Gzh 85,2). This last category further differentiates between patients for whom "a medical treatment exists" (*gso thabs yod*) and those for whom there is no treatment. The following cases are named here: those who are inevitably headed toward death, and those who bear the

---

75. Freemantle and Trungpa, *Das Totenbuch der Tibeter*, 64. Tibetan: Lhundup, *The Tibetan Book of the Dead By the Great Acharya, Shri Sing-ha*, 8,5–8: *glo gyas sa la phab nas seng ge'i 'dug stangs byas la rtsa rba rlabs brtsir ba yin te / gnyen log rtsa gnyis 'phar 'phro chad nas drag tu mnan no/*.

76. Cf. Thangka No. 47 with explanations of the *Gzh, bshad rgyud* (II), Chapter 83, in Parfionovitch and Dorje, *Tibetan Medical Paintings*, II, 265.

signs of death (i.e. those who suffer from the nine fatal illnesses). Despite the availability of therapies, the following patients should not be treated: "those who are badly disposed toward the King (*rgyal po*), toward Buddhist monk-scholars (*dge ba'i bshes*) and toward animate beings" (Gzh 85,14); those who do not remember the actions of the doctor and show him respect; those who have no possessions (*'byor ba med*), who hate living animals, who are too rushed, who do not listen to the doctor's instructions, who complain without ceasing, who destroy the Buddhist teachings or who have a bad reputation.

CONCLUSION

As is clearly shown by the final examples above, the cases from the *rGyud bzhi* reveal a tension between the ideal of codified ethics set forth by religious specialists and the practical medical ethos. In other words, it is by no means a given that a Tibetan doctor would always be called upon to help and to heal according to the self-concept of the author(s) of the standard work, the *rGyud bzhi*. The external and internal protection of socioeconomic professional interests seems to significantly shape the ethos, judging from the sources listed here. However, the cases of patients to be rejected who could nonetheless have been treated, are particularly striking, especially in the context of today's universal humanistic medical ethos. Assuming the background of a perpetrator-centered theory of karma—dominant in pre-modern contexts—it seemed entirely possible to integrate the idea that both patients and physicians were able to determine their own reality through their respective actions. On the other hand, however, it should be remembered that a primarily victim-centered concept of patients, whose protection and restoration to health is the top priority, was only institutionalized in the Western world by way of the human-rights discourse after the second World War.

In this context, it is not surprising that the Bodhisattva's special ethics of compassion do not play a significant role in the medical texts, even if their development and commentaries have increasingly been included in the area of expertise for religious specialists since the fourteenth century. It seems that the Buddhist influence on Tibetan medicine had less of an influence on the discourse surrounding proper patient care than, for instance, on the practice of therapy through "gemstone pills" (*rin chen ril bu*), which are part of the religious "Dharma medicine" (Tib. *chos sman*) and whose effectiveness is not due to the doctor's actions, but to religious acts.

BIBLIOGRAPHY

Bdud rtsi snying po yan lag brgyad pa gsang ba man ngag gi rgyud. Lhasa: Bod ljongs mi dmangs dpe skrun khang, 1982.

Benner, D. "The Medical Ethics of Professionalised Ayurveda." *Asian Medicine: Tradition and Modernity* 1 (2005) 185–203.

Bhikkhu Pāsādika. "Health and Its Significance in Buddhism." In *Health and Quality of Life: Philosophical, Medical and Cultural Aspects,* edited by Antje Gimmler et al., 147–56. Münster: Lit Verlag, 2002.

Bhikku Mettānando. "Buddhist Ethics in the Practice of Medicine." In *Buddhist Ethics and Modern Society: An International Symposium,* edited by Charles Weo-hsun Fu and Sandra A. Wawrytko, 195–213. New York: Greenwood, 1991.

Birnbaum, Raoul. *Der heilende Buddha: Heilung und Selbstheilung im Buddhismus Meditationen, Rituale, Basistexte.* Munich: Barth, 1982.

Buddhagosa, and Bhikku Ñānatiloka. *Visuddhi-magga oder Der Weg zur Reinheit: Die grösste und älteste systematische Darstellung des Buddhismus.* Uttenbühl: Jana Verlag im Buddha Haus, 1997.

Butzenberger, Klaus, and Mariana Fedorowa. "Wechselbeziehungen zwischen Buddhismus und klassischer indischer Medizin." *Sudhoffs Archiv* 73 (1989) 88–109.

Cassell, Eric J. *The Nature of Suffering and the Goals of Medicine.* 2nd ed. Oxford: University Press, 2004.

Clark, Barry, and the Dalai Lama. *The Quintessence Tantras of Tibetan Medicine.* Ithaca, NY: Snow Lion, 1995.

Clarke, G., R. T. Hall, and G. Rosencrance. "Physician-Patient Relations: No More Models." *American Journal of Bioethics* 4.2 (2004) 16–19.

Dalai Lama. "Gesundheit und Krankheit." In *Das Wissen vom Heilen,* edited by Franz Reichle, 13–22. Zurich: Oesch, 2003.

Das, Rahul Peter, and Ronald Eric Emmerick, eds. *Vāgbhaṭa's Aṣṭāṅgahṛdayasaṃhitā: The Romanized Text and Accompanied by Line and Word Indexes.* Groningen Oriental Studies 13. Groningen: Forsten, 1998.

Demiéville, Paul. *Buddhism and Healing.* Translated by Mark Tatz. Lanham, MD: University Press of America, 1985.

Edwards, Steven D. "Three Concepts of Suffering." *Medicine, Health Care and Philosophy* 6 (2003) 59–66.

Emanuel, Ezekiel J., and Linda L. Emanuel. "Four Models of the Physician-Patient Relationship." *Journal of the American Medical Association* 267 (1992) 2221–26.

Freemantle, Francesca, and Chögyam Trungpa. *Das Totenbuch der Tibeter.* Düsseldorf: Diederich, 1976.

Geertz, Clifford. "Heil/Leid." In *Wörterbuch der Religionen,* edited by Chr. Auffarth et al., 203–5. Stuttgart: Kröner, 2006.

———. "Religion als kulturelles System." In *Dichte Beschreibung: Beiträge zum verstehen kultureller Systeme.* Frankfurt: Suhrkamp, 1987. English: "Religion as a Cultural System." In *The Interpretation of Cultures: Selected Essays,* 87–125. New York: Basic Books, 1973.

Haldar, J. R. *Development of Public Health in Buddhism.* New Delhi: Indological Bookhouse, 1992.

Harvey, Peter. *An Introduction to Buddhist Ethics: Foundations, Values, and Issues.* Cambridge: Cambridge University Press, 2000.

Hilgenberg, Luise, and Willibald Kirfel. *Aṣṭāṅgahṛdayasaṃhitā: Ein altindisches Lehrbuch der Heilkunde.* Leiden: Brill, 1941.

Hinüber, Oskar von, and K. R. Norman, eds. *A Comparative Edition of the Dhammapada.* Oxford: Pali Text Society, 1995.

Honnefelder, Ludgar. "Medizinische Ethik: 2. Systematisch." In *Lexikon der Bioethik* (2000) 2:652–59.

Khangkar, Lobsang Dolma. *Lectures on Tibetan Medicine.* Compiled and edited by K. Dhondup. Delhi: Educa, 1991.

Kumar, Abhimanyu. *Ayurvedic Concepts of Human Embryology:* The Chaukhamba Ayurvijnana Studies 25. Delhi: Chaukhamba Sanskrit Pratishthan, 2000.

Lipner, Julius J. "The Classical Hindu View on Abortion and the Moral Status of the Unborn." In *Hindu Ethics: Purity, Abortion, Euthanasia,* by Harold G. Coward, Julius J. Lipner, and Katherine K. Young, 41–69. McGill Studies in the History of Religions. Albany: SUNY Press, 1989.

Mahinda, Wetera. "Medical Practice of Buddhist Monks: A Historical Analysis of Attitudes and Problems." In *Recent Researches in Buddhist Studies: Essays in Honour of Y. Karunadasa,* edited by Kuala Lumpur Dhammajoti et al., 454–66. Hong Kong: Chi Ying Foundation 1997.

Matthews, Bruce. "Post-Classical Developments in the Concepts of Karma and Rebirth in Theravāda Buddhism." In *Karma and Rebirth: Post Classical Developments,* edited by Ronald W. Neufeldt, 123–44. SUNY Series in Religious Studies. Albany: SUNY Press, 1986.

Menon, A., and H. F. Haberman. "Oath of Initiation: From the Caraka Samhita." In *Cross Cultural Perspectives in Medical Ethics: Readings,* edited by Robert M. Veatch, 130–32. Boston: Jones & Bartlett, 1989. Reprinted from *Medical History* 14 (1970) 295–96.

Meulenbeld, G. Jan. *A History of Indian Medical Literature.* Vol. Ia. Groningen: Forsten, 1999.

Meyer, Fernanad. "Introduction." In *Orientalische Medizin: Ein illustrierter Führer durch die asiatischen Traditionen des Heilens,* edited by J. van Alphen, 11–15. Bern: Haupt, 1997.

Nanayakkara, S. K. "Disease." In *Encyclopaedia of Buddhism* IV, 4 (1995) 633.

Neuhaus, Lukas. "'Ich schwöre bei Apollon dem Arzte.' Zur Bedeutung des hippokratischen Eides für die Professionalisierung des Ärztestandes." *soz:mag: Das soziologische Magazin* 4 (2003) 37–40.

Parfionovitch, Yuri, and Gyurme Dorje. *Tibetan Medical Paintings, Illustrations to the Blue Beryl Treatise of Sangye Gyamtso (1653–1705).* General editor Anthony Aris. Vol. 1. London: Abrams, 1992.

Promta, Somparn. "Law and Morality: The Buddhist Perspective." *The Chulalongkorn Journal of Buddhist Studies* 5 (1998) 3–57.

Pruett, Gordon E. *The Meaning and End of Suffering for Freud and the Buddhist Tradition.* Lanham, MD: University Press of America, 1987.

Ratanakul, Pinit. "Buddhism, Health, Disease and Thai Culture." In *A Cross-Cultural Dialogue on Health Care Ethics,* edited by Harold G. Coward and Pinit Ratanakul, 17–33. Ontario: Wilfrid Laurier University Press, 1999.

Rechung Rinpoche. *Tibetan Medicine: Illustrated in Original Texts.* Berkeley: University Of California Press, 1973.

Śāntideva. *Eintritt in das Leben zur Erleuchtung (Bodhicaryāvatāra): Lehrgedicht des Mahāyāna*. Translated by Ernst Steinkellner. Diederichs Gelbe Reihe 34. Düsseldorf: Diederichs, 1981.
Schlieter, Jens. "Endure, Adapt, or Overcome? The Concept of Suffering in Buddhist Bioethics." In *Suffering and Bioethics*, edited by Ronald M. Green and Nathan J. Palpant, 309–36. New York: Oxford University Press, 2014.
Schmithausen, Lambert. "Critical Response." In *Karma and Rebirth. Post Classical Developments*, edited by Ronald W. Neufeldt, 203–30. SUNY Series in Religious Studies. Albany: SUNY Press, 1986.
Sharf, Robert H. "Buddhist Modernism and the Rhetoric of Meditative Experience." *Numen* 42 (1995) 228–83.
Sharma, Priyavrat, ed. and trans. *Caraka-Saṃhitā: Agniveśa's Treatise Refined and Annotated by Caraka and Redacted by Dṛḍhabala: Text with English Translation*. Vol. 1–4. Jaikrishnadas Ayurveda Series 36. Varanasi, New Delhi: Chaukhambha Orientalia, 1981–1995.
Sharma, Priya Vrat. "Medicine in Buddhist and Jaina Traditions." In *History of Medicine in India*, edited by Priya Vrat Sharma, 117–35. New Delhi: Indian National Science Academy, 1992.
Sing-ha, Acharya. *The Tibetan Book of the Dead*. Sigra, Varanasi: E. Kalsang Buddhist Temple, 1969.
Soni, R. L. "Buddhism in Relation to the Profession of Medicine." In *Religion and Medicine*, edited by D. W. Millard, 3:135–51. London: SCM, 1976.
Stolberg, Michael. *Homo patiens: Krankheits- und Körpererfahrung in der frühen Neuzeit*. Cologne: Böhlau, 2003.
Tatz, Mark, trans. *Asanga's Chapter on Ethics with the Commentary of Tsong-Kha-Pa, The Basic Path to Awakening, The Complete Bodhisattva*. Studies in Asian Thought and Religion 4. Lewiston, NY: Mellon, 1986.
Tsong kha pa. *Byang chub sems dpa'i tshul khrims kyi rnam bshad Byang chub gzhung lam*. In Collected Works 2. New Delhi: N. G. Demo, 1975.
Vogel, Claus, trans. *Vāgbhaṭa's Aṣṭāṅgahṛdayasaṃhitā: The First Five Chapters of its Tibetan Version*. Wiesbaden: Steiner, 1965.
Wezler, Albrecht. "On the Quadruple Division of the Yogaśāstra, the Caturvyūhatva of the Cikitsaśāstra and the 'Four Noble Truths' of the Buddha." *Indologica Taurinensia* 12 (1984) 290–337.
Wujastyk, D. "Medizin in Indien." In *Orientalische Medizin: Ein illustrierter Führer durch die asiatischen Traditionen des Heilens*, edited by Jan van Alphen, 19–37. Bern: Haupt, 1997.
Zimmermann-Acklin, Markus. "Tugendethische Ansätze in der Bioethik." In *Bioethik: Eine Einführung*, edited by Marcus Düwell and Klaus Steigleder, 200–210. Suhrkamp Taschenbuch Wissenschaft 1597. Frankfurt: Suhrkamp, 2003.
Zysk, Kenneth G. *Asceticism and Healing in Ancient India: Medicine in the Buddhist Monastery*. Oxford: Motilal Banarsidass, 1991.

7

Emotional Affliction and Mental Illness
from a Tibetan Vajrayana Buddhist Perspective

—Martina E. Dannecker

Tibetan Buddhist teachings particularly emphasize the necessity to resolve our afflictive emotions. This represents a crucial aspect of spiritual growth. Every emotion is seen as an open-ended opportunity on the way to enlightenment. Every feeling or sensation we experience ultimately can be viewed as an expression of an enlightened state—a manifestation of the spectrum of our radiant energies. Yet, not uncommonly, emotions manifest as distorted reflections of these energies and cause mental constriction rather than expansion. And further, we can become emotionally conflicted to such an extent that we end up in a state of mental illness. Looking at emotional affliction and psychopathology in our modern day, the study of religious experience continues to have something important to contribute. This has been already suggested by prominent psychologist William James, who noted that affect generally constitutes the most essential component and healing factor in any religious experience.[1]

The religion of Buddhism and its profound understanding of meditation practice can give deeper insights into the nature of emotional experience. For the Vajrayana Buddhists, emotions are actually reflections of our awakened potentiality. Emotions, in general, are not comprehended as something which needs to be overcome as a pathological condition, but

---

1. James, *The Varieties of Religious Experience*.

rather emotions are being embraced as a spiritual path.[2] The complete unexpurgated range of what we are able to feel can be directed by moments of bliss or, on the contrary, resemble inner torture and desperation. While the focus in modern Western society has largely been on one-sided intellectual accomplishment, which may be a reason for the emotional imbalances we are increasingly encountering today, Buddhism pursues a more harmonious combination of cognitive and emotional maturity in particular. In fact, cognitive maturation does not go without emotional maturation. Depending on our level of self-awareness and our intentions, emotions can be seen as both, organizing and virtuous or disorganizing and harmful.

EMOTIONAL AFFLICTION AND THINKING PATTERNS

Within the field of cognitive science, the "emotion versus cognition" debate has dominated psychology for a long time and underestimated the influence of emotion; the discrepancy eventually has led to the realization that emotions have significant systematic effects upon cognitive processes. The importance of emotions lies in helping to structure perception as well as rational and adaptive responses to the environment. Technologically rapid and advancing neuroscientific research has discovered that emotions and cognitive activities are clearly interlinked by looking at the brain during functional MRI scanning. Current cognitive neuroscience confirms the viewpoint that a classic distinction between passion and reason is rather futile; emotion cannot be completely disentangled from cognition or vice versa. Emotions and cognitions are continually interacting in almost all mental activities and only to a certain degree is there any neurological differentiation within different centers of brain activity. Basic emotional processes are correlated with specific neurotransmitters and associated with activity in specific subcortical brain areas.[3] While we do not have a distinct cerebral "emotion center," some areas like the limbic system,[4] the basal ganglia, and the ventromedial prefrontal cortex are more active during affective episodes whereas the prefrontal cortex is predominantly an area where increased neuronal firing occurs during thinking activity. Neuroscientific research is now becoming less focused on determining specified functional localities in the brain but rather looks at the very complex neuronal connections

---

2. Dannecker, *Myogenic Transformation of Emotions*.
3. Panksepp, *Affective Neuroscience*.
4. The Limbic system is a set of evolutionarily more primitive brain structures that include the amygdala, the cingulate gyrus, the hypothalamus, and the thalamus.

between different parts of the brain, simultaneously reflecting the brain's natural plasticity.

On a physiological level, emotions can be observed through various responses of the autonomic nervous system, generally leading to classifiable types of behavior. It needs to be considered though that emotions are short-lived phenomena occurring under complex conditions. The internal experience of emotion is highly personal and often confusing, particularly because several, and often rather conflicting emotions may be experienced within the most rapid of sequence, making an objective and empirical study of emotion challenging. This leaves us with phenomenology as the most palpable way to make a clear distinction between that which is thought and felt during personal experience. Nevertheless, the empirical proof of a thinking-and-feeling amalgam within subjective experience will most likely remain physiological, neurological and, put into an evolutionary context, functionally directed towards adaptation and survival.

In Buddhist psychology, the word "emotion" does not exist in Sanskrit, Pali or Tibetan despite its rich language for describing a wide range of mental states and activities. This linguistic detail already reflects the profound Buddhist understanding that mental activity, including rational thought, is indistinguishable from any kind of feeling state, whether it is pleasure, pain, or indifference. Since there is no direct expression for emotion, the Sanskrit word *klesha* seems to be the closest to describe emotion, although it stands for negative mental or emotional factors.[5] The Buddhists generally speak of *klesha* as the three major poisons: desire (attachment, attraction, lust), aversion (hatred, anger, aggression), and indifference (ignorance, laziness, dullness). These emotional afflictions are seen as the main hindrance on the path to enlightenment. In most people they manifest as attitudinal inclinations of our personalities, and through rigid life style habits they have become mechanical rather than feeling expressions of our authentic passions. Due to deeply ingrained mental patterns (*samskara*)[6] and residual impressions (*vasana*) that form the roots of our perceptions of the world, we rarely have a clear experience free of the three poisons. In general, the term *klesha* comprises all the properties that dull, disturb, distort, agitate or excite the mind and which are the basis for unwholesome actions. Mental or emotional afflictions are entirely seen as mental factors that disrupt the equilibrium of the mind.

---

5. Dreyfus, "Is Compassion an Emotion?"
6. Terms in Italic are in Sanskrit.

Afflictive emotions often follow emotional valence which is the result of a cognitive appraisal given to external or internal events.[7] This form of valence helps us to make a distinction between positive or negative, liking or disliking, approach or withdrawal. Through valence we feel moved toward or away from things in a manner that reflects what these things or experiences mean to us personally. Feelings relate to responses of the mind when coming into contact with life situations that generate characteristics evaluated as being pleasant, unpleasant or neutral. The Buddhist psychology of the Abhidharma[8] suggests that when it comes to giving emotional value and attaching it to any content, the feeling part of our decision becomes more important than the merely cognitive meaning. In fact, there are two aspects to feeling (*vedana*): one is concrete feeling, and the other is feeling mixed up with other functions or elements such as sensation or mood.[9]

In terms of the mind's thinking patterns, Buddhist psychology distinguishes between the terms *citta* (mind) and *caitta* (mental).[10] *Citta* is the ordinary mind itself from which all the discursive and fleeting thoughts of *caitta* originate.[11] More specifically, *caitta* refers to the states of mind that are determined by events in the brain such as memory and association. These states of mind can only be determined within the human cognitive-emotive system of the brain, forming neural pathways to incorporate our world of experiences and they do not exist except within the framework of continually changing interactions of thinking and feeling. *Citta*, on the other hand, is the general sensitivity of the mind which allows us to feel and know things. It constitutes the overall mental functions of *caitta* that enable us to relate to things and to unite with the objects of experience. In other words, it divides experience into a personal and, in a sense, unique

---

7. Internal events can be seen as memories, dreams, impulses, intuitions, thoughts, and ideas.

8. The Abhidharma (compiled 300 BCE–400 CE) represents the earliest compilation of Buddhist philosophy and psychology. It is composed of the teachings and analyses concerning psychological and spiritual phenomena contained in the discourses of the Buddha and his disciples. In its systematic order it constitutes the dogmatic basis of the Hinayana and Mahayana tradition.

9. Guenther, *Philosophy and Psychology*.

10. Indian philosophy additionally distinguishes between *buddhi* and *manas*. *Buddhi* is the organ of cognition, representing rational thinking and the intellect. *Manas* is a more reactive form of mental activity which depends on the senses. It uses the senses in order to "make sense" of the impressions which enter from the phenomenal world, and then communicates those sense impressions to *buddhi*. This creates the impression of a continuous flow of our thoughts. Emotions through *manas* are more temporary responses to external stimuli whereas longer lasting mood states within *citta* are independent of them.

11. Guenther, "The Concept of Mind in Buddhist Tantrism," 263.

"sense-perception," accompanied by the conception of a "sense-field" (the relationship between subject and object) which encompasses the breadth of our conceptual capabilities. It is composed of traces and pre-dispositions that color the mind and describe our genetic brain endowment including our personality traits, emotional tendencies, mood characteristics, as well as mental abilities.

Similar to cognitive science and emotion theory, Buddhist psychology posits that emotions are interrelated with thinking patterns that support our beliefs, attitudes and desires. Thought is seen as obstructed by a veil (*citta avarana*) which results in afflictive emotions. The corresponding mental afflictions are aroused in two ways: the first is simply by a spontaneous brief event leading to a minor emotional crisis. Other mental afflictions that make up mental disorders come out of a deeper cause than simply adventitious circumstance. They come out of our genetic predilections and habitual propensities (*samskara*) within the unconscious aspect (*alaya vijnana*) of the mind, which are more difficult to remedy. In general, the identification with thoughts that arise in the mind is the main cause of worry, anxiety, fears, depression, guilt, and other emotional disturbances. Whatever mental state dominates our mind at a given moment will shape how we perceive and react to whatever is happening. Buddhist teachings often describe the mind as a monkey that jumps around creating problem after problem. If one believes that these artificially created thought forms are real, then a great deal of time and energy is expended on trying to solve all the resulting mental and emotional problems. One is kept enslaved in a state of constant motion and agitation in order to achieve what thoughts, beliefs, attitudes, and desires dictate. In essence, Buddhism expands on the materialistic and reductionist view of contemporary emotion theory by focusing on the spiritual dimension of emotional experience. Emotions looked at in this light form part of that which is fundamentally "numinous" in human nature.

WAYS OF WORKING WITH AFFLICTIVE EMOTIONS

When it comes to therapeutic methods for emotional imbalances, psychology is still engaged in a controversy between "cognitive-behavioral therapy"—meaning emotional discipline through thought structuring and reappraisal—and "catharsis," a form of emotional indulgence which involves a process of moving through affective states by entering them fully and living them out in order to eventually overcome any type of emotional inhibitions. This is widely practiced by various psychodynamic schools of therapy.

Earlier cognitive theory considered only the disruptive and disorganizing function of emotions. Emotional affliction originates from unfavorable thinking patterns that need to be corrected and adjusted.[12] More recent empirical emotion research, which has evolved further from the view that emotions are rather primitive and disruptive, continues to approve of the cognitive-behavioral approach. However, emotions are now also seen in their function as an "evolved organizer" influencing homeostatic processes of the body. In this psychoevolutionary model, emotions have an adaptive function restoring equilibrium when unexpected or unusual events create disequilibrium such that adequate functioning and survival is guaranteed.[13] Cognition functions as a participant in the emotional process, and our thinking patterns ensure that affective episodes are accordingly appraised and valued, causing adaptive behavioral reactions such as approach or withdrawal. Negative emotions are seen to off-balance homeostasis in order to force optimal survival adjustments whereas positive emotions help the bodily system to return to homeostasis through the function of "undoing".[14] Positive emotions in general tend to broaden decision making processes allowing us to recruit new ideas into an ever widening network of associations,[15] as well as improve social interactions.[16]

It is now widely believed that certain unfavorable cognitive styles enhance genetic vulnerabilities for emotional instability. In a more extreme cognitive-behavioral perspective, searching for the meaning behind a difficult life event may simply be viewed as unhelpful rumination reinforcing the negativity of our thinking patterns. However, one needs to be aware that artificially constructed positive self-statements can also strengthen the person's own negative view rather than reversing it;[17] and, for those who favor catharsis therapy, the cognitive approach can easily lead to a more or less superficial mind framing tool when the person is instructed about how one "should" be thinking and thought forms are only exchanged by more conventionally appropriate and seemingly more adaptive ones. Not uncommonly, cognitive therapy can then easily resemble some sort of clever mind

---

12. For example, Arnold, *Emotion and Personality*; Beck, *Cognitive Therapy and Emotional Disorders*; Ellis, *Humanistic Psychotherapy*.

13. Plutchik, *Emotion*.

14. As an example, people often tend to smile during or following negative emotional experiences in order to modulate their own inner experiences. See Levison and Fredrickson, "Positive Emotions Speed Recovery from the Cardiovascular Sequelae of Negative Emotions," 191–220.

15. Fredrickson, "The Role of Positive Emotions in Positive Psychology," 218–66.

16. Isen, "Positive Affect and Decision Making," 261–78.

17. Wood et al., *Should People with Low Self-Esteem Strive for High Self-Esteem?*

game which does not touch the person on a deeper level nor has the power to ultimately transform the persistent underlying emotional affliction.

The idea behind catharsis therapy is that emotional energy must be discharged or released. People may hit a pillow, for example, with the purpose of freeing up and actualizing anger. In order to unfreeze afflictive emotional states, or to break open the shell of defensive habitual patterns it is sometimes necessary to stir up emotions deliberately. Catharsis as such is not seen as attempting to change any emotion that is in the foreground but rather enhancing it, exaggerating it to the extent that it finally breaks, explodes or implodes, and depletes itself. A total convulsion of an emotional reaction, even if initially induced by pretense, is valued as profoundly therapeutic and liberating. Through this enactment often awareness about some emotion is brought to the surface which has not been there before and was only able to show itself in its extreme form. Catharsis counteracts emotional suppression which, as emotion research has been able to confirm, is harmful to our health.[18] It allows for letting the pain come through that is underneath most afflictive emotions once the steam on the surface is let off. While further emotion research, looking at short-term data, proposes that an apparently disruptive emotion like crying could be an adaptive way to receive soothing and caring through social contact,[19] catharsis therapy uses difficult emotional states as a means to enter into the deeper layers of painful feelings in order to achieve emotional homeostasis over time. The potential danger of this approach, however, is that some individuals are inclined to empower themselves with the emotion or get attached to the intense feeling and dramatic impact. In this case it only burns energy and is of no value if one becomes stuck in the "refractory period"[20] during which emotion is difficult to stop once it is initiated. When caught in this kind of an emotional grip, a person is not receptive to new information and becomes easily hung up in a vicious circle of reinforcing the old emotional pattern. Regarding a rather unfortunate possible outcome like this, the blame often falls on Western individualism for the currently prevailing tendency and approval for "acting out" emotions indiscriminatingly or the increasing encouragement of so-called "emotional ventilationism."[21]

In Tibetan Buddhism there is no conflict between the two therapeutic approaches, be it cognitive-behavioral or catharsis. Both forms of working with afflictive emotions are valid and applicable according to the rather

18. Gross and Levenson, "Emotional Suppression," 970–86.
19. Gross et al., "The Psychology of Crying," 460–68.
20. Ekman, *Emotional Awareness*.
21. Tavris, *Anger*.

unique needs of the individual. Both approaches become ineffective if not applied in a balanced way in view of the already mentioned potential pitfalls and incoherencies. With certain meditative practices or techniques, Buddhists claim that it is possible to empty the mind of all kinds of emotional affliction since those states are illnesses that can be cured and do not represent the inherently luminous nature of the mind.

For healing and transforming afflictive emotions, Tibetan Buddhism uses different methods that for ease of conceptual understanding could be described as stages applicable according to the level and temperament of the practitioner. Firstly, our cognition is addressed with the understanding that all the afflictions we experience are rooted in a fundamentally distorted way of perceiving the world. In accord with the cognitive approach, Buddhist teachings and practices repeatedly emphasize that in order to balance the emotions it is best to tame the mind. This supports the common understanding that we can influence disturbing emotional reactions through changing our thinking patterns. In order to become emotionally responsible rather than reactive one needs to become aware of the underlying thoughts and examine them objectively, which reinstates discipline and emotional self-control by means of increased mental awareness. By observing and allowing whatever thoughts arise, this method of "self-monitoring" exposes the mind's patterns and activities, predominantly by direct observation of the emotional and mental fluctuations. Once the disturbing emotion has been investigated and separated, through cognitive appraisal and through sensory awareness, emotional valence establishes the ability to apply the popular Buddhist practice of antidotes. For example in the case of anger, positive emotional states, such as cultivating tolerance and patience in the case of anger, act as a specific antidote. This means that emotional afflictions can be treated by deliberately cultivating antidotal forces like empathy, compassion, tolerance, patience, and forgiveness, using them as efficient tools to counteract negativity. The idea behind this approach is that two diametrically opposed mental processes cannot arise together toward the same object at the same time. In other words, one cannot wish to harm and benefit another person at the same instant. The more one cultivates altruistic love, the more its opposite—the wish to harm—is driven away and expected eventually to vanish. The antidotal practice of changing thoughts and attitudes in Tibetan Buddhism is only seen as a preliminary device for gaining deeper insight into the nature of the mind, which can reach as far as transforming our conditioned apprehension of the nature of reality and its illusory aspects (*maya*).

Approaching afflictive emotional states through antidotes, if turned into a rigid rule, can also create an inner conflict by over emphasizing the destruction of one's inner negativity; i.e. hate "has to" be completely destroyed and compassion created. This cuts the practitioner into two parts: the right and the wrong. When anger is dominant one is told to create the opposite, compassion, which might become a new habit. Then if one perseveres for a long time, anger might disappear and more compassion arises. Hence compassion increases, but only because one might have cultivated a habit. This demonstrates that it is relatively easy to cultivate a good habit but it is very difficult to become entirely "good" and transformed as a person.

Keeping this potential problem of antidotal practice in mind, the second stage of working with emotional affliction in Buddhist practice helps preventing from getting stuck, and should now be applied simultaneously. Instead of focusing on the exchange of maladaptive thought patterns with more adaptive ones, this next stage rather conceives of ways to make our thinking less conceptual and more flexible. This allows us "to be with" the situation instead of looking at it through different pre-formulated lenses of thought formation. The discernment between "good" and "bad" thoughts or emotions, the entire concept of positive e thinking and emotional valence becomes unimportant and can even be a hindrance since in the larger picture of universal forces no emotion is, strictly speaking, "positive" or "negative." The goal is to reach some state of transcendence of any kind of dual conceptualizations that give valence to the essentially indeterminable flow of the wide range of human experience. What ultimately counts for the Buddhists is an experiential awareness of what we think and feel in every moment and not identifying with it, instead of putting a label on it. When the habitual replacement of emotions is avoided, an inner emotional flexibility and mastery can emerge. Then, applying this to the practice of working with the antidotes the following might occur:

> When you can easily jump from the negative side of your experience to the positive, you may find that you can almost feel both at the same time—somewhat like looking into a mirror and being equally aware of your body and its reflection at the same moment. Then you may see that there is no jumping from one quality to another; there actually is only awareness itself, both within and around experience.[22]

In these first two stages of working with emotional affliction, acting out a negative emotion—even in the context of therapy and in a fictitious way—is seen as more detrimental than helpful. Expressing or acting out anger, for example, most often tries to avoid the deeper layer of the "feeling in the feeling," just as with suppression. The afflictive emotion always arises from a

22. Tarthang Tulku, *Hidden Mind of Freedom*, 54.

mind that is dissatisfied and discontent. Theravada Buddhist teacher Thich Nhat Hanh elaborates on the futile nature of catharsis: "Because you are exhausted, you will no longer have energy left to feed your anger. You may think that anger is no longer there, but that's not true; you are simply too tired to be angry."[23] The roots of anger remain untouched, and when the conditions are right, the same anger will arise again. An artificially induced release of an afflictive emotion only waters the seeds of our tendencies lying dormant in the storehouse consciousness (*alaya vijnana*). Any deliberate practice of promoting potentially harmful feelings will only encourage them to sprout. The main task is to constantly work toward building inner contentment and cultivating compassion.[24] This can be achieved through the first stage when learning to discriminate between those feelings that are harmful and those which are beneficial to our own and other being's well-being; and additionally, through the second stage, when we allow and accept feelings as they arise while also letting go of the initial discrimination—all without losing touch with the "basic goodness" of emotional experience.

The Tantrics within Tibetan Vajrayana Buddhism, on the other hand, allow intensity; they do not reject afflictive emotions, while they do not cultivate them either. It then becomes a matter of seeing things as they are—not as we would like them to be. This would represent the third stage of transforming afflictive emotions (*klesha*). The Sanskrit root of the word *tantra* means to weave and refers to the "interwoveness" and interdependence of all things which contains the dependent co-arising of phenomena (*pratityasamutpada*). In Tantrayana one purposely goes into the dark forces of difficult emotions, invoking them in order to heal and, in a sense, burn through them without any shame or guilt. A seemingly unpleasant and, thereby, evaluated as worthless or even destructive emotion can be transformed into something highly valuable. The psychology of Tantra conveys the more radical message that we do not have to escape or avoid impurity, chaos, pain, darkness, aggression, fear, and any other negative state. In fact, the more one flees these states or tries to fix them, the more one alienates oneself from the potential awakening hidden within them. The Tantrics work with the emotional reaction to difficult experiences and the resultant suffering is used as a tool for spiritual transformation. More explicitly, shock experiences, which normally increase trauma, paradoxically are considered as beneficial—if correctly executed and received—for facing the "dark side" of the personality structure and bringing the deeply ingrained negative emotions to the surface. In dealing directly with emotion and passion, a

---

23. Thich Nhat Hanh, *Anger*, 116.
24. Dalai Lama, *Awakening the Mind*.

transformative change can be elicited through evoking the extreme. This also explains why, traditionally, Tantric Buddhism represents a secret practice that is only suitable for more advanced practitioners due to risks involved which should not be underestimated by our rational thinking. The more holistic approach of Tantra could be compared to the alchemical process of fighting fire with fire, to defeat afflictive emotions with their own energy. The mind has the ability to transform any emotion into transcendental wisdom just like the alchemist is attempting to learn how to change base metal into gold. Similar to homeopathy, the alchemical component in Tantra is that the cure is similar to the disease. The very same element that causes a disease, if then utilized in a proper dose, may act as an antidote and heal it too: anger is cured with anger, desire with desire, and so on until all is eventually transmuted into wisdom. Symptoms are not suppressed but rather caused to exacerbate temporarily as a necessary step towards their complete transcendence. Moreover, Tantra offers a workable synthesis of the previously presented methods with the ability to apply both, cognitive antidotes and emotional catharsis, without their respective dangers of suppression and overextension. Tantric techniques include body gestures and postures (*mudra*), the visualization of sublime forms (e.g., an emotion is visualized as a deity), and repetition of sacred sounds (*mantra*) in order to attain purification and transformation.

The principle of Tantra is to turn a weakness like an afflictive emotion into strength while affect is explored energetically in its magical empowerment. External and internal forces which ordinarily lead to emotional pain can be used to bring about increased self-awareness and clarity instead of confusion, depression, or other kinds of emotionally difficult states. The particularly raw and unpredictable energy of emotional affliction constitutes a dynamic and direct path to transformation. The provocative energy itself becomes a means for salvation and the energy of the emotional pain is also the energy of liberation. Again, one needs to keep in mind that working with sometimes very strong negative forces implies one of the reasons why Tantra is such a fast and, if practiced incorrectly, dangerous path: first of all, there is a lot of energy involved and, secondly, one risks falling back into an even increased negativity if the right intention and attitude to bring about pure spiritual growth has not been maintained. Obviously, the path of Tantra, if pursued truthfully and sincerely, is one of the most difficult paths and requires extensive spiritual preparation and the guidance of a qualified teacher. In essence, Tantra suggests that while we are able to abide with suffering and enter into it more deeply, we can also "dance with it" and "celebrate in delight." In fact, no situation can really keep us from working with the energy of provocation and transform it into higher emotional states like equanimity, bliss, and joy; it simply becomes a matter of one's own inner flexibility. Specific Tantric practices can transform not only the nature of momentary emotional experience, but also bring about fundamental changes in more enduring traits, like shifting our so-called "happiness set-point" to a higher level which allows for more contentment in general. Buddhist Tantra could be seen as a form of therapy, not directed primarily at psychopathology, but rather at the suffering that all humans endure, and promises not only transcendence of suffering but also an enhancement of fundamental well-being.

The Tibetan Vajrayana Buddhists, altogether, are strongly aware that in dealing with emotional affliction the best approach is conceived in the path of the middle way contained in each of the three stages; this means finding a balance between allowing but not dramatizing and identifying, and healthy mental discipline but not rejecting or repressing anything that comes up emotionally.

MEDITATION PRACTICE FOR HEALING EMOTIONAL AFFLICTION

In Buddhism the practice of meditation represents the most fundamental approach for healing afflictive emotions. Moreover, continued practice allows for the development of increasingly refined and beneficial emotional awareness such as intuition, clarity, compassion, tolerance, a sense of caring, and empathy. Several neuroscientists employing fMRI scanning of the brain have discovered that experienced Buddhist meditators show increased activity in the left prefrontal lobes.[25] This area is linked to positive emotions, good mood, and improved concentration; in addition, research subjects with higher left hemisphere activity also have a tendency to spend more time on "happy" images presented to them[26] and maintain a generally more positive outlook on life. Other research suggests that meditation and mindfulness can calm the amygdala, an area of the brain associated with fear.[27] In experiments measuring physiological reactions, experienced meditation practitioners were less likely to be shocked, flustered, surprised or as angry as other subjects.[28] In connection with transcendental experiences during meditation, fMRIs demonstrate a decrease of activity in the parietal lobe which is associated with orientation. This is interpreted as a possible in-

25. For example, Lutz et al., "Long-Term Meditators Self-Induce," 16369–73.
26. Pettigrew, "Searching for the Switch," 85–118.
27. Davis, "The Role of the Amygdala in Fear and Anxiety," 352–75.
28. Goleman, *Destructive Emotions*.

dication for the often mentioned sense of oneness with the universe and a loss of the sense of self. And, similar to other skill acquisition, meditation training can induce significant changes in the brain, increasing the brain's capacity for neuroplasticity by creating new synaptic neural connections.[29] Contemporary neuroscientific research demonstrates how affect psychology is discovering by empirical means some of the more distinct features of emotion that accomplished meditation practitioners may have known for ages.

Meditation is generally used for the conscious cultivation of mental faculties, calmness, relaxation, one-pointed concentration, loving kindness, compassion, a sense of well-being, and insight into the nature of reality. Mindfulness allows an ongoing stream of feelings, which gives the awareness that emotional responses are not continuous but emerge and settle again in waves. The intention of meditation is to develop equanimity in the face of any kind of emotional intensity. Emotions can then become helpful in their function as homeostatic organizers supporting greater emotional balance and harmony. The most widely practiced method of meditation deals with cultivating mindfulness of breathing. Using the breath to come into contact with feelings can bridge the gap between any disturbing emotion and our sense of being. All Buddhist meditation practice initially focuses on the breath by gaining awareness of its rising and falling. The practice of *shamatha* helps with one-pointed concentration while the next level, *vipasyana*, is a process of holding an open space for self-arising mental, emotional and sensational phenomena. Buddhism emphasizes repeatedly that negative mental states are not an intrinsic part of the mind; they are transient obstacles that obstruct the expression of our underlying natural state of joy and happiness, our so-called "Buddha Nature." In his book, "The Art of Happiness," the Dalai Lama emphasizes that a complete insight into the ultimate nature of reality provides an antidote to all the negative states of mind. Realizing our inherent "Buddha Nature" can help us to get to the roots of reality. With the help of meditation practice one is able to cut through the illusory appearance of an emotion, eventually removing the underlying distorted state of mind. During this process of easing the habits of compulsive and erratic thinking and disturbing feelings, our attention can become intensely concentrated and one-pointed. Then, by going deeper into the meditation, the mind becomes able to free itself of all physical sense impressions, including the presence of our own body. When outer sensory distraction, discursive thinking and unbalanced feeling become absent for

---

29. Slagter et al., "Mental Training Effects Use of Limited Brain Resources"; Davidson and Lutz, "Buddha's Brain."

an extended period, the more advanced practitioner can enter a state which is experienced as joyful bliss, ecstasy, and equanimity.

So far, most meditation research has exclusively focused on the overall positive effects of meditation. Apart from hopefully tasting some transcendent happy state (*nirvana*) during the meditation, in some cases a condition could also emerge which resembles something like we are accustomed to encounter in psychopathology. In those instances there may be feelings of intense anxiety, or sudden outbursts of rage, agony, pain, and so forth coming to the surface, seemingly out of nowhere. It is important not to become too disturbed by it and to "sit with it" until the energy of it "moves through." This is a not much talked about but likewise important part of the meditation practice. It gives the practitioner the opportunity to get in touch with that which is generally repressed. In the more extreme case, some people even report psychotic-like experiences similar but not attributable to any form of a mental disorder. However, extensive meditation practice can be potentially dangerous for those whose personality structures are loosely constituted or who have repressed severe emotional problems. In such a case, the process of personal spiritual growth and change can become chaotic and overwhelming, possibly leading further to a greater crisis that continues after the meditation retreat.

The similarity of these kinds of experiences with mental disorder has led psychologists—inspired by research on spiritual emergence done by Stan and Christina Grof[30]—to come up with a diagnostic category called "Religious or Spiritual Problem" within the official categorizations for mental disorders (Diagnostic and Statistical Manual-Fourth Edition, APA 1994). Symptoms, which can also result from other spiritual practices besides meditation or even independent of it, include severe anxiety, panic, dissociation, depersonalization, altered perceptions, delusions, agitation, muscular tension or seizure-like cramps,[31] markedly illogical thinking or grossly disorganized behavior, excruciating physical pain, mania or depression, and agitated despair sometimes resulting in suicidal ideation. Physical manifestations can resemble the result of pharmacological stimulation of the central nervous system. Symptoms associated with the activation of sensitive nerves are severe headaches, bodily aches and pains, a variety of strange sensations (e.g., heat and cold, tingling), increased libido, as well as the perception of images and visions or the hearing of strange sounds.[32]

30. Grof and Grof, *Spiritual Emergency*.
31. In Hindu Tantric traditions epileptic seizures during religious experience are known as *kriya*.
32. Similarly, mystical medieval Christian literature such as "The Cloud of Unknowing" speaks of the fact that the closer the soul of the mystic gets to God the more

If psychoactive medication, like tranquilizers or antipsychotics, are being used to dampen the symptoms, very commonly the effect is to the contrary since the energetic release becomes frozen and stuck which significantly increases the person's suffering while there is no real benefit in the pharmaceutical treatment. In very exceptional and unusual cases powerful primary energy movements (*kundalini*) could have become activated.[33] In the West, most qualified meditation teachers are aware that in any of the previously described extreme and rare circumstances meditation practice needs be discontinued immediately and grounding (e.g., jogging, eating meat) has to take place until the feelings of malaise and energetic imbalance subside. The duration of the usually very terrifying experiences varies among individuals lasting from a few hours to several months or even longer. It is normally a condition that cannot be fixed and treated but merely needs to be outgrown with trust and patience; i.e., one needs to trust and allow that therapy can also happen from within and could be seen as even superior to anything that we yet know how to conduct or guide from without. Afterwards, the individual often feels strangely renewed, somewhat like being purged, which opens up some fresh space for new positive life-affirming feelings to emerge.

Meditation as a technique for spiritual growth can trigger the actualization of a person's potentialities which, as already discussed, commonly includes going through one's emotional difficulties and personal estrangement so that one can gain greater emotional maturity and awareness. It becomes a matter of learning how to tolerate the intensities of pleasure and pain. By being present to that which is in the moment, one becomes less and less emotionally affected by the ups and downs of life. Accepting the way things are helps one to relinquish the conditioned habit of trying to understand and analyze. Once one ceases to try to change and fix emotional affliction, there is the possibility that the suffering eases as well; "the way out" of mental and emotional suffering becomes "the way through." Letting

---

darkness and confusion arises. The mystical experience entails that one has to be stripped away of every idea, every intellectual conception, before one can approach the light which is surrounded by the darkness of utter confusion, dissatisfaction, and pain. In alchemy this condition is termed the "nigredo" state which is necessary for the alchemical process of transmutation during which active imagination is applied in order to enter into a "voluntary psychosis."

33. Most traditional Tibetan teachers avoid talking of *kundalini* experiences since it is part of the more esoteric Tantric teachings and kept secret. It is also considered temporary phenomena with a tempting illusory quality (*mara*) that should not get too much attention and only distracts the meditator from one-pointed concentration. Additionally, according to the Tantric tradition, whether one deals with a full *kundalini* awakening can only be perceived by a qualified teacher whose own *kundalini* has been awakened.

go of identifying with any emotional contraction allows for an internal shift. Afflictive emotions then may become self-liberating when the mind enters a state of apprehending the nature of emptiness (*sunyata*). Eventually the meditator is able to experience that emotions have no inherent substance. There is no more feeling, feeler, and felt-about. All the arising and vanishing of emotional states is "emptiness dancing with emptiness" when mind becomes as infinitely vast as the open sky. The greater the passions, the more intense the thinking, the more powerful becomes the realization of the ultimate nature of reality (*dharmakaya*). Emotional upset is now seen as a disguise of "non-dual energy wisdom," not in any way apart from the *dharmakaya*. This ulterior outlook often described by the Dzogchen or Mahamudra tradition within Tibetan Vajrayana Buddhism could be seen as the fourth and final stage of emotional transformation—although in view of emotion as an expression of openness mind and emptiness, there ultimately is no gradual approach.

MENTAL ILLNESS SEEN WITHIN THE LARGER PICTURE OF TIBETAN BUDDHISM

In its "nature versus nurture" debate psychology has come to the conclusion that different people may be genetically equipped with some vulnerability for mental illness. At the same time the environment can trigger those otherwise possibly latent predispositions through stressful events. Individuals with typically stronger left-sided prefrontal activation may recover more quickly from negative affect or stress than their right-activated counterparts who might become more vulnerable to mental and emotional instability. One could say that psychopathology begins to manifest when there is emotional dysregulation instead of regulation; "madness" as an affective phenomenon is always related to exceptionally strong states of emotion.

The contemporary challenge becomes how much we can see through the various connotations, spectrums, and complexities that mental illness represents. From a more materialistic viewpoint, most mental health professionals still view psychopathological conditions as an almost inalterable state of predominantly inherited imbalances in the brain chemistry. The brain, in a mechanical way treated similarly to the motor of a car, is supposed to become rebalanced through the treatment of drugs. Once the oil is changed, for example, the motor is expected to run "smoothly" again. In the same way, the patient on psychoactive drugs is expected to function "normally" again. The psychiatrist draws a linear model forecast of the illness' expected trajectory, which is logically enlightening and satisfying. It seems like a simple—or, perhaps, simplistic—solution which gives assurance that a certain problem can be fixed and the solution realistically applied to something which in actuality, however, still remains largely incomprehensible and fundamentally mysterious despite our technological advances. In addition, mental illness is extremely threatening to any individual and society at large which increases the desire for a quick and easy cure. Through psychopathological diagnosis the subjectivity of the so-called "insane" individual is categorized by an objectivity formed within the reductionist tool box of what is available and conceivable to psychiatry. In this respect, psychopathological diagnosis is not neutral or non-contextual but reflects values, expectations, standards, and the respective thinking frame of the judging authority. By means of rather rigid standardized cognitive-behavioral therapy methods and prescription drugs the patient is rendered compliant and "adjusted," generally understating medication side effects and denying potential complications during future withdrawal.[34] In this respect, much of mainstream psychiatry reminds of an image of the magician's apprentice: he has learned from his master how to call the ghosts, but does not know how to get rid of them again. In fact, we really do not yet know exactly and in detail how the medications work in the brain and what long-term effects might still come to the surface when chemically altering a person's dopamine and serotonin neurotransmitter levels, for example. The duration of the drug consumption could in the future easily be close to a life-time if one takes into account that more and more children are already being diagnosed for needing psychochemical treatment.

In a Buddhist view, the expression of emotional affliction through mental illness becomes an ultimate demonstration of the wheel of existence (*samsara*) when life is understood as continuous suffering—whether through pleasure and attachment (*sukha*) or pain and aversion (*dukkha*)—until we come to the point of liberation. A schizophrenic person who is lost in the unreality of his hallucinations touches the most basic nature of illusionary human experience (*maya*). In some paradoxical way, the "insane"

---

34 The side effects of psychoactive drugs can be devastating. While antidepressants are known for potentially causing suicidal thoughts and generally dull the emotions, antipsychotics (also called neuroleptics, which means "brain-seizuring") are now more commonly and indiscriminatingly used for any form of personal crisis that might be diagnosed as an agitated depression due to surfacing emotional disturbances such as tension, fear and sadness. The extrapyramidal effects in the brain cause movements and facial expressions to become stiff while there are uncontrollable, repetitive twitching and tremors (tardive dyskinesia) besides some nervous movement agitation in the limbs (akathisia) which resembles the familiar rocking movements of the so-called "insane" in psychiatric institutions. Withdrawal symptoms from any psychoactive drug can be very severe for more sensitive people.

person could be seen as even closer to truth and more perceptive of the human condition in its existential uncertainty. Through the illness he has been stripped off his filters that keep the ordinary image of a conventional "self" sustained such that we can continue to function in our established and habitual social roles. On the other hand, the mentally ill can also become identified with the diagnosed "illness" resulting in helplessness and dependency over time. Emotional pain then turns into a reference point, something that gives proof that one exists. In the extreme form this is expressed by the borderline disorder, when incurring cuts on parts of the body allows the person to have a sense of being, an identity by means of the self-afflicted pain, or an unpleasantly felt self-definition in an increasingly unpredictable and impalpable world. It gives the mind a justification by demonstrating to the external environment "I hurt, therefore I am," reassuring that the experience of emotional affliction is at least something comfortingly familiar. What we often see as therapeutic alleviation when talking about our struggles to mental health professionals, the Buddhist perspective may also consider the potential danger in tending our pain excessively, to the degree of even cultivating it through continuously "processing" feelings and talking about it.

Tibetan Buddhism offers the possibility of widening the understanding of mental health. Mental disorders are accepted in their enigmatic nature while the insubstantiality of labeling in form of diagnostic categories is recognized. Seen in a larger picture, human beings go through cycles concerning their physical and emotional energies, and there are times for great health, activity and productivity as well as there are times when things come to a halt, all of it depending on the individual conditions and circumstances (*karma*). Many mental illnesses are often created through fighting against the cycles of low energy, which are vital for regeneration. In this sense, being "depressed" could instead be understood as becoming "de-pressured," and the need to take a "deep rest." The intelligence of the body, the wisdom of organismic self-regulation, may take over as a self-protective measure in order to force the person to retreat, so that the necessary regeneration can take place. Accordingly, Vajrayana Buddhists often prefer to look at the energetic physical manifestation of the illness rather than what it is called or what it means. And they have also a more transcendental way of looking at mental illness: if one is trapped in a nightmare there will probably be a stronger motivation to awaken than someone who is just caught in the ups and downs of an ordinary dream. It takes the person out of the collective mindset almost by force. Mental and emotional suffering can then become a great awakener eventually producing more refined and exalted feeling states like depth, humility, compassion, and inner peace. Going through the pains of mental illness can show a person what is unreal and real in life, what is superfluous and what ultimately matters. Seen from this transpersonal position, conditions are always empty—which is neither positive nor negative—and each emotional experience whether good or bad, in an ultimate sense, can only be positive. Through inner spiritual growth, emotional expansion happens and imbalanced mental states can be overcome.

Unfortunately, the way we are treating mental illness in modern utilitarian society is representative of how we have become alienated from religion and lost depth. Science and technology have become humanity's foundation for faith. Confirming the predominant materialistic world view, neuroscience explains that religious sentiment is merely a property of the brain and part of our general brain chemistry. Religious experience sometimes hard to tell apart from mental illness is usually not something that is valued or even taken into consideration. Those who used to be highly esteemed as religious and mystical saints in ancient times or may still be appreciated as shamanic healers in some indigenous cultures are in modern society rather denigrated as useless and possibly crazy. In this sense we have not evolved very far from the medieval inquisition and its witch hunting atrocities. However, today through globalization we should increasingly be tolerant and open enough to bring rational science and the typically discredited mystical side of religion together. Each human life could be seen as a spiritual adventure and, in Buddhist terms, a unique meeting with our own "Buddha Nature," with that which is divine within and without. Religious experience, whether it manifests as a blissful opening or rather resembles periodical mental illness, is our unique expression of who we are. The religion of Buddhism can give us a perspective through which we may eventually be able to move beyond suffering in the face of emotional afflictions and mental instability. Seeing the enormous value of religion in dealing with illness, a profound religion like Tibetan Buddhism, if carefully treasured and preserved from extinction, can still teach us: that there is wisdom in the universe, something larger to live for, and that in unity we can reach for global transformation and happiness.

BIBLIOGRAPHY

Arnold, Magda B. *Emotion and Personality*. Vols. 1 and 2. New York: Columbia University Press, 1960.

Beck, Aaron T. *Cognitive Therapy and the Emotional Disorders*. New York: Plume, 1984.

Dalai Lama. *Awakening the Mind, Lightening the Heart*. The Path to Enlightenment Series. San Francisco: HarperSanFrancisco, 1995.

Dalai Lama, and Howard C. Culter. *The Art of Happiness: A Handbook for Living.* New York: Riverhead, 1998.

Damasio, Antonio R. *Descartes' Error: Emotion, Reason, and the Human Brain.* New York: Penguin, 1995.

Dannecker, Martina E. *Myogenic Transformation of Emotions: A Dialectical Inquiry into Western Psychotherapy and Buddhist Psychology.* Cologne: Lambert Academic, 2009.

Davidson, Richard J., and Antoine Lutz. "Buddha's Brain: Neuroplasticity and Meditation." *IEEE Signal Processing Magazine* 25 (2008) 171–74.

Davis, Michael. "The Role of the Amygdala in Fear and Anxiety." *Annual Review of Neuroscience* 15 (1992) 352–75.

Dreyfus, Georges. "Is Compassion an Emotion? A Cross-Cultural Exploration." In *Visions of Compassion: Western Scientists and Tibetan Buddhists Examine Human Nature,* edited by Richard J. Davidson and Anne Harrington, 31–45. Oxford: Oxford University Press, 2002.

Ekman, Paul, ed. *Emotional Awareness: Overcoming the Obstacles to Psychological Balance and Compassion: A Conversation between the Dalai Lama and Paul Ekman.* New York: Henry Holt, 2008.

Ellis, Albert. *Humanistic Psychotherapy: The Rational-Emotive Approach.* Edited by Edward Sagarin. New York: McGraw-Hill, 1988.

Fredrickson, Barbara L. "The Role of Positive Emotions in Positive Psychology: The Broaden-and Build-Theory of Positive Emotions." *American Psychologist* 56 (2001) 218–26.

Goleman, Daniel. *Destructive Emotions: How Can We Overcome Them? A Scientific Dialogue with the Dalai Lama.* New York: Bantam, 2003.

Grof, Stanislav, and Christina Grof, eds. *Spiritual Emergency: When Personal Transformation Becomes a Crisis.* A New Consciousness Reader. Los Angeles: Tarcher, 1998.

Gross, James J, and Robert W. Levenson. "Emotional Suppression: Physiology, Self-Report, and Expressive Behavior." *Journal of Personality & Social Psychology* 64 (1993) 970–86.

Gross, James J., Barbara L. Fredrickson, and Robert W. Levenson. "The Psychology of Crying." *Psychophysiology* 31 (1994) 460–68.

Guenther, Herbert V. "The Concept of Mind in Buddhist Tantrism." *Journal of Oriental Studies* 3 (1956) 263.

———. *Philosophy and Psychology in the Abhidharma.* 3rd ed. Berkeley: Orient Book Distributors, 1976.

Isen, Alice M. "Positive Affect and Decision Making." In *Handbook of Emotions,* edited by M. Lewis and J. M. Haviland, 261–78. New York: Guilfords, 1993.

James, William. *The Varieties of Religious Experience: A Study in Human Nature.* New York: CreateSpace Independent Publishing Platform, 1890/1958.

Levenson, Robert W., and Barbara L. Fredrickson. "Positive Emotion Speed Recovery from the Cardiovascular Sequelae of Negative Emotions." *Cognition and Emotion* 12 (1998) 191–20.

Lutz, Antoine, Lawrence L. Greischar, Nancy B. Rawlings, Matthieu Ricard, and Richard J. Davidson. "Long-Term Meditators Self-Induce High-Amplitude Gamma Synchrony during Mental Practice." *Proceedings of the National Academy of Sciences* 101 (2004) 16369–73.

Nhat Hanh, Thich. *Anger: Wisdom for Cooling the Flames.* New York: Riverhead, 2001.

Panksepp, Jaak. *Affective Neuroscience: The Foundations of Human and Animal Emotions.* Series in Affective Science. New York: Oxford University Press, 1998.

Pettigrew, John D. "Searching for the Switch: Neural Bases for Perceptual Rivalry Alternations." *Brain and Mind* 2 (2001) 85–118.

Plutchik, Robert. *Emotion: A Psychoevolutionary Synthesis.* New York: Longman Higher Education, 1980.

Slagter, Helene A., Antoine Lutz, Lawrence L. Greischar, Andrew D. Francis, Sander Nieuwenhuis, James M. Davis, and Richard J. Davidson. "Mental Training Effects Use of Limited Brain Resources." *PLoS Biol.* 5.6 (2007) e138, 1–8.

Tarthang Tulku. *Hidden Mind of Freedom.* Nyingma Psycholoogy Series. Berkeley: Dharma, 1981.

Tavris, Carol. *Anger: The Misunderstood Emotion.* New York: Simon & Schuster, 1989.

Wood, Joanne V., Danu B. Anthony, and Walter F. Foddis. "Should People with Low Self-esteem Strive for High Self-esteem?" In *Self-Esteem Issues and Answers: A Sourcebook of Current Perspective*, edited by M. H. Kernis, 288–97. New York: Psychology Press, 2006.

Part 3

Religion, Illness, and Care of the Sick in the Old Testament and Judaism

8

Written on the Body
Body and Illness in the Physiognomic Tradition of the Ancient Near East and the Old Testament

—Angelika Berlejung

INTRODUCTION

Physicality is one of the basic human experiences that is always felt as an individual experience but that affects everyone. The same is true for the functions and malfunctions of the human body that significantly determine each person's life and rhythms. Nonetheless, the understanding and perception of one's own body[1] and its functions and malfunctions, as well as the process of defining images of illness and health, are by no means timeless "anthropological universals." Rather, there are always cultural constructs that take on different forms according to the historical and social conditions. These cultural constructs do—when seen in retrospect—go back to the people who jointly created them. However, they also—looking forward—exert a constant conditioning influence on people's actions.

---

1. On the changing construction of the body in Western cultures, see Synnott, *Body*; Synnott, "Tomb," 79–110. On body constructs in the Old Testament, see Hedwig-Jahnow research project, *Körperkonzepte*.

All persons within a cultural system[2] have the same interpretive patterns and internal cultural guidelines, which come from the same cultural symbolization process and with which they were confronted as soon as they were born. These guidelines (mainly structures of common interpretation and evaluation) are acquired over the course of their lives, through enculturation,[3] so that from childhood on they are equipped with a suprasubjective frame of reference and set of values within which their imaginative, intellectual, emotional and linguistic world as well as their sphere of action will move ever afterward. When members of a group and a culture (= a system of signs and contexts for action) who have received the same cultural guideline training communicate with one another, this takes place on the basis of their shared frame of reference, which each party implicitly assumes that the other will know and acknowledge.

Particularly with regard to the human body, its functions and malfunctions, a cultural system assumes a large number of implicit axioms. Therefore it is not surprising that in the Ancient Near East and in the Old Testament, there is no fundamental discussion that explains or reflects on the concepts of the body, illness or health. Ancient Near Eastern (and thus Old Testament) authors and editors, in writing about the human body or about sickness and health, could assume that the implicit meanings and values that they naturally associated with these topics were equally familiar to their readers (= members of their culture and era). From their perspective, explicit explanations of what lay behind a description of the human body as "sick," "healthy," "beautiful," "ugly," "fat," "thin," or even just "tall" or "short," were unnecessary. These self-evident facts may have been accepted without question and generally known during their specific era and cultural context, but they do pose the occasional problem for us. For instance, we are forced to ask when people of that time considered a/their body to be "healthy" or "sick," and to what extent these classifications affected their behavior.

Against the background of these preliminary remarks, the present article will focus on teasing out the cultural guidelines and patterns that affected behavior in Ancient Near Eastern culture (primarily in the first millennium BCE) with regard to the human body. These implicit bodily concepts and established standards of bodily perception were the primary things that determined body image for men and women, and thus of course also their lives, their identities and their self-image as well as their understanding of illness and health. It should be noted here that "body image is part of a person's identity, and constitutes his entire relationship with his

---

2. See Malina, *Welt*, 23. Similarly, Steger, "Einleitung," 11–14.
3. On this term, see Harris, *Kulturanthropologie*, 21–24.

own body. It also includes the internal representation of a person's own figure, in other words the mental image that a person has of his physical appearance. This 'bodily schema' does not need to be identical with the objective body; rather, it is one's own perception of the body."[4]

The starting point for the following investigation is the physiognomic tradition of the Ancient Near East and the Old Testament. Since this tradition had a strong interest in precisely observing the human body, it represents a rich and definitive source for investigating concepts, perceptions and evaluations of the body as well as its classification of bodies as "healthy" or "sick."

The following investigation is thus based on (1) the "physiognomic omens"[5] of Mesopotamia, which make the human body the starting point and the medium for divinatory practices, and (2) the few Old Testament and apocryphal texts that assume knowledge of physiognomic ideas. The primary focus will be on sources that discuss illness and death. In addition, in terms of bodily malfunctions, we will also look at the inability to conceive or give birth, which—just like an illness—resulted in serious social consequences.

THE ANCIENT NEAR EAST

General Statements about Gods, Illness, and Patient Treatments in Ancient Mesopotamia

When a person in the Ancient Near East was afflicted by an illness, this was generally ascribed to an intervention by a divinity, or by evil demons or spirits of the dead that had infiltrated his body and wanted to drag him away to the underworld.[6] However, the demons and spirits of the dead (also stars and planets[7]) were not self-determined; they acted as executors of

---

4. Quotation translated; German original in Daszkowski, *Körperbild*, 9.

5. These omens were published by Böck, *Morphoskopie* (see also the review by Heeßel, "Review," 575–79; ibid., *Divinatorische Texte*, No. 49–54). A short summary of the physiognomic literature in Mesopotamia is provided by Popovic, *Reading*, 72–85.

6. Cf., e.g., Farber, *Beschwörungsrituale*, 144f.:68–92; 148f.:128–132 (AIIa); Scurlock, *Means*; Scurlock and Anderson, *Diagnoses*, 10–12.

7. On the astral-astrological aspect of the etiology of illness, see Heeßel, "Astrological Medicine."

divine orders.[8] Those who had been struck down by illness,[9] then, had been condemned by the gods, who used this method to punish human failings (intentional or not) as well as negligence (for instance in the cultic care of gods of the upper world and the underworld or familial spirits of the dead). However, divine anger or a destructive judgment could be changed.

There was still the possibility of turning to the gods of the heavens and the underworld[10] as well as the spirits of the dead in the event of a legal dispute, in order to convince them to revise their previous judgment and take back their orders. Specifically, they were asked to render a new judgment for the patient and to call off the demon or spirit who had been sent.[11] Gods and spirits (possibly from one's own family) who had passed a destructive judgment on someone and "set a demon on his heels" could in some cases be satisfied with presents, prayers and the provision of a sacrificial substitute.[12]

Through corresponding rituals and prayers, the sick person could influence the gods and spirits to his benefit, so that they would issue a new verdict for him[13] and so that the "evil" spirits of the dead could be taken back to the underworld and kept safely there:

> "The evil that is in my body, my flesh, my fibers, is given over to Namtaru, the Wazir of the underworld.
>
> May Ningišzida the "seat-bearer" (= minister) of the wide underworld strengthen their (= the demons who bring the evil) guards/prison!

---

8. See, for instance, explicitly Farber, *Beschwörungsrituale*, 146f.:94–103 (AIIa). There are also cases where witchcraft was believed to be responsible for such processes. However, witches and sorcerers could only be effective if they first incited the gods against the patient/their victim and the gods had distanced themselves from the person; see Schwemer, *Rituale*, 1–4; Abusch, *Witchcraft*, 30–48; Heeßel, "Diagnosis," 99.

9. Similar ideas applied to the suffering of a miscarriage or death in childbirth. Here, too, there were often considered to be demons or witches who worked against a person; see, e.g., Schwemer, *Rituale*, No. 41. In these contexts, the "Guideline for the Art of Incantation" (KAR 44 and duplicates) mentions the groups of texts that should be applied to protect pregnant women from premature labor, to ease difficult births and to protect the mother and child from the demoness Lamaštu; see Farber, *Schlaf*, 4; Farber, *Lamaštu*; on the topics of miscarriage and infertility, see Stol and Wiggermann, *Birth*, 27–33, 33–37.

10. Divine pairs of judges are Šamaš and Gilgameš (VAT 8910), Šamaš and Pabilsag (W 22758/2), Ištar and Dumuzi (K 2001+), primordial gods and Sîn (VAT 13653) as well as Aššur and Šamaš (K 1152).

11. See Zgoll, "Toten." These connections were drawn out somewhat unclearly by Frey-Anthes, *Unheilsmächte*, 75–80.

12. E.g., a goat. Cf. Tsukimoto, *Totenpflege*, 125ff, 151ff.

13. See Maul, *Lösung*, 87f.

> May Biti, the senior gatekeeper of the underworld, [lock up] before (or behind) them!
>
> Grip him tightly (= the demon) and take him down to the land from which there is no return!"[14]

Upon instructions from a god, the demons who were in pursuit of human beings could also be given a substitute animal, which was identified through corresponding rituals with the sick person.[15] The substitute animal was then killed and buried according to the rules for human burial, and thus sent to the realm of the dead in place of the sick person.

The *āšipu* and *asû* were responsible for treating the illness,[16] and the treatment could include two phases: the magical/ritual phase and the medical/therapeutic phase.[17] The goal of the first phase was to eliminate the divine/demonic causes of the illness as well as the gods' desire to do harm. Only then could the sick person be successfully freed from his illness and its acute symptoms, through corresponding prescriptions and cures.

Still, these procedures could only be used once the effects of a divine judgment—which was in turn due to a disrupted relationship with the god—were already visible due to the outbreak of an illness and the corresponding diagnoses of symptoms in the body.[18] In addition, however, there were also efforts to recognize threatened illnesses and thus divine determinations even before any symptoms presented themselves. Like the question of whether a man would ever sire children (especially sons) or a woman would ever bear children (especially sons), this was less a matter of medical diagnostics than a form of divining the future that used a wide range of practices in addition to physiognomics.[19]

---

14. E.g., Tsukimoto, *Totenpflege*, 161ff. (VAT 8910:9–13 and duplicates); Scurlock, *Means*, 351ff., No. 85. Similarly, Farber, *Beschwörungsrituale*, 150f.:140–48 (AIIa).

15. E.g., Tsukimoto, *Totenpflege*, 133.

16. As an introduction, see Scurlock and Anderson, *Diagnoses*, 8–10.

17. Maul, "Lösung," 79–90. The fundamental necessity of combining both treatment phases in each case is disputed by Schwemer, *Rituale*, 4. In his opinion, invocation rituals and medicines have an "initially complementary effect, depending on the diagnosis" (ibid.), and one form of treatment alone can also suffice.

18. Worth mentioning here is the series on symptoms of illness, SA.GIG, *sakikkû* or *enūma ana bīt marṣi āšipu illaku* (= "When the exorcist visits the home of a sick person"). On the topic of diagnoses and prognoses in Mesopotamian medicine, see also Scurlock and Anderson, *Diagnoses*, as well as the articles in Finkel and Geller, *Disease*. On the ideas that were behind diagnoses and divination, see Heeßel, "Diagnosis," 99ff.

19. By no means are only physiognomic omens used to divine the future of an illness or a birth; see, e.g., Heeßel, *Divinatorische Texte*, p. 30f.:Rs. 5; 35/38:Rs. IV 3; 35/39:Rs. IV 15.23f.; 36/39:Rs. V 9 (*šumma ālu*); Heeßel, "Diagnosis," 100; Maul, *Omina*, 45–88.

The Mesopotamian Physiognomic Omens

The oldest examples of physiognomic omens come from the early second millennium BCE. The material for the present series was (re-)organized and summarized in the late second millennium BCE, with 27 tablets and the title Šumma alamdimmû (= "if the distinctive form").[20]

These omens begin—in keeping with the conventions for omen texts—with a conditional phrase (šumma "if..."). In this protasis, the signs that can be recognized in the body are clearly formulated. This is followed by the apodosis, which includes an interpretation of the diagnosed signs. As typical examples, here are the first two lines of the series šumma alamdimmû, tablet II:[21]

> 1. "If a man's cowlick is turned to the right, then his days will be short." (i.e. he will live to be 50)
>
> 2. "If a man's cowlick is turned to the left, then his days will be long." (i.e. he will live to be 70)

Today, the relationship between the protasis and the apodosis is often difficult for us to see right away. In some cases, it seems to be defined by the principles of analogy, association or inversion.[22] In addition, the protasis can also compare a characteristic or part of the human body with an animal. In these cases, the apodosis seems to include a characteristic of the compared animal that is culturally seen as "typical," and transfers it to the person. In addition, generalizations play a large role. This is particularly the case when physical signs of affects (such as joy, sorrow or anger) are not seen as temporary, but as an outward sign of the person's ongoing disposition.[23]

The tablets are gender-specific, dealing separately with the bodies of men and women. In the main series šumma alamdimmû and the sub-series šumma liptu, the body is systematically checked from top to bottom. Certain signs in the body, but by no means all, are classified by the exorcist as being relevant for the prognosis. These can be interpreted in two ways: first, the signs allow conclusions to be drawn about the person's character, habits or behavior; second, they provide information about the person's future and the course of his or her life. In addition, the prognoses for illnesses, fertility and birthing conditions as well as types of death play a large role here.

---

20. On the details of the historical tradition, see Heeßel, *Divinatorische Texte*, 9f.; Heeßel, "Neues."

21. Böck, *Morphoskopie*, 72–73.

22. Ibid., 38–40.

23. Ibid., 114–15:102.

When it comes to questions about patterns of bodily concepts and bodily perceptions, the *protases* of the omens are particularly informative, since they include a clearly systematized and detailed display of the body. The *apodoses*, on the other hand, feature a wide range of topics that were considered useful knowledge about a person. There is a great deal of material here about which implicit values and maxims determined the thoughts and actions of people in the Ancient Near East.[24] The most common topics, which will be developed as dichotomies, are the hope for a long life, joy, profit, success, dignity, wealth, satisfaction and health—contrasted with the fear of a short life, grief, loss, failure, indignity, poverty, dissatisfaction and illness. The goal was to learn more about one's future good or bad reputation, future children or childlessness, and the intact nature or disruption of one's relationship with the gods.

The apodoses of the omens reflect the individual Mesopotamian life experience, but also the supra-individually established orientations and expectations that shaped the lives of the men and women of the time. In addition, it is easy to see which threats the individual saw in his/her life: "evil" spirits of the dead (see above), angry gods, various illnesses, premature forms of death (for men: accidents, murder, execution, animal bites, war, starvation) and childlessness. However, the loss of life and limb were not the only problem; other concerns were the loss of name, honor, reputation, happiness, satisfaction, possessions, family, home or the favor of the king. With regard to fellow human beings, people feared not only assaults on their own bodies and possessions, but also envy and defamation.

The apodoses of the physiognomic omens are based on *deterministic ideas* and can thus be seen as providing information about character-related conditions or future developments in the life of the person being examined—things *that cannot be changed*. The skilled exorcist can recognize and interpret the signs so that the examinee or the person ordering the examination will understand later what sort of character is involved and what can be expected. In this way, a kind of personal and life profile is created that includes the person's future destiny as well as future illnesses, offspring and the manner of death.

There are no means available within physiognomics to influence the statements about future disasters in such a way that they will *not* occur. However, the Mesopotamian cult and ritual structure does offer helpful tools for the worst disasters that are predicted in advance,[25] which could be

---

24. As in ibid., 3. See also Guinan, "Behavioral Omens," 11; Kraus,"Sittenkanon," 82; Oppenheim,"Omenliteratur," 202.

25. See Guinan, "Head," 18–19; Maul, "Babylonians," 123–29; see also the connection between physiognomic omens and medical therapeutic prescriptions in Heeßel,

used in an attempt to counteract them. The situation is somewhat different for characteristics that have been diagnosed in a person. Here, there does not seem to have been any option to interfere by way of a ritual or the like. This is precisely why we must assume that physiognomics played an important role in helping to determine character and human understanding, and that its findings were highly relevant in shaping human interactions.

The tablets for the physiognomic omens are separated by gender. Thus there are some tablets that deal exclusively with male or female bodies. This alone shows that the texts are based on the construct of gender difference rather than the construct of gender equality. The apodoses are particularly informative when it comes to defining the content of this gender-specific construct. In the interpretations of bodily signs that are given for men or women as a gender group, parameters are established: where the apodoses make predictions for the future, the gender-differentiated omens define the gender-differentiated actions and expectations, in that a man's or woman's life can be classified as compliant with the system and thus "successful" and "accomplished" (or not, as the case may be). On the other hand, if bodily signs are interpreted in relation to the existence of certain character traits, then gender-specific character stereotypes are also applied and stabilized. Implicit ideas about the (gender-differentiated) ideal way of life for a man's or woman's (equally gender-differentiated) ideal character can be seen in the apodoses.

Most of the physiognomic omens are dedicated to the male body. Generally, it is assumed that these omens were used for filling jobs and granting promotions at court.[26] The group of omens dedicated to the female body is much smaller. For the most part, their main use seems to have been in searching for a bride. What all of these areas of application have in common is that physiognomics were used to promote human understanding, and were also intended to say something about a person's future and impact on his or her surroundings. The goal was to avoid bringing a disruptive factor into one's house or the court—in the form of a new family member or court administrator—if at all possible. Instead, one wanted to find people who would stabilize the existing social system. Fundamentally, of course, it cannot be ruled out that a person might have asked for an individual examination in order to learn more about his future life. Perhaps concerned (upper-class) parents also presented their children to the priests for a diagnosis.

Choosing a partner, filling open jobs and other personnel issues were the main areas of application for physiognomics, and not just during the

---

"Warzen" (BM 108872+).

26. For instance in Böck, *Morphoskopie*, 55–59.

pre-Christian era. Physiognomic texts from Qumran,[27] classical antiquity,[28] the Talmudic[29] and later epochs[30] all demonstrate that people of various eras wanted to improve their understanding of the human condition using physiognomics, and to protect themselves against unwelcome surprises from the people around them.

Bodily Concept and Bodily Perception in the Physiognomic Omens

The human body as a medium for divining the future leads us to a field that cannot always be clearly differentiated from physiognomics. Particularly when it comes to recognizing signs of future illnesses, birthing difficulties or infertility, there is a certain proximity to medicine,[31] since medical diagnosticians analyze, interpret and make predictions using physical signs as indicators of latent or emerging ailments. For physiognomicians, however, physical ailments and childlessness were written on a person's body right from the start; so they examined the body not for signs of existing illnesses (medical connections between protasis and apodosis are rarely even hinted at), but for what had already been programmed as its future life:

> "If he has sparse/disorderly hair on his head, his days are short, he will be infected."[32]

Since the activities of a physician (see above) as well as those of a physiognomician fell within the same area of responsibility—that of the *āšipu* ("exorcist/incantation priest")—this person could ultimately use whatever he deemed appropriate according to the time, case and diagnosis.

27. See also Berlejung, "Physiognomik," 20ff., and recently Popovic, *Reading*, 17–67.237–239; idem., "Reading the Human Body and Writing in Code," 271ff.

28. See, for instance Förster, *Scriptores Physiognomonici*; Degkwitz, *'Physiognomonica'*; Barton, *Power*, 95–131; Sassi, *Science*, 34–81.

29. Scholem, "Fragment," 175–93. On the Hebrew text, see Scholem, "הכרת פנים," 459–95; also Grünwald, "Fragments," 306–19; Schäfer, *Geniza-Fragmente*, No. 12. See also Greenfield and Sokoloff, "Omen Texts," 201–214. Also interesting are the physiognomics of Bar Hebraeus from the thirteenth century A.D.; see Furlani, "Physiognomik," 1–16, reprinted in Wallis Budge, *Stories*, 177–85.

30. Lavater, *Fragmente*. For an analysis of this work, see i.a. also Pestalozzi and Weigelt, *Antlitz*; Percival and Tytler, *Physiognomy*.

31. For instance in Böck, *Morphoskopie*, 83:114. The close relationship between physiognomics and medicine holds true in later epochs as well; see, e.g., Barton, *Power*, 133–68; Gerabek, "Physiognomik," 1157–58; Müller-Jahncke, "Signaturenlehre," 1330–31.

32. Böck, *Morphoskopie*, 78–79:80.

The basis of physiognomics is the conviction (which applies to divination as a whole) that experts are able to recognize signs, and that these have a direct meaning and a clear cause. Within physiognomics, a sign can have two possible causes: first, the bodily sign can arise because the person's inner character has brought forth an external sign on his or her body, which then indicates the character. Another possibility is for a divinity to mark the determination of fate on a person's body so that the bodily sign contains and permits a future prognosis for that person. Both models for explaining the causes of a sign are closely related to the basic principles of physiognomics—the abovementioned determinism and the conviction that the person's external appearance corresponds to his or her internal state. The physiognomy expert (as part of the profession of the *āšipu*) can thus draw conclusions about a person's fate, as well as his or her innermost being and character, based on external signs on the body. Thus, in Ancient Near Eastern anthropology, the gods were believed to care about the life path of each individual person and to inscribe this on the person's body. In addition, the person is considered to be a psychosomatic unit in which physicality, emotionality, character, reason, internal and external being all belong together.[33] Human beings "do not *have* bodies, they *are* bodies."[34] Based on this concept, which is also familiar in the Old Testament, it follows that any damage or limitation of the body (illness, handicap, injury, inability to give birth or conceive a child) represents a damage or limitation of the person and his or her vitality.

With regard to the perception of the human body, the protases of the physiognomic omens indicate the cultural guidelines that determined what was to be perceived in a human body (selection), and how (categorization).

In the omens, the human body is generally described from top to bottom. An internal bodily hierarchy can be observed, which ascribed particular value to the head and the front of the body. For physiognomicians, physical peculiarities were of especial interest, since only the deviations from the average, regular body and the presence of skin markings needed to (or could) be interpreted, and were included in the interpretation.[35] However, what was considered "average" was a cultural and time-dependent measure that is nearly impossible for us to understand with any precision

---

33. As already stated in Asher-Greve, "Body," 8–37.

34. Translated ccording to the German original in Frevel and Wischmeyer, *Menschsein*, 27.

35. Regularity, perfect physical shape, even rows of teeth and an absence of marks on the body were required if a person wanted to enter into cultic service; see Borger, "Weihe," 163–76; Lambert, "Qualifications," 149:30–35; van der Toorn, *Sin*, 29–33; see also Lev 21:20.

today, and thus we cannot implement it in a model of the "normal" standard human body.

The ideal of feminine beauty, as far as can be determined from the physiognomic omens,[36] simply shows in a very basic sense that fat arms,[37] very large breasts,[38] long hands, toes and genitals,[39] a very fat bottom,[40] very thick labia and large calves[41] were valued, although "fat," "long" and "large" were very different from our current parameters in some cases. Other rules applied for men, even if a belly[42] and a plump chin[43] were fundamentally desired, since for them the important thing was not just these outward signs of being well-fed and wealthy, but also and primarily the thickness of their hair. A thick head of hair and a red and/or long face,[44] red hair,[45] shaggy hair on the cheeks,[46] and an extraordinarily large upper cheek area[47] were among the external bodily signs that produced a positive interpretation. A "fullness" in the body correlated to a certain extent with a person's "fullness of vitality." This also corresponds to the positive role that the color red plays in the context of physiognomics, showing that colors also had certain values for the body. Red was considered to be a sign of vitality and strength, so it is not surprising that omens diagnosing this color in the body or as a hair color in the protasis also have a positive apodosis.[48] One exception to this are red marks on the skin or swellings, which could have a medical/diagnostic cause. In addition, skin markings were not necessarily negative; it simply depended where they were located and what they looked like. For instance, it was considered to be a good sign if a man had an *umṣatu* mole on the right side.[49]

---

36. In summary, see Berlejung, "Frau," 59.
37. Böck, *Morphoskopie*, 156f.:88, 92, 94, 97.
38. Ibid., 160–61:156.
39. Ibid., 156–57:102; 167:233; 164–65:201.
40. Ibid., 164–65:205.
41. Ibid., 165:208, 210.
42. Ibid., 120–21:47.
43. Ibid., 106–7:8.
44. Ibid., 78–79:73.75; 108–9:2; 114–15:93.
45. Ibid., 80–90:95.
46. Ibid., 104–5:61.
47. Ibid., 104–5:88.
48. Böck, *Morphoskopie*, 76–77:55, 65; 78–79:75; 80–81:87, 89, 95; 85:140; 110–11:61; 114–15:93; 168–69:248; 265:23; 280–81:3–4; 312–13:34, 40, 44. Exceptions: ibid., 112–13:85; 114–15:101; 162–63:185.
49. Böck, *Morphoskopie*, 114–15:111.

The following context is also relevant for the perception of the body: the individual male and female body parts were associated with the answers to various questions. In the female body, for instance, the breasts, navel and labia were said to provide information about whether the woman was fertile and would give birth. In the male body, the chest and navel[50] only provided information about comparable issues if there were moles in these areas (see 2.4.). Here, it was primarily the penis that was said to provide information about the man's ability to procreate, and whether he would sire male or female children.[51]

Bodily perception is determined through the physiognomic omens (as in other forms of divination) by using the principle of binarism.[52] The examined bodies are classified and described using the categories of top-bottom, front-back, right-left. This information was also associated with value judgments, since "right" was considered positive, as the *pars familiaris*, and "left" had a negative connotation, as the *pars hostilis*.[53] Binary classifications also played an important role with regard to light-dark as well as bright-gloomy. In particular, a person's face and eyes, if they were considered to be shining brightly, were seen as a sign that the person was to be judged positively. A figure of light could not be expected to have dark thoughts! Instead, according to the physiognomic line of thought, these were ascribed to people whose body, face or eyes were perceived as being "gloomy."

Finally, the forehead should be mentioned separately, since the Mesopotamian physiognomicians considered it to be a key body part. They could use it to identify symbolic signs (usually cuneiform characters—protasis), which provided information about a wide range of topics relating to the character, life path and illnesses of the examinee (apodosis):[54]

> "If the EN or RI or HU character is drawn there, the man will be epileptic . . .
>
> If the UR or IB character is drawn, ditto."[55]

The forehead was also an essential body part in the Old and New Testament (Exod 13:9, 16; 28:38; Deut 6:8; 11:18; Ezek 9:4.6; Rev 7:3; 9:4), so it could

---

50. The navel provided information about the person's general condition, health/illness, satisfaction/dissatisfaction, worries, wealth or power; see Böck, *Morphoskopie*, 120f.:50–58.
51. Böck, *Morphoskopie*, 122f.:84–88; 124f.:89.
52. On the binary structure of divination, see Guinan, "Perils," 229ff.
53. See Guinan, "Symbolism," 5–10; Starr, Rituals, 15–24.
54. Böck, *Morphoskopie*, 92:76–96f.:133.
55. Ibid., 94f.:86f.

be marked with signs. In this context, however, the signs were not given to people at birth, but were written on the fateful spot later.

Gender-differentiated Images of Illness and the Body in the Physiognomic Omens

The best thing that a man or woman could hope for in life, and part of leading a successful, ideal life, was a long healthy life with economic security, social status, blessed harmony with the gods,[56] and a stable, lasting and child-filled marriage with the prospect of a prosperous estate. The counterpart to all these hopes, in turn, was one's worst fear. Each person's life line was drawn between these two extreme poles, and could be traced according to the bodily omens. Illness, premature (= early) death and childlessness limited the fullness of the life that the gods had intended for people, and attempts were made to seek out their causes and eliminate them where possible.

Within the physiognomic omens, the cause of an illness like childlessness was not interesting in and of itself. The goal was simply to determine *whether* the examined human body displayed a certain sign, which was then to be interpreted according to the specialized literature or tradition such that the examinee's childlessness or illness or early death was foretold as part of his or her destiny. This implicitly assumes the abovementioned idea that the gods had made decisions about the person's life and inscribed these on his or her body in the form of signs. Thus the individual person's future could be divined based on his or her body; future employers or spouses could then respond accordingly, and turn to the experts for help (see above).

The following compilation mainly includes the omens whose apodosis deals with illness, premature death, difficulties in giving birth and in conceiving; since the tablets are separated by gender, it makes sense to look at them in a gender-differentiated way.[57] Once again, it should be noted that, other than a few exceptions, the omens that predict illness in the apodosis do not list any physical signs in the protasis that would suggest a medical diagnostic cause. There are hardly any symptom-related connections between bodily signs (protasis) and illness (apodosis) in this corpus.

---

56. With regard to the man: Böck, *Morphoskopie*, 78f.:73, 75; 80f.:95; 86f.:146f. With regard to the woman: Böck, *Morphoskopie*, 156f.:82f, 85f., 88, 92, 94, 97, 102; 158f.:142f. passim.

57. The following overview is based on the edition on the omens by Böck, *Morphoskopie*. For a detailed description and interpretation of the omens for women, see Berlejung, "Frau," 32–38, 42ff.

General Life Expectancy and Manner of Death

Life expectancy is often projected for men and women in the omens, generally by stating that they will have a "long" or "short" life. For men, this information can even be provided in absolute numbers, with specific months or years of life.[58] The differences between the men's and women's tablets are especially noticeable when it comes to the types of death, which are largely differentiated by gender. According to the tablets, women generally die in childbirth or of pregnancy complications and within the domestic context, which represents the framework for their lives.[59] For men, on the other hand, the apodoses of the omens describe many types of death that predict an early, unnatural demise outside the house. For instance, death can occur through a spell,[60] murder[61] or execution.[62] This finding can be explained by the fact that in Ancient Near Eastern society, men were the ones who represented the family in the outside world, and were subject to different dangers than women due to their professional lives and military service. Thus men are much more likely than women to experience situations of conflict and competition,[63] which can have a fatal outcome. This differentiation between their everyday lives is reflected by the possible manner of death and the omens.

Illnesses

In addition to many other questions, the physiognomic omens were meant to provide information about whether the man or woman being examined would become sick; some apodoses actually name the specific illness and/or its outcome. As stated earlier, the abovementioned bodily signs are rarely connected with the medically relevant symptoms of a potentially latent or even existing illness. Another fundamental problem here, of course, is that the Akkadian description of an illness does not always correlate clearly with the terminology of modern medicine. In addition, many of the apodoses

---

58. Böck, *Morphoskopie*, 84f.:126, 129–131; 92f.:56, 58.

59. See also Fischer, "Ist der Tod nicht für alle gleich?"

60. Death through a spell: Böck, *Morphoskopie*, 114f.:96f.; 188f.:72. On spell-related illness, see Maul, "Lösung."

61. Böck, *Morphoskopie*, 294f.:80, 90; 142f.:193; 92f.:59; 94f.:89; 206f.:36.

62. Ibid., 94f.:117; 308f.:12.

63. See Neumann, "Kultur und Mentalität," 36f.

remain fairly general and simply predict "illness"[64] or "health."[65] For mental illness, there is also the problem that the boundaries between character traits and diagnoses are largely dependent on cultural norms and perspectives. For instance, it is impossible to determine the extent to which a prediction that a person (male or female) will experience worry, affliction, misery, grief, unease and dissatisfaction[66] can be interpreted as meaning "depression" in the sense of an illness. Even if the omen's apodoses emphasize that this emotional state is common or constant within the person, that by no means indicates a concrete illness. A person who constantly laments and complains, for instance, can also simply be a "whiner" who makes life difficult for those around him. Based on the physiognomic omens, it can be seen clearly that each case is less about the individual's condition and personal suffering than it is about evaluating the person's social acceptability.

In comparing the illness-related apodoses in the omens for men and women, it is abundantly clear that illnesses take up very little space in the women's omens.[67] No specific illnesses are named, and only in one case is a demon attack mentioned. Only the following omens are worth mentioning:

> "If they (a woman's hands) are narrow, she will struggle (*muš-tam-ri-[ṣ]a-at*) (poss. in relation to birth?)"[68]; "If it (a woman's breast) is hard and swollen, then she is sick[ly]"[69]; "If they (a woman's toes) are separated, she will be seized by the *alû* demon;[70] she will have no friend or helper"[71]; "[If a *kittabru* mole] is located on the front between her arms, right and [left], she will expe[rien]ce a severe illness."[72]

The illnesses described in the omens' apodoses for men are very different. Here it is noteworthy that very specific illnesses are named. Specifically,

---

64. Mann: ibid., 198f.:72f; 276f.:11; 309:15 (TBP 32).

65. Mann: ibid., *Morphoskopie*, 84f.:124, similar ibid., 96f.:127; 104f:63; 290f.:13.

66. With regard to the man: ibid., 108f.:4; 146f.:7; 174f.:16; 198f.:59f.; 206f.:46; 212f.:1f.; 220f.:70. With regard to the woman: ibid., 156f.:107, 112; 158f.:118; 164f.:199f; 166f.:215.217; 230f.:14, 20–22; 232f.:25, 30, 36.

67. Similar findings arise from the series of medical diagnostic texts; see Heeßel, *Unterschied*, 17–23.

68. See Böck, *Morphoskopie*, 156f:101; similar ibid., 158f.:132; 250f.:11. In my opinion, there is no support for the very tendentious translation by Böck, "hypochondriac."

69. Ibid., 160f.:146.

70. The reading is unclear.

71. Ibid., 168f.:244.

72. Ibid., 232f.:33.

these involve the following omens; the last two (twitching) could also refer to a symptom-related diagnosis of an incipient illness:

> "If the hair on his forehead grows downward to the *abbuttu* headdress, he has a rash (skin illness) (*rišûtu*)"[73]; "If a *kittabru* mole is found on his top and bottom lips, he will suffer paralysis of the mouth (KA.DIB.BI.DA)"[74]; "If the Ú sign is drawn (on his forehead), he will [die] of *ašû* illness"[75]; "If the GÌR, UG, PAN/ AS or GIM sign is drawn (on his forehead), the man will die from *rībtu* illness"[76]; "If the NA/BA or MA sign is drawn (on his forehead), the ma[n's] family will [suffer] from *li'bu* illness / alternative: the man will suffer from *li'bu* illness"[77]; "[I]f the man has an *umṣatu*-mole on the right side of his head, he will face worry, sickness and *di'u* illness / alternative: he will be robbed of his manhood (*dūtu*)"[78]; "If he has scorpion feet, . . . he will die of dropsy . . ."[79]; "If he looks at the ground while walking, his days will be long, he will become blind (?)"[80]; "If a muscle in his anus twitches, then he will suffer anal illness"[81]; "if the vein in the ball of his right foot twitches, he will contract *sagallu* illness (= a severe leg illness)."[82]

In addition to the more general predictions of future illness or sickliness,[83] there are also specific threats of demon attacks:

73. Ibid., 82f.:114.
74. Ibid., 216f.:31.
75. Ibid., 94f.:105.
76. Ibid., 96f.:126.
77. Ibid., 96f.:132.
78. Ibid., 184f.:1.
79. Ibid., 266f.:31; similar, ibid. l. 32.
80. Ibid., 274f.:118 similar, ibid., 276f.:16.
81. Ibid., 266f.:25.
82. Ibid., 270f.:65.

83. Ibid.: "If the hair on his head is sparse, his days will be short, he will become infected" (78f.:80); "If his right temple is slack, he will [be gripped by / experience] a serious illness]" (92f.:66 similar, ibid., 214f.:18; 220f.:75); "If the BE character is shown (on his forehead), the man will experience illnessess" (94f.:120, similar ibid., 121:59; 174f.:24); "If his jaws are loose and his face has yellow [dots, he will die in the prime of life]" (102f.:44); "If his navel has collapsed, he is sick[ly]" (120f.:53, similar ibid., 311:11); "If his body is constantly brimming with strength, he will be gripped by a serious illness" (137:91); "If they (*umṣatu*-moles) cover his ankles, he will be confin[ed to bed]" (192f.:146 similar 266f.:26); "If a *umṣatu*-mole is located in the middle of his penis, death and illness will grip him, death . . ." (298f.:52).

"If it (the *umṣatu*-mole) is on the back *dito* (= right side) of his head, then the Saghulhaza demon will defeat him and make him die"[84]; "If the SAG sign, then a dead person (= the spirit of the dead) will seize him."[85]

The above mentioned reservation applies to the man's mental illnesses. The following omen could potentially be related to depression:

"[If] they (*umṣatu*-moles) spread on the back of his head, then misery (*ašuštu*) over himself will constantly seize him."[86]

Male Ability to Procreate and Female Fertility

A person's reproductive capability was and still is very significant for maintaining and perpetuating the social system. Thus it is not surprising that the omens were used in an attempt to gain clarity early on about whether the examinee would fulfill his or her duties in this regard. Fundamentally, the goal was to determine whether the examinee would be able to conceive a child[87] and/or give birth. Within the patrilinear society, it was very important to know whether the man would sire an heir to continue the family line and name. Omens for women that discuss the future existence of an heir have not been found in the corpus thus far. The answer to this question was expected to be provided by the man's body. Overall, the sex of the child was clearly ascribed to the man, whose body was already said to provide details about his future offspring. Answers to the basic question about bearing an heir and children in general were sought in signs that could be read from the man's head, face, hair, penis, veins, fingers, and feet. Other interpretable signs included moles on the cheek, penis, chest, navel, lower body or entire body. The corresponding apodoses stated:

"He will have many sons"[88]; "he will not have a son"[89]; "he will have a daughter"[90]; "he will have a legitimate heir (*ap-lum*

---

84. Ibid., 184f.:7.
85. Ibid., 294f.:75.
86. Ibid., 184f.:10; similar, ibid., 186f.:51.
87. Ibid., 160f.:158–162; 162f.:170; 163:187; 164f.:191.193–96.
88. Ibid., 76f.:62; 86f.:152; 122f.:77; 137:89; 175:31.
89. Ibid., 278f.:13.
90. Ibid., 196:30.

ki-nu)"[91]; "he will not have an heir"[92]; "this man will sire men"[93]; "he will sire a full heir"[94]; "this man will sire women / alternative: his wife will bear women"[95]; "he will have sons and daughters"[96]; "he will have neither sons nor daughters"[97]; "his wife will bear sons and he will not send her away."[98]

Pregnancy and Birth

Naturally, this is a female-specific topic that is largely (with one exception[99]) missing in the apodoses for male omens. In the apodoses for female omens, prognoses regarding the course of pregnancy and birth for the examinee play a central role. The ideal was to learn that the woman would have unproblematic pregnancies and births. Miscarriages and complications during birth were feared. The woman's belly, breast, nipples, navel and labia were the locations for clear signs that would answer these questions:

> "If she holds her belly, she will not be one of those with an easy [bir]th"[100]; "If a woman's breast looks like that of Belet-ili/balaṭi, she will become pregnant and have a miscarriage; her breasts are the food of the god"[101]; "If a woman's nipples are white/yellow, she will (not) terminate a pregnancy"[102]; "If a woman's nipples are black/dark, she will not terminate the pregnancy"[103]; "If they (the nipples) are small, she will not terminate the pregnancy"[104] "If a woman's navel is hard, she will have a difficult birth"[105]; "If

---

91. Ibid., 270f.:68, similar, ibid., 286f.:24.
92. Ibid., 108f.:6 (tablet VIII).
93. Ibid., 122:84f.; 124f.:89.
94. Ibid., 266f.:31.
95. Ibid., 123:86.
96. Ibid., 220f.:67; 221:78; 222f.:85.87.
97. Ibid., 228f.:131.
98. Ibid., 176f.:50.
99. Ibid., 94f.:97.
100. Ibid., 156f.:104.
101. Ibid., 160f.:162ab.
102. Ibid., 161:163f.
103. Ibid., 161:165f.
104. Ibid., 162f.:168. See further ibid., l. 169.
105. Ibid., 163:188. Similar, ibid., l. 190.

it (a woman's navel) is soft, she will terminate the pregnancy"[106];
"If they (the labia) are narrow, she will have a difficult birth."[107]

Family Destiny and Family Illness

The apodoses for male omens are not just focused on the man's own fate. The body of the head of the family also contains signs that provide information about the life expectancy, activities and fortunes of his heir (specifically named), his other sons and his daughters (including adopted children). This topic does not appear in the female omens. The body of the father/head of the family was expected to provide information about the children's future and their health. The mother's body did not play any role in this context. This is certainly related to the patrilinear and patriarchal structure of the Ancient Near Eastern family, which physiognomicians considered to be written on the man's body and inscribed in the person's nature. The body of the male head of household not only bore the signs of his own fate, but also indicated everything that affected his offspring, his father, his brothers, his wife and his slaves. Consequently, the signs of future illness in the family were expected to be found on the man's body (and not on the body of the future patient). The entire family's life and future, including those of its dependents, were written on the body of the man of the house.

In summary, with regard to the bodily images and images of illness within the physiognomic tradition of omens, it can be said that the category of "gender" played a very important role in these, since the bodies in the male and female gender groups were investigated separately, and since the interpretations of the apodoses differed significantly from one another, at least to some extent based on gender. The examinee's illness or state of health and his or her capacity to reproduce played an important, but by no means exclusive role.

Certain questions were only associated with male bodies (information about male honor or dignity, social status, name, career, results during conflicts [e.g., rebellions] or competitive situations [e.g., legal proceedings], the maintenance and fate of the household, the gender of the children, the existence of an heir, the fate of the family, staff and offspring as well as any adopted children), while others were only associated with female bodies.[108] For women, the omens were primarily intended to determine their chaste-

---

106. Ibid., 163:189. See also ibid., 164f.:192.196a; 166f.:222.
107. Ibid., 165:209.
108. See Berlejung, "Frau," 42–50, 52–55.

ness, fertility, childbearing ability, reticence, careful budgeting, obedience, dutifulness and influence on their husband and in-laws. Thus in physiognomics, signs were written on the male body that were relevant and informative for the future life of a man, while the signs written on the female body offered prognoses for a "typical female" biography associated with the roles of wife and mother. Thus physiognomics had a stake in reinforcing the dichotomy of maleness and femaleness, along with their idealizations and established system-appropriate role distributions, as being natural and "written on the body" according to the gods' instructions. From these texts, it is easy to see how social conventions can take on the character of quasi "natural categories."[109] In the omens, the human body—within which, with which and through which lifelong socialization takes place—becomes a medium for social control and for stabilizing the existing orders and hierarchies.[110]

With regard to the image of illness in physiognomic tradition, the omens have an extraordinary interest in possible male illnesses, which are very clearly differentiated. The omens for women leave little space for this topic, and hardly go beyond general determinations such as "sick" or "sickly." On the other hand, the female omens are much more numerous and detailed when it comes to fertility, the progress of pregnancy and childbearing capacity. Thus an analysis of the illnesses and clinical patterns in the physiognomic omens necessarily creates the impression that the goal was more to evaluate whether a person would fulfill his or her specific gender-related roles within society and his or her environment in a successful, socially acceptable way, rather than to prevent personal suffering. In addition, it seems as though general medical terms were used in examinations of the male body, while examinations of women mainly analyzed gynecological aspects. Women's bodies were also expected to show general indications of their state of illness or health, but here the main goal was to predict reproductive capability. Furthermore, signs of a woman's future illness or early death could be inscribed on her husband's body, since the bodily signs of the head of the family could also include illnesses and early deaths of his family members. In addition, the omens by no means described all of the illnesses that faced people of this era.

From the above, it can be seen that sickness and health, the ability to conceive and bear children, and the body image of men and women were integrated into an interactive network of relationships within the

---

109. On this, see Bourdieu, *Herrschaft*, 19ff.

110. See also Müller, "Natur," 52–59; Guinan, "Constructions," 61–68; Guinan, "Auguries," 38–55; Synnott, *Body*, 262ff.; Freund, "Society," 148ff.

physiognomic omens, which incorporated and perpetuated the cultural guidelines of their time. Thus it is not surprising that the interpretation of omens was relevant to the behavior of all the participants, and that future relationships (whether in marriages or employment situations) were shaped accordingly, or in some cases not entered into at all.

OLD TESTAMENT AND APOCRYPHA

Yahweh, Illness, and the Treatment of Patients in the Old Testament and the Apocrypha

The Old Testament's position on illness and the treatment of patients must be seen within the context of the worldview and constructs of illness in the Ancient Near East. In the Biblical texts, religious, social and biological aspects are more important than medical details. Illness is seen as a "disruption of the God-given integrity of human life and a disruption of the God-given, inherently good order."[111] It is a limitation of human vitality, a state of powerlessness and weakness, that leads toward death and can be interpreted as distance from God (cf. Ps 88 and Lamentations). At the same time, however, it isolates the patient from his social partners and thus disrupts or destroys relationships.

As in the Mesopotamian context (see above), illness is associated with God's actions, which are intended to punish people through illness for their failings, often described as "sin" (e.g., Pss 38:5–9; 41:5; Job 4:7–9; 1 Kgs 17:17f.; Isa 53:3–5). It was also possible to ascribe the illness to a personified evil power[112] (see the evil spirit in 1 Sam 16:14ff.; Satan in Job 2:5–7), which could, however, only affect a person if Yahweh had withdrawn his protective presence, thus giving his permission for the illness to set in. In this context, the illness can also (assuming the connection between action and condition) be seen as a pedagogical tool that God uses to temporarily punish individuals (Ps 32:10; 2 Chr 21:15–20; Num 12:10) or the people as a whole (see plagues and childlessness: Exod 23:25f.; plagues: Lev 26:25; Num 14:12; Deut 28:21f., 27–29; 1 Kgs 8:37) for their failings. Its outbreak is the expression of a disrupted relationship between God and man. At the same time, the illness has a social dimension, since the interaction of a sick person with his or her environment (and vice versa) is different than that of a healthy person. Isolation is often associated with illness. On occasion, there

---

111. Frevel, "Krankheit/Heilung," 284.

112. On the problem of illness-bringing demons in the Old Testament, see Frey-Anthes, *Unheilsmächte*, 81–102.

is also mention of the "social death" of the patient, who is considered dead to his fellow man while he is still living (Ps 38:12; 88:9, 19; Job 2).[113] The Old Testament frequently emphasizes the fact that the patient suffers due to the changed behavior of his environment and its self-imposed distance from him. Physical suffering is often so closely associated with emotional suffering that the illness and its social consequences blend into one another.

From the priestly point of view, illness can be associated with impurity and thus cultic prohibitions: Lev 13f. lists a broad spectrum of skin anomalies (not leprosy!) that have cultic consequences. In these contexts, the diagnosis of existing symptoms is logically made by the priests. Very little is known about the existence of the medical profession. Healers could be prophets (Is 38:1; 2 Kgs 1; 2 Kgs 4f.; 20:1–11 et al.), but also wise men and women as well as midwives. However, since the cause of the illness was primarily located in a disrupted relationship with God, the patient was primarily interested in turning to Yahweh through prayer, lamentation and sacrifice in order to heal the illness. Theologically speaking, this can be taken further in the Old Testament to mean that only Yahweh was to be addressed as a healer and physician (Num 12:13; Hos 5:13; 1 Sam 6; Ps 103:3; 147:3; Job 5:18; especially Exod 15:26, "I am the Lord who heals you," also seen in Is 30:26; Jer 33:6; Hos 6:1), so that a competition arises between Yahweh's healing abilities and those of medical specialists (2 Chr 16:12).[114]

Like illness, childlessness was also considered a form of divine punishment (Gen 16:2; 20:18; 30:2; Exod 23:26; 2 Sam 6:23). Since infertility was generally seen as a female problem (Gen 11:30; 25:21; 29:31; 1 Sam 1:5–6 et al.), it was the woman from whom Yahweh withdrew his blessing in this way, and who then had to try to change God's mind in her favor (1 Sam 1:9ff.; intercession by the man: Gen 25:21). Difficulties in childbirth were known and feared as a possible cause of death for both mother and child, although one could ask Yahweh in advance whether the pregnancy and birth would go well (Gen 25:21–26).[115] Childlessness harmed not only a wife's social status within her family (1 Sam 1:5f.), but also her relationship with her husband, who according to the polygamous system described in the narrative texts of the Old Testament was permitted to take another wife who could bear him children.

The Old Testament texts generally focus on illness and childlessness as the consequence of a disrupted relationship with God, and offer possible

---

113. On this topic, see Hasenfratz, *Toten*, 87–88.

114. See Frevel, "Krankheit/Heilung," 286. On the topic of illness, cf. ibid., 284–288; Avalos, *Illness*; interesting from a paleopathological perspective: Zias, "Death," 147–59.

115. On infertility in the OT, see Grohmann, *Fruchtbarkeit*, 294–305. On miscarriage, see ibid., 269–71.

methods—in psalms, prayers and exemplary stories—for "healing" this relationship. Thus the main goal is to demonstrate helpful possibilities for dealing with illness and childlessness, and to posit and reinforce the idea that maintaining an intact relationship with God is the best possible method for preventing personal disaster.

The texts have no interest in recognizing the divine will in terms of a person's illness or health in advance if the person does not yet exhibit any symptoms. However, Yahweh could foretell the blessing of children as part of a personal revelation (e.g., Abraham) or a prophetic vision (e.g., Hos 1; Isa 7–8), even if the outward signs and physical condition of the future child-bearer (e.g., Sarah's age) completely contradicted this.[116] Similarly, this was true for prophetic statements (creating "miracles" in unity of action with Yahweh) about future healing or spontaneous illness where the person (body) in question had shown no signs of either healing or sickness (2 Kings 5). According to the Old Testament view, Yahweh—as the God of illness and healing, of the blessing of children and childlessness—could always decide what he wanted to give whom and at what time. The idea that a person's fate was determined right from the start and written in signs on his body is not found here. In the Old Testament, the concept of illness and health as consequences of a disturbed or intact relationship with God had less to do with the idea of divine determinism over an entire human life (as in physiognomics) than with a connection between actions and consequences (*Tun-Ergehen-Zusammenhang*) that constantly provides new choices for people as well as for God (e.g., turning back, regret, forgiveness, and re-building the relationship with God).

Physiognomics in the Old Testament and the Apocrypha

Within the Old Testament and the Apocrypha (jointly referred to as OT [LXX scope] in the following), there are only a few texts that use the principles of physiognomic thought. Like the Mesopotamian physiognomic omens, they assume that a sign and its direct meaning, in other words the interior and exterior, correspond to one another, and that an outward sign on a person's body could be used to draw conclusions about his or her inner state (Sir 19:29f.!). However, there are important differences with Mesopotamian physiognomics: first, significant linguistic differences can be seen, since the Biblical texts are not formulated in the conditional phrases that are

---

116. On pregnancy and birth in the OT, see Kunz, "Vorstellung"; Grohmann, *Fruchtbarkeit*, 132–40.

so common in the omens.¹¹⁷ Second, the principle of determinism applies only to a limited extent within the Old Testament. Thus bodily signs can be interpreted in such a way that their bearers' character is established and labeled as "positive" or "negative" for the significant people in his or her environment. In other words, physiognomic examinations can promote human understanding and be used to adapt one's behavior to this knowledge. However, what the texts do not include is the idea of the body as a divination medium for predicting the future. Therefore the goal is not to identify future events, illnesses or childlessness in advance, but to classify the person in question. Naturally these things are related to some extent, since "positive" people were expected to experience equally positive events, circumstances and results, and therefore a shared future would not hold any "unpleasant surprises." However, the relevant Biblical texts use physiognomics less to determine future predestined illnesses and fates than to analyze character and promote human understanding. As a result, they are a valuable source for the implicit cultural guidelines regarding bodily conception and perception.

Bodily Conception and Perception in Old Testament Texts with Physiognomic Principles

The conception and perception of the body in the Old Testament is situated within the context of Ancient Near Eastern ideas: It assumes the psychosomatic unity of the body and "spirit,"¹¹⁸ the Ancient Near Eastern conventions regarding the hierarchy and perception of the body ("top/front" above "bottom/behind"; "right" vs. left"), the validity of the category of "gender" (including as a mechanism for assigning status) and binariness.

Ideals of beauty are generally implicitly assumed, for both men and women; in the descriptive passages of the Song of Songs, which describe the ideal physiognomy of a woman (Sg 4:1–7; 6:4–7; 7:2–10) and a man (Song 5:10–16), they are made more explicit. The bodies of both are generally described from the top down in these songs (as in Song 4:1–7; 6:4–7; 5:10–15; not Song 7:2–10), which corresponds to the standard Ancient Near Eastern direction of the gaze (see above). In these texts, too, the culturally defined hierarchy of the body applies, in that the head and front of the body are given greater recognition than the back and the rest of the body. Fullness, hair growth, regularity, the presence of shining light (face/eyes) and the "red-colored" indication of vitality are among the implicit parameters that

---

117. On this discussion, see Berlejung, "Frau," 60f.; Berlejung, "Physiognomik," 14f.
118. As already stated by Frevel, "Körper," 280; Meier, "Beziehungsweisen," 185–87; Schroer and Staubli, *Körpersymbolik*, 27f.; Frevel and Wischmeyer, *Menschsein*, 27–38.

apply when thick hair, even rows of teeth, a flawless shape, round navel and buttocks (Song 7:2f.), a tall, even stature, gleaming eyes, hair like purple (Song 7:5) and full breasts characterize feminine beauty for the author. According to the physiognomic ideal of the correspondence between the internal and external condition, the text also leaves no doubt that the bride's external beauty corresponds to her flawless character (Song 5:2; 6:9). Also in keeping with the Ancient Near Eastern convention (cf. David in 1 Sam 16:12; 17:42) is the ideal of beauty that appears in the description of the groom: he is described as red,[119] with gleaming eyes, dark, dense curls, and a tall stature (Song 5:10–12). Thick hair and the color red are also considered in the Old Testament (2 Sam 14:26; Eccl 11:10; Song 4:1; 5:10; 6:5; Ezek 16:7) to be indicators of a person's vitality, which are positively associated with youth and beauty. Gray hair, on the other hand, is an outward sign of advanced age, but also "inner" wisdom (Prov 16:31; 20:29).

The front of the head, especially the mouth and eyes, is carefully observed because it stands for the person's communicative and social dimension. Tightly closed eyes or lips are interpreted as signs of deceitful intent (see Prov 6:12–14; 10:10a; 16:30; Ps 35:19):

> When someone starts winking/presses together the eyes, he has something bad in mind, and no one can stop him from going through with it. (Sir 27:22)

An even, open gaze, on the other hand, is associated with an honest character that is not planning anything evil (Prov 4:25). The eyes and face are considered a "mirror" for the "internal" thoughts, feelings and intentions. They also indicate outward signs of joy, fear, worry and anger, which were interpreted not only as the person's momentary internal state, but also as his fundamental disposition (Gen 31:5; Job 9:27; Sir 25:23).

Just as in Mesopotamian physiognomics, the perception of the body that underlies Old Testament texts focuses on the binary nature of light and darkness in conjunction with the face and eyes. Since physiognomics is based on the principle that the inner state corresponds to the outer state, light thoughts belong with a radiant face just as dark thoughts belong with a fallen countenance (Gen 4:5–7). Thus it is the radiance of the face or eyes that reveals the person's love of life, vitality or even benevolence to the observer (Prov 15:13.30; 16:15a; Gen 29:17; Sir 26:4). Accordingly, this radiance is interpreted as an outward sign of a person who is to be judged positively.[120] The true beauty of a "good" woman also comes from within

---

119. Ibid., 114f.:93 (*alamdimmû* VIII): "If it [his face] is red, he is a man of God, he will become rich, his wealth will grow."

120. Ibid., 114f.:102; 280f.:7.

(Sir 26:16–18) and has an outward effect: she brightens her surroundings and can be compared with a lampstand or the rising sun.

Wicked women, on the other hand, should be easily recognized by their frowning faces:

> The wickedness of the woman changes her outer appearance and darkens her face (until she looks) like a bear [variant: makes her husband's appearance dark, so that it resembles a bear]. (Sir 25:17)

The variant text demonstrates that the "diagnosis" of a bad woman is unrelated to the individual psychological dimension, the question of why this person is bad or what made her the way she is, let alone considerations about how one could help her. Instead, it is based on an interest in protecting the social environment, in this case a potential husband, from such wives. A person's evil nature causes others to suffer, and the darkness in her face can be transferred to them. In a certain sense, the darkening of the face as well as its lightening is presented as something that significantly affects the social environment and is in a sense "contagious." The effects that women (whether wives or daughters) have on their social contexts ("constellations") and on the persons associated with them (husband, father, brother) are the main focus of Sirach 25–26.

This also applies to Sir 26:9, which says that the shamelessness of a woman can be recognized by her bold and flirting eyes. One gaze at a woman's shamelessly raised eyes, or at her dark or shining face, is said to be enough for a man to find out what kind of woman she is. Then he can easily conclude how she will behave in the future, which in turn reveals what his life would be like by her side ... Ultimately, the goal of these texts is to use signs on the body, along with facial expressions and gestures, to identify women who might destabilize the applicable role, honor, status and hierarchy assignments—as quickly as possible. The warnings about aggressively raised eyes and dark faces are intended to be used by men so that they know to stay away from women who bear these signs. On the other hand, women who put on this type of face know that they are quickly headed for a social no-man's land, while modestly lowered eyes in an otherwise radiant face have a positive connotation; this is desired by the social environment and likely also rewarded. In dealing with people in general, tightly closed eyes and lips were clearly associated with deceitfulness. These contexts affected actions as well, in that people distanced themselves from others with these traits because they feared evil from them. Conversely, it is also possible that a person might tightly close his eyes and lips in order to intentionally convey reluctance, deceit, or similar emotions in the sense of a threat.

A person might consider his or her own body and body language to be a way of communicating and constructing his or her own "social self" (status, honor, dignity). However, the body and body language are also media for social control (by others). Naturally, this requires the culturally conditioned body signals and their associated meanings to be controlled and known. Old Testament texts that express the bodily conceptions and perceptions in the Old Testament show that, for these Biblical texts, being human included "the individual's complete integration into social contexts ("constellations") and/or a "bond" with others (principle of "connectivity")."[121] The body was seen as the center of all potential human relationships and interactions. As dyadic[122] people, women and men oriented their body image, body language and bodily perception toward what others expected of them; in this regard, their entire relationship with their bodies was largely constructed by others.[123]

Gender-differentiated Images of Illness and the Body in Old Testament Texts with Basic Physiognomic Principles

The ideal that underlies these Old Testament texts—for women and men alike, just as described above in 2.4 for Mesopotamia—included the hope of a long, healthy life, economic security, a stable, lasting marriage with many children, and the prospect of an estate (for an example, see the depiction of Job's still-intact situation). An intact relationship with God was the foundation for and a constant part of such a life. The opposite of this ideal was the worst outcome, something to be feared, avoided and lamented (once again, see Job).

In contrast to the physiognomic omens of Mesopotamia, though, the Old Testament did not share the view that each person's life line was written on his or her own body; the body was not believed to bear signs of how a person's life would develop, whether he or she would suffer illnesses or childlessness later in life or would live a healthy life surrounded by offspring.

In this regard, it was not possible to divine the future based on a person's body. Signs of illness could only be diagnosed after the outbreak of the illness (Leviticus 13); the only possible prognosis for the future was

---

121. Similarly stated in Di Vito, "Anthropology," 221–25, 234ff.

122. On dyadism, see Malina, *Welt*, 67–84; Neyrey, "Dyadism," 53–56; Neumann, "Kultur und Mentalität," 38–40.

123. On this connection which still applies today, see Daszkowski, *Körperbild*, 67ff.; Synnott, *Body*, 36f., 73–102 (regarding ideals of beauty), 262ff.; Freund, "Society," 135ff.; Bourdieu, *Herrschaft*, 17ff.

whether the disease would end well or badly (cf. e.g., 2 Kgs 20:1–7)—or, in the priestly sense, could be classified as pure or impure.

However, signs could certainly be made out on a person's body that would illuminate his or her character and social behaviors. Insincerity, dishonesty and deceit were especially undesirable (Prov 6:12–14; 10:10a; 16:30; Sir 27:22), since they caused suffering and conflict and could harm those nearby or the person's supervisor/king in the court. For women, wickedness and shamelessness (Sir 25:17; 26:9) were other feared vices that were said to be identified by way of external signs.

From this, it becomes clear that the interpretive framework for physiognomic signs on the male or female body was neither particularly subtle nor personalized. Instead, it perpetuated stereotypes whose profiles had been socially established and evaluated, and which were known to everyone. The individual person whose physiognomy was being observed was supposed to be assigned to one of the stereotypes that were established for the respective gender according to the culture and the time. This would in turn make it easier to judge an unknown person as quickly as possible so that one could behave appropriately toward him right from the start, and either seek out or avoid his company. The main goal, in other words, was to correctly judge a person's influence over his social surroundings (in advance, if possible). Since men in the Ancient Near East had different social spheres and interaction partners than women did, the opportunities for positively or negatively influencing one's social environment also differed by gender. People expected as well as feared different behaviors from men than from women.

The stereotypes that were available for men and for women were based on the gender-specific division of labor, which intended men to represent the family's interests outside the home while women were responsible for the inside.[124] To this was added the gender-specific moral division of labor, which assigned honor to the man (on risks to the man's honor, see, for instance, Sir 26:5.28), and shame(fulness) to the woman. For women, according to Sir 25:13–26:18[.19–27], there were two main stereotypes that could be assigned to the individual woman as a representative of her gender group: the ideal woman was modest, loyal, radiant, quiet, reticent, hardworking and clever in the household. Her opposite was shameless, promiscuous, malicious, dark, chatty, offensive, argumentative and disobedient. A woman could have a significant impact on her social environment (= family and husband) through her dark face, her eyes (Sir 26:9.11), and her mouth and/or idle talk (Sir 25:20; 26:6.27).

---

124. For a summary, see Frevel, "Frau/Mann," 188f.

As a representative of his gender group, a man also fell within the spectrum of two stereotypes: according to conventional wisdom, the ideal man (Sir 19:29f.) was a wise man, with all of the attributes that went along with it (see also Dan 1:3f.). In addition, there was the stereotype of the picture-perfect "successful man" (David in 1 Sam 16:18) who illuminates his social environment (supervisors, colleagues) through his intact relationship with Yahweh, and whom people wish to be near. These positive stereotypes were counterbalanced by the negative stereotype of the heretic, liar and conspirator who would bring trouble to the people around him (Prov 6:12–14; 10:10; 16:30; Sir 27:22)—to whom the seven "detestable things" largely apply (Prov 6:16–19). The weapons with which men can damage their social environment, like those of women, are their faces/eyes and mouths (see especially bearing false witness). In addition, however, their hands also come into play, since they can use these to inflict physical violence on innocent persons (Prov 6:17; Ps 5:7; Genesis 4).

SUMMARY

What, then, does all this say about the topic of this volume, "religion and the treatment of illness"?

It is clear that a diagnosis of illness was what primarily brought about social consequences in the ancient Near East and the Old Testament, which then made people consider how this blow of fate could be explained and/or avoided if possible. Since a healthy and functional body was considered to be "natural" and "God-given," a sick body was generally seen as the result of a disrupted relationship with God.

In addition, the Mesopotamian physiognomic tradition of interpreting omens attempted to discover signs of an illness before it broke out, or to evaluate a person's ability to sire or bear a child in advance. This information was used to determine whether the examinee would be able to fulfill his or her gender-specific roles within the social structure, and whether he or she would "function" in a socially acceptable and successful way. In general, discussions about body and illness as well as offspring were the expression and part of a specific field of reference. The following standards applied:

1. The appearance of the human body and/or signs on the body had an effect on behavior. In other words, if a person was diagnosed by physiognomics as currently healthy but already within the orbit of a certain illness or an early death, then the consequence was probably that he would not be given the desired position at court. If a man was

diagnosed as being unable to procreate or a woman was infertile, it can be assumed that his or her value on the marriage market was severely limited.

2. From point 1 it can be seen that even when people were still healthy, they were treated as sick by their social interaction partners. This was similar for limitations involving a person's reproductive capabilities.

3. The signs on the body were considered to have been inscribed by the gods and legible to their representatives. However, as a rule they could not be changed. Therefore these omens sometimes provided an explanation for why certain illnesses were/would be experienced, but no method for curing them. They were also able to say in advance whether a certain illness would end in death or recovery, but this too simply had to be accepted. The same was true for the determination as to whether a person would have children or not.

4. However, omens are used to learn about the future so that one may take action in the present. They allow people to make judgments about others and interact with them based on a pre-established trust or distrust (created by the omens). That way, they have a clear guideline for the future. The person who is examined by way of omens can also arrange his current life in such a way that certain signs of illness can be observed and potentially prevented. This particularly applies to all the cases where a very specific illness has been predicted. Such knowledge about the future was not seen fatalistically, but was meant to influence behavior. People were supposed to take action! The most important and central measure was for the affected person to strengthen the relationship with his or her personal god or with the god who was considered responsible for the outbreak of a specific illness. Sacrifices and prayers were the appropriate means for repairing a disrupted relationship with the divine. Medical treatments could only help as a secondary step. In addition, there were ritual tools (namburbi) for certain ailments that were able to prevent the predicted misfortune. Naturally, in order for a future to be adjusted in this way, the event had to be correctly diagnosed in the present.

5. Furthermore, the "*ahû* omens"[125] show that one sign could well have multiple contradictory meanings. In other words, divination was rarely completely clear, which also left room for hope.

---

125. These are tablets or lines of text that are not included in a standard series and include alternative or additional interpretations or excursions.

Some selected (and late) Old Testament texts also show a tendency to read signs on a person's body as predicting the person's future social behavior and his or her character traits. However, what is missing from these texts is any attempt to discover signs of an illness before its outbreak or to evaluate a person's ability to conceive or bear children in advance. Here, the discussions about the body and illnesses as well as offspring were also embedded within specific fields of reference, but the diagnosis was performed retroactively, and in the monotheistic context the cause and the remedy were both sought in Yahweh. Illnesses could only be defined after their outbreak, and at that point an expert made a prognosis about whether they were treatable and survivable or untreatable and deadly (or, within the priestly context, pure or impure). The decision about how a diagnosed illness or inability to bear children would turn out was always made by Yahweh.

Thus for the Ancient Near East as well as the Old Testament, it can be said that the most important way to prevent illness was to maintain an intact relationship with the divine!

BIBLIOGRAPHY

Abusch, Tzvi. *Mesopotamian Witchcraft: Toward a History and Understanding of Babylonian Witchcraft Beliefs and Literature.* AMD 5. Leiden: Brill, 2002.

Asher-Greve, J. M. "The Essential Body: Mesopotamian Conceptions of the Gendered Body." In *Gender and the Body in the Ancient Mediterranean*, edited by M. Wyke, 8–37. Oxford: Blackwell, 1998.

Avalos, Hector. *Illness and Health Care in the Ancient Near East: The Role of the Temple in Greece, Mesopotamia, and Israel.* Harvard Semitic Monograph 54. Atlanta: Scholars, 1995.

Barton, Tamsyn S. *Power and Knowledge: Astrology, Physiognomics, and Medicine under the Roman Empire.* The Body, in Theory: Histories of Cultural Materialism. Ann Arbor: University of Michigan Press, 1994.

Berlejung, Angelica. "Frau nach Maß: Physiognomische Omina für die Frau als Quellen für Überlegungen zur Mentalität und Kultur der altorientalischen Gesellschaft im 1. Jt. v.Chr." In *Sara lacht . . . Eine Erzmutter und ihre Geschichte: Zur Interpretation und Rezeption der Sara-Erzählung*, edited by R. Kampling, 27–63. Paderborn: Schöningh, 2004.

———. "Physiognomik im Alten Testament, den Apokryphen und Qumran." *Leqach* 6 (2005) 7–25.

Böck, Barbara. *Die babylonisch-assyrische Morphoskopie.* Archiv für Orientforschung Beihefte 27. Vienna: Selbstverlag des Instituts für Orientalistik der Universität Wien, 2000.

Borger, R. "Die Weihe eines Enlil-Priesters." *BiOr* 30 (1973) 163–76.

Bourdieu, Pierre. *Die männliche Herrschaft.* Frankfurt: Suhrkamp, 2005 [1998].

Budge, E. A. Wallis, ed. *The Laughable Stories: Collected by Mâr Gregory John Bar-Hebraeus, Maphrian of the East from A.D. 1264 to 1286*. 1897. Reprinted, Piscataway, NJ: Gorgias, 2003.

Daszkowski, Alexandra. *Das Körperbild bei Frauen und Männern: Evolutionstheoretische und kulturelle Faktoren*. Marburg: Tectum, 2003.

Degkwitz, A. "Die pseudoaristotelischen 'Physiognomonica' Traktat A: Übersetzung und Kommentar." PhD diss., University of Freiburg, 1988.

Di Vito, R. A. "Old Testament Anthropology and the Construction of Personal Identity." *CBQ* 61 (1999) 217–38.

Ebeling, Erich. *Keilschrifttexte aus Assur religiösen Inhalts*. Wissenschaftliche Veröffentlichung der Deutschen Orient-Gesellschaft 28, 34, Leipzig: Hinrichs, 1915–1923 (= KAR)).

Farber, Walter. *Beschwörungsrituale an Ištar und Dumuzi: Attī Ištar ša harmaša Dumuzi*. Akademie der Wissenschaften und der Literatur. Veröffentlichungen der Orientalischen Kommission 30. Wiesbaden: Harrassowitz, 1977.

———. *Lamaštu: An Edition of the Canonical Series of Lamaštu Incantations and Rituals and Related Texts from the Second and First Millennia B.C.* Mesopotamian Civilizations 17. Winona Lake, IN: Eisenbrauns, 2014).

———. *Schlaf, Kindchen, schlaf! Mesopotamische Baby-Beschwörungen und -rituale*. Mesopotamian Civilizations 2. Winona Lake, IN: Eisenbrauns, 1989.

Finkel, I. L., and M. J. Geller, eds. *Disease in Babylonia*. Cuneiform Monographs 36. Leiden: Brill, 2007.

Fischer, I. "Ist der Tod nicht für alle gleich? Sterben und Tod aus der Genderperspektive." In *Tod und Jenseits im alten Israel und in seiner Umwelt. Theologische, religionsgeschichtliche, archäologische und ikonographische Aspekte*, edited by Angelika Berlejung and Bernd Janowski, 87–108. FAT 64. Tübingen: Mohr/Siebeck, 2009.

Förster, Richard. *Scriptores Physiognomonici. Graeci et Latini*. 2 vols. Bibliotheca Scriptorum Graecorum et Romanorum Teubneriana. Leipzig: Teubner, 1893.

Freund, P. E. S. "Bringing Society into the Body: Understanding Socialized Human Nature [1988]." In *The Body: Critical Concepts in Sociology*, Vol. 2: *Sociology, Nature and the Body*, edited by Aberdeen Body Group, 133–55. London: Psychology Press, 2003.

Frevel, C. "Frau/Mann." In *Handbuch theologischer Grundbegriffe zum Alten und Neuen Testament*, edited by Angelika Berlejung and C. Frevel, 188–90. Darmstadt: Wissenschaftliche Buchgesellschaft, 2006.

———. "Körper." In *Handbuch theologischer Grundbegriffe zum Alten und Neuen Testament*, edited by Angelika Berlejung and C. Frevel, 280–84. Darmstadt: Wissenschaftliche Buchgesellschaft, 2006.

———. "Krankheit/Heilung." In *Handbuch theologischer Grundbegriffe zum Alten und Neuen Testament*, edited by Angelika Berlejung and C. Frevel, 284–88. Darmstadt: Wissenschaftliche Buchgesellschaft, 2006.

Frevel, Christian, and Oda Wischmeyer. *Menschsein*. NEB Themen 11, Würzburg: Echter, 2003.

Frey-Anthes, Henrike. *Unheilsmächte und Schutzgenien, Antiwesen und Grenzgänger. Vorstellungen von "Dämonen" im alten Israel*. OBO 227. Göttingen: Vandenhoeck & Ruprecht, 2007.

Furlani, G. "Die Physiognomik des Barhebräus in syrischer Sprache I." *ZS* 7 (1929) 1–16.

Gerabek, W. E., "Physiognomik." In *Enzyklopädie Medizingeschichte*, edited by B. D. Haage et al., 1157–58. Berlin: de Gruyter, 2005.

Greenfield, J. C., and M. Sokoloff. "Astrological and Related Omen Texts in Jewish Palestinian Aramaic." *JNES* 48 (1989) 201–14.

Grohmann, Marianne. *Fruchtbarkeit und Geburt in den Psalmen*. FAT 53. Tübingen: Mohr/Siebeck, 2007.

Grünwald, I. "Jewish Physiognomic and Chiromantic Fragments." *Tarbiz* 40 (1970–1971) 306–19.

Guinan, A. K. "Auguries of Hegemony: The Sex Omens of Mesopotamia." In *Gender and the Body in the Ancient Mediterranean*, edited by Maria Wyke, 38–55. Gender and History. Oxford: Wiley-Blackwell, 1998.

———. "The Human Behavioral Omens: On the Threshold of Psychological Inquiry." *BCSMS* 19 (1990) 9–14.

———. "Left/Right Symbolism in Mesopotamian Divination." *SAAB* 10.1 (1996) 5–10.

———. "The Perils of High Living: Divinatory rhetoric in *Šumma Ālu*." In *DUMU-E2-DUB-BA-A: Studies in Honor of Ake W. Sjöberg*, edited by H. Behrens, D. Loding and M. T. Roth, 227–35. Occasional Publications of the Samuel Noah Kramer Fund 11. Philadelphia: University of Pennsylvania Museum Publications, 1989), 227–235.

———. "A Severed Head Laughed: Stories of Divinatory Interpretation." In *Magic and Divination in the Ancient World*, edited by L. Ciraolo and J. Seidel, 7–40. AMD 2. Leiden: Brill, 2002.

———. "Social Constructions and Private Designs: The House Omens of *Šumma Ālu*." In *Houses and Households in Ancient Mesopotamia, Papers Read at the 40e Rencontre Assyriologique Internationale, Leiden, July 5–8, 1993*, edited by Klaas R. Veenhof, 61–68. PIHANS 78. Leiden: Nederlands Historisch-Archaeologisch Instituut te Istanbul, 1996.

Harris, Marvin. *Kulturanthropologie: Ein Lehrbuch*. Frankfurt: Campus, 1989.

Hasenfratz, H.-P. *Die Toten Lebenden: Eine religionsphänomenologische Studie zum sozialen Tod in archaischen Gesellschaften. Zugleich ein kritischer Beitrag zur sogenannten Strafopfertheorie*. Beihefte der Zeitschrift für Religions- und Geistesgeschichte 24. Leiden: Brill, 1982.

Hedwig-Jahnow-Forschungsproject, ed. *Körperkonzepte im Ersten Testament. Aspekte einer Feministischen Anthropologie*. Stuttgart: Kohlhammer, 2003.

Heeßel, N. P. "Astrological Medicine in Babylonia." In *Astro-Medicine: Astrology and Medicine, East and West*, edited by Anna Akasoy et al., 1–16. Micrologus' Library 25. Florence: SISMEL edizioni del Galluzzo, 2008.

———. "Diagnosis, Divination and Disease: Towards an understanding of the rationale behind the Babylonian Diagnostic Handbook." In *Magic and Rationality in Ancient Near Eastern and Graeco-Roman Medicine*, edited by H. F. J. Horstmanshoff and M. Stol, 97–116. Studies in Ancient Medicine 27. Leiden: Brill, 2004.

———. *Divinatorische Texte I. Terrestrische, teratologische, physiognomische und oneiromantische Omina*. WVDOG 116 (= KAL 1). Wiesbaden: Harrassowitz, 2007.

———. "Neues zu Esagil-kīn-apli. Die ältere Version der physiognomischen Omenserie alamdimmû." In *Assur-Forschungen: Arbeiten aus der Forschungsstelle "Edition literarischer Keilschrifttexte aus Assur" der Heidelberger Akademie der*

Wissenschaften, edited by Stefan M. Maul and N. P. Heeßel 139-87. Wiesbaden: Harrassowitz, 2010.

———. Review of B. Böck, *Die babylonisch-assyrische Morphoskopie*. BiOr 61 (2004) 575-79.

———. "Der verschwiegene Unterschied. Die Geschlechterdifferenz in medizinischen Texten aus dem Alten Mesopotamien." In *Krankheit und Heilung: Gender—Religion—Medizin*, edited by B. Heininger and R. Lindner 9-24. Geschlecht—Symbol—Religion 4. Berlin: LIT Verlag, 2006.

———. "Warzen, Beulen und Narben. Eine Sammlung medizinischer Rezepte und physiognomischer Beobachtungen aus Assur gegen Gesichtsmale." In *Studies in Ancient Near Eastern World View and Society: Festschrift für Marten Stol*, edited by R. J. van der Spek, 161-71. Bethesda, MD: CDL Press, 2008.

Kraus, F. R. "Ein Sittenkanon in Omenform." ZA NF 9 (1936) 77-113.

Kunz, A. "Die Vorstellung von Zeugung und Schwangerschaft im antiken Israel." ZAW 111 (1999) 561-82.

Lambert, W. G. "The Qualifications of Babylonian Diviners." In *Festschrift für Rykle Borger zu seinem 65. Geburtstag am 24. Mai 1994: Tikip santakki mala bašmu*, edited by Stefan M. Maul, 141-58. Cuneiform Monographs 10. Groningen: Styx, 1998.

Lavater, Johann Caspar. *Physiognomische Fragmente, zur Beförderung der Menschenkenntnis und Menschenliebe*. Leipzig: Weidmanns Erben & Reich, Steiner, 1775-1778.

Malina, Bruce J. *Die Welt des Neuen Testaments: Kulturanthropologische Einsichten*. Stuttgart: Kohlhammer, 1993.

Maul, Stefan M. "How the Babylonians Protected Themselves against Calamities Announced by Omens." In *Mesopotamian Magic: Textual, Historical, and Interpretative Perspectives*, edited by Tzvi Abusch and Karel van der Toorn, 123-29. Ancient Magic and Divination 1. Groningen: Styx, 1999.

———. "Die 'Lösung vom Bann': Überlegungen zu altorientalischen Konzeptionen von Krankheit und Heilkunst." In *Magic and Rationality in Ancient Near Eastern and Graeco-Roman Medicine*, edited by H. F. J. Horstmanshoff and M. Stol, 79-95. Studies in Ancient Medicine 27. Leiden: Brill, 2004.

———. *Omina und Orakel*. RLA 10. Berlin: de Gruyter, 2003-2005.

Meier, C. "Beziehungsweisen. Körperkonzept und Gottesbild in Ps 139." In *Körperkonzepte im Ersten Testament: Aspekte einer Feministischen Anthropologie*, edited by Hedwig-Jahnow-Forschungsprojekt, 172-88. Stuttgart: Kohlhammer, 2003.

Müller, K. E. "Die Natur der Geschlechter: Zur Ethnologie des Geschlechtskonflikts." In *Die Braut: Geliebt, verkauft, getauscht, geraubt. Zur Rolle der Frau im Kulturvergleich*, edited by G. Völger and K. von Welck, 1:52-59. Ethnologica Neue Folge 11. Cologne: Rautenstrauch-Joest-Museum für Völkerkunde, 1985.

Müller-Jahncke, W.-D. "Art. Signaturenlehre." In *Enzyklopädie Medizingeschichte*, edited by W. E. Gerabek et al., 1330-32. Berlin: de Gruyter, 2005.

Neumann, K. "Kultur und Mentalität." In *Handbuch theologischer Grundbegriffe zum Alten und Neuen Testament*, edited by A. Berlejung and C. Frevel, 35-42. Darmstadt: Wissenschaftliche Buchgesellschaft, 2006.

Neyrey, Jerome H. "Dyadism." In *Handbook of Biblical Social Values*, edited by John J. Pilch and Bruce J. Malina, 53-56. 2nd ed. Peabody, MA: Hendrickson, 2002.

Oppenheim, A. L. "Zur keilschriftlichen Omenliteratur." Or NS 5 (1936) 199-228.

Percival, Melissa, and Graeme Tytler, eds. *Physiognomy in Profile: Lavater's Impact on European Culture*. Newark: University of Delaware Press, 2005.

Pestalozzi, Karl, and Horst Weigelt, eds. *Das Antlitz Gottes im Antlitz des Menschen: Zugänge zu Johann Caspar Lavater*. Arbeiten zur Geschichte des Pietismus 31. Göttingen: Vandenhoeck & Ruprecht, 1994.

Popovic, Mladen. *Reading the Human Body: Physiognomics and Astrology in the Dead Sea Scrolls and Hellenistic-Early Roman Period Judaism*. Studies on the Texts of the Desert of Judah 67. Leiden: Brill, 2007.

———. "Reading the Human Body and Writing in Code: Physiognomic Divination and Astrology in the Dead Sea Scrolls." In *Flores Florentino: Dead Sea Scrolls and Other Early Jewish Studies in Honour of Florentino García Martínez*, edited by Anthony Hilhorst et al., 271–84. JSJSup 122. Leiden: Brill, 2007.

Sassi, Maria Michela. *The Science of Man in Ancient Greece*. Translated by Paul Tucker. Chicago: University of Chicago Press, 2001.

Schäfer, P. *Geniza-Fragmente zur Hekhalot-Literatur*. Texte und Studien zum antiken Judentum 6. Tübingen: Mohr/Siebeck, 1984.

Scholem, G. "Ein Fragment zur Physiognomik und Chiromantik aus der Tradition der spätantiken jüdischen Esoterik." In *Liber Amicorum: Studies in Honour of Prof. Dr. C. J. Bleeker, Published on the Occasion of His Retirement from the Chair of the History of Religions and the Phenomenology of Religion at the University of Amsterdam*, 175–93. Studies in the History of Religions 17. Leiden: Brill, 1969.

Scholem, G. "הכרת פנים—Physiognomy and Chiromancy." In *Sepher Assaph* [FS Simha Assaf], edited by J. Klausner et al. 459–95. Jerusalem: Mosad ha-Rav Kuk, 1953. (Hebrew)

Schroer, Silvia, and Thomas Staubli. *Die Körpersymbolik der Bibel*. Darmstadt: Wissenschaftliche Buchgesellschaft, 1998.

Schwemer, D. *Rituale und Beschwörungen gegen Schadenzauber*. WVDOG 17 (= KAL 2). Wiesbaden: Harrassowitz, 2007.

Scurlock, JoAnn. *Magico-Medical Means of Dealing with Ghosts in Ancient Mesopotamia*. Ancient Magic and Divination 3. Chicago: University of Chicago Press, 1988.

Scurlock, JoAnn, and Burton R. Anderson. *Diagnoses in Assyrian and Babylonian Medicine: Ancient Sources, Translations, and Modern Medical Analyses*. Urbana: University of Illinois Press, 2005.

Starr, Ivan. *The Rituals of the Diviner*. BibMes 1. Malibu, CA: Undena, 1983.

Steger, Florian. "Einleitung. Kultur: ein Netz von Bedeutungen." In *Kultur: Ein Netz von Bedeutungen. Analysen zur symbolischen Kulturanthropologie*, edited by Florian Steger, 11–22. Würzburg: Königshausen & Neumann, 2002.

Stol, M., and F. A. M. Wiggermann. *Birth in Babylonia and the Bible: Its Mediterranean Setting*. Cuneiform Monographs 14. Leiden: Brill, 2000.

Synnott, Anthony. *The Body Social: Symbolism, Self and Society*. London: Routledge, 1993.

———. "Tomb, Temple, Machine and Self: The Social Construction of the Body." *British Journal of Sociology* 43 (1992) 79–110.

Toorn, Karel van der. *Sin and Sanction in Israel and Mesopotamia: A Comparative Study*. Studia Semitica Neerlandica 22. Assen: Van Gorcum, 1985.

Tsukimoto, A. *Untersuchungen zur Totenpflege (kispum) im alten Mesopotamien*. AOAT 216. Neukirchen-Vluyn: Butzon & Bercker, 1985.

Zgoll, A. "Die Toten als Richter über die Lebenden. Einblicke in ein Himmel, Erde und Unterwelt umspannendes Verständnis von Leben im antiken Mesopotamien." In *Tod und Jenseits im alten Israel und in seiner Umwelt: Theologische, religionsgeschichtliche, archäologische und ikonographische Aspekte*, edited by Angelika Berlejung and Bernd Janowski, 567–82. FAT 64. Tübingen: Mohr/Siebeck, 2009.

Zias, Joseph. "Death and Disease in Ancient Israel." *BA* 54 (1991) 147–59.

9

"Heal me, for I have sinned against you!" (Psalm 41:5MT)

On the Concept of Illness and Healing in the Old Testament

—Bernd Janowski

PRELIMINARY COMMENTS

Anyone attempting to make a contribution to the topic of "Religion and Illness" must first name the methodological premises and conceptual implications under which he plans to approach the topic.[1] This applies to Biblical scholarship just as to any other area of humanities or cultural studies. Let us begin with the term "illness." Its lack of specificity clearly makes it seem unsuitable for academic linguistic use:

> For the same word, illness, should not be used without differentiation in order to describe the state of being ill, the symptoms of illness, the difference between health and illness in the 'concept of illness,' and should not be used to mean the same thing as the 'illness presentation.' Furthermore, 'illness' can refer to the

---

1. The following statements refer to the arguments in my essay Janowski, "Heile mich, denn ich habe an dir gesündigt!" (Ps 41,5): Zum Konzept von Krankheit und Heilung im Alten Testament, 47–66, and expand on these.

aspect of the patient (his condition), the aspect of the doctor (the diagnosis) and the aspect of society (the patient's level of distress and need for assistance), which involves a different side of the phenomenon each time, with different characteristics. Finally, the term 'illness' appears in other intellectual contexts (theology, philosophy, etc.) where it does not refer to anything medical.[2]

In order to clarify the term "illness," therefore, distinctions have been suggested that account for the *pathological diagnosis*, in other words: the demonstrable disorganization of the bodily structure and function, the *subjective condition of the patient*; the sufferer's feeling of being sick, and the *clinical picture*; the respective clinical unit. In this schema, people are considered to be ill if they "require help due to a loss of coordinated interactions between the physical, mental or psychophysical functional elements of the organism, either in a subjective or a clinical sense."[3]

This brings up the question of the meaning that the sufferer assigns to the illness. Since we only consider something to be "meaningful" if it has significance for something else within a certain context,[4] it is important how this context is defined and/or viewed: as a religious, philosophical, psychoanalytical, medical or psychosomatic context. Whichever aspect is dominant as an interpretive framework in the individual context, "the way in which we think and talk about illness and healing is embedded within a large number of contexts; and in some respects, despite endless mental efforts over the last few millennia, it is still full of mysteries."[5] What is clear here is that the terms illness and healing, or health, ultimately do not describe a purely biological circumstance. Rather, they are a social construct whose plausibility depends on the interactions between descriptive and normative aspects as well as existential and value judgments, for individuals as well as for society as a whole.[6]

That brings us to the second key concept, namely "religion." If, following J. Habermas,[7] we assume the expressive potential of religious language—which Habermas says must be made accessible to secular society through a process of "redeeming deconstruction" in order to overcome

2. Rothschuh, "Krankheit," 1186 (1184–90).
3. Ibid., 1187.
4. Cf. ibid., 1189–90.
5. Ibid., 1190.
6. See Körtner, "Mit Krankheit leben," 1275 with reference to von Engelhardt, *Krankheit, Schmerz und Lebenskunst*, 7; Etzelmüller, "Der kranke Mensch," 163–76; and Schramme, *Krankheitstheorien*.
7. See Habermas, *Glauben und Wissen*, 20ff.

"Heal me, for I have sinned against you!" (Psalm 41:5MT)   175

the one-sidedness of a purely secularist consciousness and its "enlightened self-interest"[8]—then post-secular society in particular could regain an understanding of pre-modern, religiously determined concepts of illness and healing, even if most of its members are distanced from these concepts. However one defines the start of the modern era in epochal terms,[9] the adjective "pre-modern" always refers to a stage before the start of the modern era and its rational ideas about God, human beings and the world. The following will discuss the logic and the unique understanding of this pre-modern idea of illness and healing based on the example of the Old Testament.

ILLNESS AND HEALING IN THE OLD TESTAMENT

Illness as a Subject of Old Testament Anthropology

The interpretation of illness and healing "is always based on a certain anthropology, or teaching about human beings"[10] that, based on the witness of the Old Testament, can be described as a *constellative anthropology*. I have sketched out its contours elsewhere based on the aspects of the "whole human being," "social sphere" and "perception of the world," and have attempted to define them through their relationships with one another.[11] The people of ancient Israel always move within all three contexts simultaneously—the *individual*, the *social* and the *symbolic* context—although the emphasis varies depending on the literary profile and historical location of the text sources:

* *The whole human being: the body/'soul' connection*

    Old Testament anthropology is primarily characterized by the *correlation between bodily organs and vital functions*. Since the body is the human being's anchor in the world, the Old Testament concept of the person relies not just on the physical sphere, but also on the social sphere.

* *The social sphere: the constellative concept of the person*

    The characteristics of Old Testament anthropology also include an understanding of the *community focus of Hebrew thinking*, according to

---

8. Habermas, *Glauben und Wissen*, 23, 24.
9. Cf. Graf, "Art. Neuzeit I," 254–59.
10. Rothschuh, Krankheit, 1190.
11. Cf. Janowski, "Der Mensch im alten Israel," 143–75; Janowski, *Konfliktgespräche mit Gott*, 430–31; and Janowski, "Anthropologie des Alten Testaments," 535–55.

which the behavior of the individual is consistently seen in relation to the social context in which it occurs.

* *Perception of the world: the system of religious symbols*

Every religion, including the religion of ancient Israel, uses a *system of symbols or a worldview* with which it claims the authority to structure reality as a whole and to provide interpretations that individuals can use to shape their lives.

In attempting to define the specific Old Testament concept of illness and healing, together with its anthropological dimensions, we encounter a fundamental problem, namely the question of the *criteria for defining texts about illness and healing*, and particularly the Old Testament psalms that have to do with illness and healing.[12] In order to answer this question, K. Seybold[13] defined four aspects that provide a complex picture of illness and healing in ancient Israel. These are as follows:

- *Linguistic elements*

  Terms relating to illness and healing, such as ^{a}ḥālāh "to be/become weak, sick," kā'ab "To experience pain, to suffer," ṣāla' "to limp, to be lame," etc., and ḥājāh qal./pi./hif. "to be revitalized, to heal," as well as ḥālam "to become strong, to strengthen," rāpā' "to heal," etc.

- *Forms of belief*

  Certain ideas about life and death, the *Sheol* motif, residual magical beliefs, correlation between sin and punishment, etc.

- *Social implications*

  Isolation, rejection, ostracism, hostility, cultic impurity, etc.

---

12. See Seybold, *Das Gebet des Kranken im Alten Testament*, 98ff., 123ff., 153ff., 169–70, subdivided into *Psalms with a definite reference* (Pss 38; 41; 88; Ps III [syr.3 = 11QPsa 155]), *Psalms with a likely reference* (Pss 30; 39; 69; 102; 103; Isa 38:9–20) and *Psalms with an uncertain reference to illness or healing* (Pss 6; 13; 32; 51; 91), cf. also Seybold and Müller, *Krankheit und Heilung*, 11–79; Wolff, *Anthropologie des Alten Testaments*, 209ff.; Scharbert, "Krankheit II," 680–83; Oeming, "Mein Herz ist durchbohrt in meinem Innern," 5–28; Oeming, *Das Buch der Psalmen*, Psalm 1–41, 75–76; Briend, *Krankheit und Heilung im Alten Testament*, 84–85; Ebner, "Krankheit und Heilung," III1730–31; Otto, "Magie—Dämonen—göttliche Kräfte," 208–25; Frevel, "Krankheit / Heilung," 284–88; Beyerle, "Medizin—Phänomene im Alten Israel und im antiken Judentum," 45–78; and Ruwe and Starnitzke, "Krankheit / Heilung," 315–20.

13. Seybold, *Das Gebet des Kranken im Alten Testament*, 17ff., 165–66, cf. also Achenbach, "Zum Sitz im Leben mesopotamischer und altisraelitischer Klagegebete II," 584ff.

- *Religious practices*

  Incantations, oracle consultations, prayers for the sick, penitential rites, cultic healing practices, etc.

According to Seybold, the fact that a relatively clear picture of the patient's situation can still emerge is because

> ... the patient's particular physical, mental, social and religious situation brought forth and developed certain linguistic expressions, fixed beliefs and behaviors *in praxi* that assumed a downright stereotypical character through usage and custom, and gained a normative influence (to the point of institutionalization). The conventionalized typology thus replaces the missing conceptual clarity, and is beneficial particularly with regard to the Psalms, since it accommodates the peculiarities of these texts.[14]

Thus there is a kind of *basic pattern for the course of illness and healing* that is based on a combination of the abovementioned individual elements, and that can be represented as a characteristic ideal using texts such as Ps 6 (KE = *Klagelied des einzelnen* [individual's lament]),[15] 30 (DE = *Danklied des einzelnen* [individual's song of thanks]), 38 (KE),[16] 41 (DE with a citation from a KE, see below), 69 (DE), 88 (KE), 102 (KE) and 116 (DE) (Fig.1). This sketch shows the main line of interpretation for Old Testament illness and healing: the *guilt/sin* or *punishment/illness relation*, and the *forgiveness/healing relation*.[17] Within this overall framework, there are a few special features that occur in various combinations in many psalms: the *description of suffering* (A—C: divine punishment due to "sin," fall, deterioration of life), the *Sheol motif* (D: distance from God, social disintegration, proximity to the underworld) and the *healing process* (C'—A': revitalization, return to life, cultic restitution), shown schematically here:

---

14. Seybold, *Das Gebet des Kranken im Alten Testament*, 167–68; cf. Seybold, *Die Psalmen*, 133; and Gerstenberger, "Krankheit," 542–43.

15. On Ps 6, see Kuckhoff, *Psalm 6 und die Bitten im Psalter*.

16. On Ps 38, see ibid., 173ff; and Zernecke, *Gott und Mensch in Klagegebeten aus Israel und Mesopotamien*, 194ff.

17. Cf. Seybold, *Gebet des Kranken*, 170.

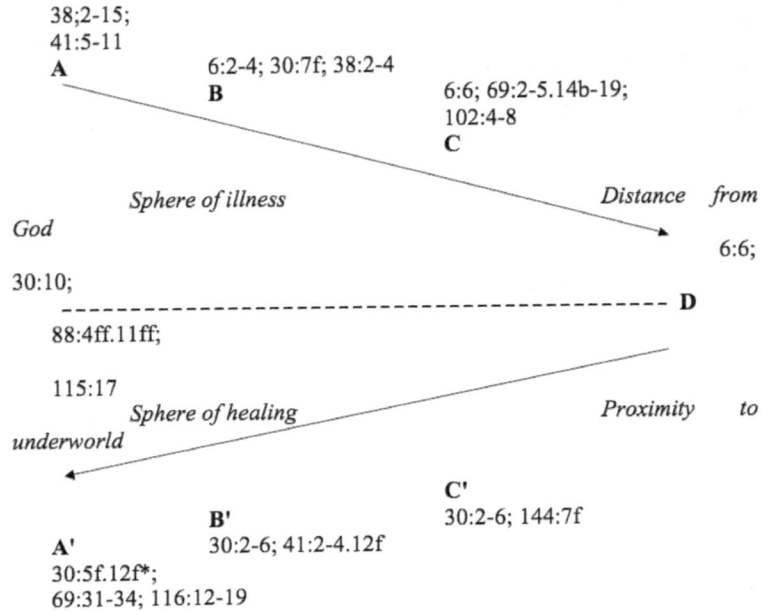

Fig.1: Ideal course of illness and healing

Since the experience of illness and healing is integrated into an *overall framework of religious existential understanding,* Seybold can be said to posit a "conventionalized typology."[18] This typology provides a "replacement for a lack of conceptual clarity"[19] and is shown to be beneficial because it accounts for the linguistic and motif-related peculiarities of the psalms on illness and healing. Some striking examples of this are the depictions of suffering in Ps 38:2–8 and Ps 102:1–7, where *emotional suffering* and *physical distress* are closely related:

> 2 For Your arrows have sunk deep into me,
> And Your hand has pressed down on me.
>
> 3 There is no soundness in my flesh because of Your indignation;
> There is no health in my bones because of my sin.
>
> 4 For my iniquities are gone over my head;
> As a heavy burden they weigh too much for me.

---

18. Ibid., 168.
19. Ibid.

> 5 My wounds grow foul and fester
> Because of my folly.
>
> 6 I am bent over and greatly bowed down;
> I go mourning all day long.
>
> 7 For my loins are filled with burning,
> And there is no soundness in my flesh.
>
> 8 I am benumbed and badly crushed;
> I groan because of the agitation of my heart. (Ps 38:2–8)
>
> 1 Hear my prayer, O Lord,
> And let my cry come to You.
>
> 2 Do not hide Your face from me in the day of my trouble;
> Incline Your ear to me;
> In the day that I call, answer me speedily.
>
> 3 For my days are consumed like smoke,
> And my bones are burned like a hearth.
>
> 4 My heart is stricken and withered like grass,
> So that I forget to eat my bread.
>
> 5 Because of the sound of my groaning
> My bones cling to my skin.
>
> 6 I am like a pelican of the wilderness;
> I am like an owl of the desert.
>
> 7 I lie awake,
> And am like a sparrow alone on the housetop. (Ps 102:1–7)[20]

In particular, the lament of impermanence in Ps 102:3–5 vividly shows how various images of the body flow together to create an overall impression:

> "Here, the terms ʿṣm (bones as scaffolding and the central support system), lb (heart as the emotional and rational center), bśr (skin as a visible sign of human beings' vulnerability) act as partial components of a linguistically and intellectually well-defined image of the *person as a whole*."[21]

Attempting to derive a precise diagnosis of an illness from this seems inappropriate. Instead, the goal is to provide a "subjective understanding

---

20. Cf. Brunert, *Psalm 102 im Kontext des Vierten Psalmenbuches*, 113ff.
21. Ibid., 115.

of disrupted life,"²² in other words, an overall image of the subject of impending death, which is not composed of the semantic content of the basic anthropological terms "bones," "heart" and "skin," but of a targeted combination thereof. According to this understanding of illness, the experience of healing is also expressed not through medical terminology, but as a spatial return to life, a "bringing the soul up from the grave" (Ps 30:3) by YHWH.

The second problem, in addition to the criteria for defining the psalms of illness and healing, regards the question of the supplicant's "*actual suffering.*"²³ Here, too, as demonstrated by Ps 38 and Ps 108, we discover a lack of terminological clarity. Instead, as first noticed by H. Gunkel, there is a great deal of uncertainty, even contradiction, in the supplicant's depiction of illness and agony:

> No *specific situation* for the one praying is clear from the portrayals of mortal distress. They are too generally maintained. Seldom is it clearly expressed whether sickness, misfortune, or persecution from enemies have created the problem. More commonly, the images of the complaint contradict one another and do not allow themselves to be coordinated into one self-contained situation. For example, *within a single context*, the singer of Ps 22 asks for liberation from wild animals and deliverance from the sword that persecutes him. He believes himself to be already in the underworld, then he sees that wild animals have been turned loose on him that want to rob him of his life. Then he speaks of himself as one who is deathly ill whose belongings are divided by those who survive him."²⁴

In many psalms of lamentation, the enemy's actions are listed side by side with references to illness,²⁵ accusations,²⁶ the supplicant's own guilt,²⁷ poverty²⁸ and social disintegration,²⁹ so that it is often difficult to decide "whether the sufferer is sick, depressed, captured, embattled or threatened."³⁰

---

22. Ibid., 116.

23. On the following, see Crüsemann, "Netz," 157–64; and Janowski, "Die 'Kleine Biblia,'" 134ff.

24. Gunkel, *Introduction to Psalms*, 134.

25. Cf. Pss 6; 13; 22; 42/43; 69; 102; 109 passim.

26. Cf. Pss 3; 4; 5; 7; 17; 26; 27; 57; 63; 69 passim.

27. Cf. Pss 6; 38; 51; 69; 88; 143 passim.

28. Cf. Ps 22; 31; 38; 69; 88 passim.

29. Cf. Ps 22; 35; 69; 88; 102; 109 passim.

30. Seybold, *Psalmen*, 133.

The "discontinuity of the images"[31] often makes it impossible to identify the "particular distress"[32] of the patient.

Nonetheless, the various impressions of the experiencing self are combined into a unified whole. Gunkel described this process as follows:

> The poet does not place as much weight on a completely faithful reflection of the external circumstances as he does on communicating the internal circumstances, by expressing the impressions which the external events release in him. He wants to "pour out his sorrow before YHWH." (Ps 102:1. Cf. also Ps 42:5) He reaches for images that powerfully and poignantly reflect his pain and distress, his abandonment, and his betrayal. He appropriates an image as an expression of his feeling to the extent that it appropriately suggests the mood of his spiritual condition. If one image does not suffice, then he multiplies images unconcerned about whether their appearances agree as long as they shock and provoke with their burning colors. In other words, they provide a dynamic impression of what is occurring in his soul."[33]

F. Crüsemann took up this topic once again, posing the question, widespread since H. Gunkel's article, about the "actual distress" of the supplicant and making the thesis of the "non-monocausal view of suffering" plausible:

> Perhaps the way in which the laments describe the distress are more realistic than the assumption of a single cause. The texts that only include one factor, whether it be illness or an accusation, are more marginal forms and are correspondingly rare, while the confusing multiplicity of factors is more the norm according to which the genre is oriented. Perhaps the effect and utility of the texts is related to precisely this non-monocausal view of suffering, even in the present day.[34]

Thus *illness* consists not only of bodily suffering but also of social suffering: of contempt,[35] disintegration and loneliness, in short, the destruction of the supplicant's living environment. Accordingly, *health* represents the balance that the individual must restore again and again in dealing with the world around him and the challenges that it poses—if this is even possible! What the Old Testament concepts of health and illness share, however, is not just

---

31. Gunkel, *Introduction to Psalms*, 134.
32. Ibid.
33. Ibid.
34. Crüsemann, "Netz," 160.
35. On social disregard in ancient Israel, see Janowski, Konfliktgespräche mit Gott, 196ff.

the interaction between subject and environment, but also the classification of this interaction within the theological concepts of the YHWH faith. This context is made particularly clear based on the example of Ps 41.[36]

Psalm 41 as an Exemplary Text

To the Chief Musician. A Psalm of David.

1 Blessed is he who considers the poor;
  The Lord will deliver him in time of trouble.

2 The Lord will preserve him and keep him alive,
  And he will be blessed on the earth;
  You will not deliver him to the will of his enemies.

3 The Lord will strengthen him on his bed of illness;
  You will sustain him on his sickbed.

4 I said, "Lord, be merciful to me;
  Heal my soul, for I have sinned against You."

5 My enemies speak evil of me:
  "When will he die, and his name perish?"

6 And if he comes to see me, he speaks lies;
  His heart gathers iniquity to itself;
  When he goes out, he tells it.

7 All who hate me whisper together against me;
  Against me they devise my hurt.

8 "An evil disease," they say, "clings to him.
  And now that he lies down, he will rise up no more."

9 Even my own familiar friend in whom I trusted,
  Who ate my bread,
  Has lifted up his heel against me.

10 But You, O Lord, be merciful to me, and raise me up,
   That I may repay them.

11 By this I know that You are well pleased with me,
   Because my enemy does not triumph over me.

---

36. On Ps 41 see most recently Janowski, *Konfliktgespräche mit Gott*, 174ff.; also Bauks, *Feinde des Psalmisten und die Freunde Jobs*, 84ff.; and Kuckhoff, *Psalm 6 und die Bitten im Psalter*, 176ff., 184ff., 192ff. passim.

12 As for me, You uphold me in my integrity,
And set me before Your face forever.

13 *Blessed be the Lord God of Israel*
From everlasting to everlasting!
Amen and Amen.

At its core, Psalm 41 is a lament stylized as an individual's prayer to the Lord, YHWH (vv. 4–10), which is framed on one side by a wisdom-based, parenetic sentence (vv. 1–3) and on the other by an avowal of thanks (vv. 11–12). While vv. 2–4 mainly speak of YHWH in the 3rd person—although v. 2b // v. 3b switch to a form of direct address, in other words the prayer form—vv. 12–13 look ahead to the supplicant's healing and cultic restitution, including elements of an individual prayer of gratitude. The look back on his distress, introduced with a citation formula (v. 4aα) and concluding with a plea (vv. 4–10), not only includes two citations from the enemy (vv. 5b, 8)—it is also framed by the echoing supplication "Lord, be merciful to me!" (vv. 4a, 11a). A schematic analysis produces the following overview:

> *Heading*
> To the Chief Musician. A Psalm of David.
> *Wisdom-based, parenetic sentence*
> 1   General beatitude
> 2–3   Explication with regard to
>   2   Enemy persecution
>   3   Illness
> *Lament followed by request*
> 4aα   Citation formula
> ab.b   Request and confession of sin
> 5–9   Description of distress (= enemy-related complaint)
> 10   Request and desire for compensation
> *Avowal of thanks*
> 11   Confidence in being heard
> 12   Cultic reintegration
> *Final doxology* for the 1st Psalm of David (Pss. 2–40)
> 13   *Blessed be the Lord God of Israel*
>   *From everlasting to everlasting! Amen and Amen.*

The circumstance of illness forms the background of Ps 41. However, the entire psalm was clearly not written from a sickbed, only the middle section, namely the lament in vv. 4–10. The location of the entire psalm can thus be determined from the sections vv. 1–3 and vv. 12–13 that frame this lament, according to which the psalm was presented (in the temple?) *after* the supplicant had been healed (vv. 3b, 12). Thus the patient's healing took place during the time between the prayer of supplication on the sickbed (vv. 4–10)[37] and the public presentation of the entire psalm (vv. 1–12) to the cultic community. The supplicant's situation when he speaks this psalm is described by vv. 12–13 and particularly by v. 12b ("before your face"). Thus the supplicant is in a *"cultic situation . . . in which the deity, who is considered to be present, and a listening community can be addressed without the address and format of a prayer."*[38] The subject of this address is made clear by the lament in vv. 4–10, thanks to the correlation between *sin and illness* as well as between *physical sphere and social sphere.*

Religious Aspects of Illness

At the center of Ps 41 is the explicit lamentation (vv. 4–10), which begins with an introductory citation (v. 4aα) and includes two requests: one for mercy (v. 4aβ // v. 10aα) and the other for healing (v. 4 b):

> I said, "Lord, be merciful to me;
> Heal me/my life (*nefeš*), for I have sinned against You."

Other lamentations also include requests for healing;[39] Ps 6:1–3[40] is especially interesting because its request shows that "healing" (*rp'*) does not simply refer to binding up wounds, but to "reviving" body and soul:

> 1 O Lord, do not rebuke me in Your anger,
>   Nor chasten me in Your hot displeasure.
> 2 Have mercy on me (*ḥnn*), O Lord, for I am weak,
>   Heal me (*rp'*), O Lord, for my bones are troubled (*bhl* nif.)!
> 3 My soul also (*nefeš*) is greatly troubled (*bhl* nif.),
>   But You, O Lord—how long?

In Psalm 104, too, the hiding of the divine face leads to a sense of "being troubled" (*bhl* nif.)[41] among all living creatures, and to the withdrawal of life-giving breath. In the final summarizing section (vv. 27–30), YHWH is

---

37. Cf. the reference to the "bed of illness" in v.4a.
38. Seybold, *Gebet des Kranken*, 109 (emphasis original).
39. Cf. Ps. 6:3; 30:3; 60:4; 107:20; 147:3 passim.
40. On this text and on the question of a *cultic* space in life for the lamentations, see Achenbach, "Zum Sitz im Leben mesopotamischer und altisraelitischer Klagegebete," II.584ff.
41. Cf. Janowski, *Konfliktgespräche mit Gott*, 62ff. The idea that the turning away of the divine face results in the start of chaos ("deathly silence") as well as the dissolution of all social bonds ("protective roof") is also a topos of Mesopotamian prayer literature, cf. ibid., 63–64.

praised as a giver of life; in other words, the experience is expressed that providing nourishment ("food," vv. 27–28) and making life possible ("breath/spirit," vv. 29–30) are gifts of the Creator God:

> 27 These all (animals and people) wait for You,
>   That You may give them their food in due season.
> 28 What You give them they gather in;
>   You open Your hand, they are filled with good.
> 29 You hide Your face (*str* hif.), they are troubled (*bhl* nif.),
>   You take away their breath, they die and return to their dust.
> 30 You send forth Your Spirit, they are created;
>   And You renew the face of the earth.

The theme of "life granted by God" can already be found in v. 14 (grass for the cattle and plants for the service of man) and in v. 21 (young lions "roar after," or seek, their food from God). In addition, vv. 27–30 use the image of a creaturely longing to describe the dependency of people and animals on the life-giving God who provides his creatures with all that is necessary for life (food and breath). The aspect of "spirit" (*rûaḥ*)—Gen 2:7 also refers to "the breath of life" (*nᵉšāmāh*) in a similar fundamental context—is associated with God's face here, which brings death when it is hidden (V. 29)[42] and life for all creatures when it is shown (v. 30).[43] According to Ps 41, this experience of death can only be overcome through an act of "healing," a "revitalization" or a *return to life*.[44] "Since illness was seen as the process of being gripped by death, healing is a return to life"[45]—and it is a return that can only be brought about by "YHWH the healer"—"I am the Lord who heals you (Israel)" (Ex 15:26).[46]

With the confession of sin in Ps 41:4bβ—"Heal my soul, for I have sinned against You"[47]—the supplicant indicates that he is aware of sin as the cause of illness. Perhaps he is familiar with the rule:

---

42. On v. 29a, in addition to Ps 13:2, also compare Pss 10:1; 30:8; 44:25; 69:18; 88:15; 143:7 passim; on vv. 29b–30, cf. Ps 146:4; Job 10:12; 12:10; and 34:14–15.

43. On the connection between the "breath of life" and "vitality," see Wolff, *Anthropologie des Alten Testaments*, 96ff.

44. Cf. Ps 41:2a: *ḥjh* pi. "preserve, keep alive"!

45. Lohfink, "Gott, Gesellschaft und menschliche Gesundheit," 126 Note 102, cf. also Niehr, "JHWH als Arzt," 11f.

46. Cf. Deut 32:29f; 1 Sam 2:6; Hos 6:1; and Lohfink, "Gott, Gesellschaft und menschliche Gesundheit," 121ff and Brown, "*rp*," 623–24.

47. Cf. 2 Sam 12:13; and Job 33:27–28.

He who covers his sins will not prosper,
But whoever confesses and forsakes them will have mercy. (Prov 28:13)[48]

Social Aspects of Illness

The subsequent description of the enemy in Ps 41:5–9 is in many ways reminiscent of Job 19:13–20, where Job's illness is described not only as physical suffering (cf. v. 17 and v. 20),[49] but also as a physical and social affliction that is reinforced by the behavior of the "in group," his familiar circle of family and friends:[50] neighbors become strangers, and friends become enemies. Even Job's nearest and dearest, his wife and his children as well as his servants, keep their distance and avoid contact with the oppressed man:

> 13 He (God) has removed my brothers far from me,
>   and my acquaintances are completely estranged from me.
> 14 My relatives have failed,
>   and my close friends have forgotten me.
> 15 Those who dwell in my house, and my maidservants,
>   Count me as a stranger;
>   I am an alien in their sight.
> 16 I call my servant, but he gives no answer;
>   I beg him with my mouth.
> 17 My breath is offensive to my wife,
>   And I am repulsive to the children of my own body.
> 18 Even young children despise me;
>   I arise, and they speak against me.
> 19 All my close friends abhor me,
>   And those whom I love have turned against me.
> 20 My bone clings to my skin and to my flesh,
>   And I have escaped by the skin of my teeth. (Job 19:13–20)[51]

The enemies who appear in Ps 41:6–10 and try to make the supplicant's suffering definitive belong to different groups:

First there appear the 'ôyᵉbîm enemies. Their opposition to the supplicant is heightened to a deadly enmity, which is primarily expressed through

---

48. Cf. Hossfeld and Zenger, *Psalmen I*, 263 (Hossfeld).

49. Cf. also Lang, "Ein Kranker sieht seinen Gott," 138f.

50. Cf. Pss 27:10; 31:12; 35:13–14; 38:10–15; 41:6–7, 10; 55:14–15; 69:9; 88:9, 19 passim.

51. Translation Ebach, *Streiten mit Gott*, 151f; on this text, see also Seybold, "Gebet des Kranken," 51ff.

the *annihilating word*. The enemy's citation in v. 5b ("When will he die, and his name perish?") formulates a double death wish: the *damnatio vitae* and the *damnatio memoriae*. The physical death of the supplicant is to be exceeded and sealed by the vanishing of his "name" from the social memory of the community. In Egypt, too, the image of death through social isolation is contrasted with the image of life through social connectivity. This image of life, according to J. Assmann,

> can best be reconstructed from two maxims already mentioned at the outset of this book. One of them reads, "One lives, if another guides him" and refers above all to life *before* death. The other is, "One lives, if his name is mentioned," and it refers above all to life *after* death. But both refer to a single concept of life, one that is based on the principle of social "connectivity." A solitary person is not capable of life, that is, alive in the full sense of the word. There must be someone else to take him by the hand and guide him. By the same token, he is also not dead, so long as there are others to mention his name, so long as the bond of connectivity is not broken."[52]

According to Ps. 41:6 ("And if he comes to see [me] . . ."), neighbors and/or relatives (?) appear to be paying a sick visit. This enemy does three things: his heart, the central human organ,[53] speaks falsehoods and "gathers iniquity," in other words, incriminating material, and takes it out into the world[54] to be told on the streets. Verses 8–9, which completes the previous description of the enemy, is formulated with great sensitivity toward (social) psychological processes. For upon closer inspection, the "evil disease" that the enemies ascribe to the patient is in fact coming from them. In Prov 6:12–15, we read how this mechanism works:

> 12 A worthless person, a wicked man,
>   Walks with a perverse mouth;
> 13 He winks with his eyes,
>   He shuffles his feet,
>   He points with his fingers;
> 14 Perversity is in his heart,
>   He devises evil continually,

---

52. Assmann, "Death and Salvation in Ancient Egypt," 39, 73ff. Just as naming is a creative and possessive or acknowledging act, the loss of the name is equivalent to erasing all memories of its bearer; cf. Keel and Schroer, *Schöpfung. Biblische Theologien*, 135.

53. Cf. Janowski, *Konfliktgespräche mit Gott*, 166ff.

54. It is important to note the contrast between "his heart" (*inside*) and "goes out" (*outside*).

> He sows discord.
> 15 Therefore his calamity shall come suddenly;
> Suddenly he shall be broken without remedy.[55]

With the appearance of the "own familiar friend" who "ate my bread," the description of the enemy reaches its height, introduced by the word "even." The "familiar friend," or the one with whom the supplicant previously lived in *shalom*,[56] was the one whom the supplicant trusted and with whom he shared meals. This person has now "lifted up his heel" against him. The terrible nature of this breach of trust is emphasized by Job 19:19, and particularly by the "friend laments" in Ps 55:12–15 and Sir 37:2:

> All my close friends abhor me,
> And those whom I love have turned against me. (Job 19:19)

> 12 For it is not an enemy who reproaches me;
> Then I could bear it.
> Nor is it one who hates me who has exalted himself against me;
> Then I could hide from him.
> 13 But it was you, a man my equal,
> My companion and my acquaintance.
> 14 We took sweet counsel together,
> And walked to the house of God in the throng. (Ps 55:12–14)[57]

> The sorrow when a close friend becomes an enemy
> Is almost like mourning for a friend who has died. (Sir 37:2)[58]

The description of the enemy in Ps 41:5–11, which represents a small *phenomenology of social death*,[59] is extremely dramatic. It begins with the an-

---

55. Furthermore, despite the differences between the Book of Job and the psalms on illness in the Psalter, Job 2:11–13 clearly shows how the visitors in Ps 41:6–9 should behave: Job's three friends "made an appointment together to come and mourn with him, and to comfort him (Job)" (v. 11). Even from far away, they looked up "(12) and did not recognize him, (and) they lifted their voices and wept; and each one tore his robe and sprinkled dust on his head toward heaven (13). So they sat down with him on the ground seven days and seven nights, and no one spoke a word to him, for they saw that his grief was very great." Cf. the interpretation by Lohfink, "Klageriten," 263ff.

56. Cf. Jer 20:10; 38:22; and Obad 7.

57. Translation by Hossfeld and Zenger, *Psalmen 51–100*, 94 (Hossfeld). On the term "friend lament," cf. Hossfeld and Zenger, *Psalmen 51–100*, 97, 100 (Hossfeld); and also Keel, *Feinde und Gottesleugner*, 132ff., as well as Bauks, *Feinde des Psalmisten*, 76ff.

58. Sir 37:1–6 also discusses table fellowship, but this disintegrates in the time of need: "Some friends are happy for you when everything is fine, but when you have trouble they turn against you" (v. 4).

59. On the term "social death," see Janowski, *Konfliktgespräche mit Gott*, 47–48.

nihilating death wish from external "enemies" (v. 6), but then focuses on an individual visitor (a neighbor or family member?) who exploits the supplicant's helplessness (v. 7) and accompanies this person from the sickbed out into the street, where people have already begun to destroy the victim by ganging up on him and declaring a downright death sentence (v. 8f). As if that were not enough, the familiar friend then appears, standing out from the crowd of enemies because he was part of the oppressed person's immediate circle (table fellowship)[60] and has now become the greatest threat to him. This *contrast between intimate closeness and greatest threat* is introduced in v. 9 with the heightening particle "even":

> "enemies," neighbor(s), relatives
> 5   death wish: "When will he die . . . ?"
> 6   visit to the patient: speaking lies // gathering iniquity
> 7   collaboration: whispering // devising hurt
> 8   death sentence: "An evil disease . . ."
> *Trusted friend*
> 9aα   Even my own familiar friend
>   ab.b   Who ate my bread

According to Ps 41:8, the enmity against the patient is expressed as "hatred," which is also enacted through a conspiracy: "all" who hate him whisper against the sick supplicant and devise harm against him. The details of this harm are specified in the death sentence in v. 8, with the unusual phrase "an evil disease,"[61] which "clings" to the patient like a liquid. Just as in Ps 18:4–5, this evokes the image of a person who has already entered the underworld and experienced its life-destroying power:

> 4 The *pangs of death* surrounded me,
>   And the *floods of ungodliness* made me afraid.
> 5 The *sorrows of Sheol* surrounded me;
>   The *snares of death* confronted me.[62]

In light of this lament, the declaration of death in Ps 41:9 indicates that, in the eyes of his enemies, the supplicant has already been caught up in the chaotic "floods of ungodliness" (Ps 18:4b) and is surrounded on all sides.[63]

---

60. The aspect of social intimacy and its abuse, in addition to the abovementioned texts, is also mentioned in Ps 35:13–14, cf. Jer 20:7–18 passim; cf. Bail, *Gegen das Schweigen klagen*, 171ff.

61. Cf. Pss 18:5 and 101:3.

62. On the topic of chaos in Ps 18:5–6, cf. Adam, *Der königliche Held*, 55ff.

63. The feeling of being surrounded and besieged by enemies, caught as if in a net, is typical of the experiences of suffering described in the individual lamentations; cf. Lamp and Tilly, "Öffentlichkeit als Bedrohung," 51–52.

Since the word *bᵊlijja'al*, as shown by the semantics in Ps 18:4–5, has a *relationship to the chaotic*, it is often used for things that are hostile to God and harmful to society.[64]

A parallel passage on this *cosmic dimension of illness* can be found in the famous bronze tablet from Assyria (Fig. 2),[65] according to which the patient was subject to the effects of demonic forces and hoped that good would win out over evil in battle. These and similar representations are derived from a specific concept of illness and healing based on the close correlation between magical/religious and medical/therapeutic aspects, one that is particularly distinguished by its worldview-like dimension and its focus on the relationship between the sick person and the gods.[66]

---

64. On the significance of *bᵊlijja'al* cf. Otzen, "belija‚ al," 55 nn. 37–39.

65. The illustration comes from Janowski, *Konfliktgespräche mit Gott*, 191. On the Lamaštu amulet, see also Pezzoli-Olgiati, "Die Gegenwelt des Todes," 387ff.

66. Cf. Maul, "Die 'Lösung von Bann,'" 79–95; also Achenbach, "Zum Sitz im Leben mesopotamischer und altisraelitischer Klagegebete I," 367ff.

"*Heal me, for I have sinned against you!*" *(Psalm 41:5MT)* 191

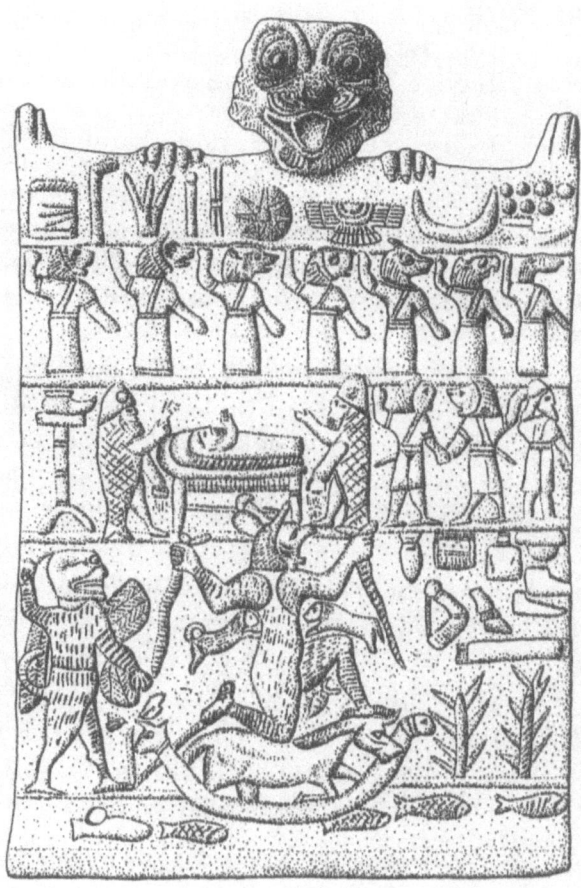

Fig. 2: Assyrian *Lamaštu* **amulet (early first millennium BCE)**

Description of the amulet: In the *middle row*, we see the patient—an adult male—lying on his sickbed, his hands raised to the great gods represented in the *top row* together with their symbols: *Anu* (horned hat), *Ea* (ram's head), *Adad* (bundle of lightning bolts), *Marduk* (digging stick), *Nabu* (writing utensil), *Ištar* (star of Venus), *Šamaš* (winged sun), *Sîn* (crescent moon) and *Sebettu* (seven-pointed star). At the head and foot of his bed are two exorcists (*āšipu*) dressed in fish masks and holding cleansing vessels, into which they are clearly dipping clusters of plants in order to sprinkle the patient. The entire event —as indicated by the oil lamp at left—is probably taking place at night. The significance of the scenery is explained by the *bottom row*: *Lamaštu* the demoness of fever, wearing a lion's head, with two-headed snakes in each hand and the unclean animals, a pig and a dog, at her breasts, is threatened by the demon *Pazuzu* and sent away from the patient's presence on a boat, to traverse the Ulaja River and go out onto the ocean (known as a travel scene). She is kneeling on an onager (a type of wild donkey), which is standing in a reed boat with upward-curving animal-shaped protomes. The gesture of banishment (raised right hand) is echoed in the second and third rows by cult actors wearing animal masks, and thereby reinforced. The head of the apotropaic demon *Pazuzu* peers over the *top edge* of the amulet and is shown once again in the bottom row as he banishes the fever demoness.

As we can see, the *symbolism of animals* plays a central role in the Mesopotamian healing process:

> Clean (edible) animals seem to represent the positive powers, while unclean (inedible) animals represent the negative. It should be noted that every culture has developed its own criteria for cleanliness. However, some animals, like the demons themselves, have an ambivalent character and embody both powers (lion, snake).[67]

In addition, exorcists appear in fish costumes and lion masks, while other figures mediate between the world of the upper gods (top row) and the world of the people (middle row). Even the illness is represented as a chimera with an animal form (the fever demoness *Lamaštu*). Finally, the *cosmic aspect of the representation* is important in our context, because the patient's case

> draws wide circles on Earth, in two lower realms and one upper realm of the world (this was formerly known as a 'Hades relief'); sets actions in motion that begin in the social, cultic/ritual realms and affect the entire inhabited world, gods, demons; sparks battles in the in-between areas where spirits fight over the patient, and only the intervention of the Ea priests, enforcing the powers of the upper world, can save him.[68]

From here, let us return to Ps 41: the plea in v. 10 begins with a double invocation, "But you, Lord" and continues with a plea for mercy ("may you have mercy on me," cf. v. 4a) and for revitalization ("raise me up").[69] However, what is unusual and singular is the final request that the supplicant be able to settle his accounts with his enemies (v. 10b). With regard to the

---

67. Staubli, "Biblische Speisetabus," 52; cf. also Janowski and Neumann-Gorsolke, "Reine und unreine Tiere," 214–18.

68. Seybold and Müller, *Krankheit*, 24 (Seybold).

69. Cf. the contrasting formulation from the mouths of the "haters" in v. 8b: "he will never get up from the place where he lies."

issue of revenge, I mentioned the fine line between an *assumption of revenge* and a *refusal of revenge* that exists in the psalms of lamentation. Here, this line is crossed in the direction of the supplicant's self-empowerment to take revenge. Thus it contradicts the otherwise closely followed warning in Prov 20:22:

> Do not say, "I will pay you back for this wrong (*šlm* pi.)!"
> Wait for the Lord, and he will avenge you.[70]

However, as if this wish for revenge had caught in his throat, the supplicant admits in v. 11, "I know that you are pleased with me, for my enemy does not triumph over me." He thus also acknowledges that the enemy's end may have completely different reasons than he could have imagined in his time of distress.[71]

SUMMARY

Based on selected Old Testament psalms about illness and healing, we have sketched out the expressive potential and individual conceptions that, as indicators of religious language, are obligated to follow a pre-modern but not irrational logic. This logic centers around the concept of a "constellation," which in turn refers to the complex relationships and fundamental situations that give human life its meaning and direction. Three aspects are relevant for our topic and should once again be emphasized.

Relationship with God and Self

The Old Testament concept of illness and healing, as shown in the example of Ps 41, has both a religious and a social dimension. The *religious dimension of illness* can be seen from the fact that "sin," which the ill supplicant acknowledges before God in Ps 41:4, signifies the disruption and reversal—the Old Testament refers to "error"[72]—of balances that are necessary for life. The criterion of what is necessary for life can be found in Israel's fundamental

---

70. Cf. also Pss 31:24; 62:13; 94:23; and 109:15, 20.

71. This touches on the question of how the end of the heretic/enemy is represented in the individual lamentations. As a rule, the answer is that the heretics/enemies are destroyed by the self-destructive nature of their actions, while YHWH rescues the just from their distress/death; see Sticher, "Rettung der Guten durch Gott," 26–27.

72. *ḥāṭā'* "to fall into error," *ḥaṭṭā't* "error"; on this and the other sin-related terms in the Old Testament, cf. Janowski, *Ein Gott, der straft und tötet?*, 236ff.

conviction that "life is constitutively bound to YHWH,"[73] a conviction that shapes all statements about existence and is specified differently according to the situation.

Bodily Sphere and Social Sphere

In contrast to the moralization of an understanding of sin that is dissociated from the relationship with the self and with society,[74] in an Old Testament understanding the problem of sin is not limited to the individual person, but always relates to the person's social context. This *social dimension of illness* can be seen in the correlation between the bodily and social spheres, in the fact that the social realm—as is vividly shown in Ps 41:5-9—is shaped by a conflict structure that must be dissolved in order for healing to take place and justice/communal loyalty to be restored.

Life and Death

Finally, a fundamental question regards medical diagnosis and treatment, for which no clear terminology is defined in the Old Testament.[75] Instead, a "conventionalized typology"[76] is assumed that always refers to the overall framework of a religious approach to existence. The focus is not on the exact "scientific" diagnosis of illness, but on the "subjective perception of a disrupted life,"[77] in other words the experience of the threat of death, which means a definitive separation from YHWH, the God of life. This *concept of life and death* is the experiential and interpretative horizon within which all experiences of illness are able to build a bridge to an understanding of life that has not been entirely lost even in our post-secular society.

BIBLIOGRAPHY

Achenbach, R. "Zum Sitz im Leben mesopotamischer und altisraelitischer Klagegebete I." *ZAW* 116 (2004) 364–78.

———. "Zum Sitz im Leben mesopotamischer und altisraelitischer Klagegebete II." *ZAW* 116 (2004) 581–94.

73. Leuenberger, "Ausformungen," 366.
74. See also von Soosten, "Die 'Erfindung' der Sünde," 87–88.
75. Cf. Seybold, *Gebet des Kranken*, 168.
76. Ibid.
77. Brunert, *Psalm 102*, 116.

Adam, K.-P. *Der königliche Held: Die Entsprechung von kämpfendem Gott und kämpfendem König in Psalm 18*. WMANT 91. Neukirchen-Vluyn: Neukirchener, 2001.
Assmann, J. *Death and Salvation in Ancient Egypt*. Translated by David Lorton. Ithaca, NY: Cornell University Press, 2005.
Bail, U. *Gegen das Schweigen klagen: Eine intertextuelle Studie zu den Klagepsalmen Ps 6 und Ps 55 und der Erzählung von der Vergewaltigung Tamars*. Gütersloh: Gütersloher, 1998.
Bauks, M. *Die Feinde des Psalmisten und die Freunde Jobs: Untersuchungen zur Freund-Klage im Alten Testament am Beispiel von Psalm 22*. SBS 2003. Stuttgart: Kohlhammer, 2004.
Beyerle, St., "'Medizin'—Phänomene im Alten Israel und im antiken Judentum." In *Gesundheit: Humanwissenschaftliche, historische und theologische Aspekte*, edited by M. Roth and J. Schmidt, 45–78. Leipzig: Eva, 2008.
Briend, J. "Krankheit und Heilung im Alten Testament." *WUB* 18 (2000) 84–85.
Brown, M. L. "*rp*". In *ThWAT* 7 (1993) 617–25.
Crüsemann, F. "Im Netz: Zur Frage nach der 'eigentlichen' Not in den Klagen der Einzelnen." In *Kanon und Sozialgeschichte: Beiträge zum Alten Testament*, edited by F. Crüsemann, 157–64. Gütersloh: Gütersloher, 2003.
Ebach, J. *Streiten mit Gott: Hiob, Part 1: Hiob 1–20*. Kleine Biblische Bibliothek. Neukirchen-Vluyn: Neukirchener, 1996.
Ebner, M. "Krankheit und Heilung III." In *RGG4* 4 (2001) 1730–31.
Engelhardt, D. von. *Krankheit, Schmerz und Lebenskunst: Eine Kulturgeschichte der Körpererfahrung*. Munich: Beck, 1999.
Etzelmüller, G. "Der kranke Mensch als Thema theologischer Anthropologie." *ZEE* 53 (2009) 163–76.
Frevel, C. "Krankheit / Heilung." In *Handbuch theologischer Grundbegriffe zum Alten und Neuen Testament*, edited by A. Berlejung and C. Frevel, 284–88. 2nd ed. HGANT. Darmstadt: WBG, 2009.
Gerstenberger, E. S. "Krankheit." In *NBL* 2 (1995) 542–44.
Graf, F. W. "Neuzeit I." In *RGG*^{4} 6 (2003) 254–59.
Gunkel, H. *Introduction to Psalms: The Genres of the Religious Lyric of Israel*. Completed by Joachim Begrich. Translated by J. D. Nogalski. Mercer Library of Biblical Studies. Macon, GA: Mercer University Press, 1998.
Habermas, J. *Glauben und Wissen*. Frankfurt: Suhrkamp, 2001.
Hossfeld, F.-L., and E. Zenger. *Die Psalmen I: Psalm 1–50*. NEB 29. Würzburg: Echter, 1993.
———. *Psalmen 51–100*. HThK.AT. Freiburg: Herder, 2000.
Janowski, B. "Anthropologie des Alten Testaments: Grundfragen—Kontexte—Themenfelder." *ThLZ* 139 (2014) 535–55.
———. *Ein Gott, der straft und tötet? Zwölf Fragen zum Gottesbild des Alten Testaments*. Neukirchen-Vluyn: Neukirchener Theologie, 2013.
———. "Freude an der Tora. Psalm 1 als Tor zum Psalter." *EvTh* 67 (2007) 18–31.
———. "'Heile mich, denn ich habe an dir gesündigt!' (Ps 41,5): Zum Konzept von Krankheit und Heilung im Alten Testament." In *Krankheitsdeutung in der postsäkularen Gesellschaft: Theologische Ansätze im interdisziplinären Gespräch*, edited by G. Thomas and I. Karle, 47–66. Stuttgart: Kohlhammer, 2009.

———. "Die 'Kleine Biblia': Die Bedeutung der Psalmen für eine Theologie des Alten Testaments." In *Die rettende Gerechtigkeit*, edited by B. Janowski, 125–64. Beiträge zur Theologie des Alten Testaments 2. Neukirchen-Vluyn: Neukirchener, 1999.

———. *Konfliktgespräche mit Gott: Eine Anthropologie der Psalmen*. 4th ed. Neukirchen-Vluyn: Neukirchener, 2013.

———. "Der Mensch im alten Israel: Grundfragen alttestamentlicher Anthropologie." *ZThK* 102 (2005) 143–75.

Janowski, B., and U. Neumann-Gorsolke. "Reine und unreine Tiere." In *Gefährten und Feinde des Menschen: Das Tier in der Lebenswelt des alten Israel*, edited by B. Janowski et al., 214–18. Neukirchen-Vluyn: Neukirchener, 1993.

Keel, O. *Feinde und Gottesleugner: Studien zum Image der Widersacher in den Individualpsalmen*. SBM 7. Stuttgart: Katholisches Bibelwerk, 1969.

Keel, O., and S. Schroer. *Schöpfung: Biblische Theologien im Kontext altorientalischer Religionen*. 2nd ed. Göttingen: Vandenhock & Ruprecht, 2008.

Körtner, U. H. J. "Mit Krankheit leben: Der Krankheitsbegriff in der medizinischen Diskussion." *ThLZ* 130 (2005) 1273–90.

Kuckhoff, A. *Psalm 6 und die Bitten im Psalter: Ein paradigmatisches Bitt- und Klagegebet im Horizont des Gesamtpsalters*. BBB 160. Göttingen: Vandenhoeck & Ruprecht, 2011.

Lamp, E., and M. Tilly. "Öffentlichkeit als Bedrohung: Ein Beitrag zur Deutung des 'Feindes' im Klagelied des Einzelnen." *BN* 50 (1989) 46–57.

Lang, B. "Ein Kranker sieht seinen Gott." In *Wie wird man Prophet in Israel? Aufsätze zum Alten Testament*, edited by B. Lang, 137–48. Düsseldorf: Patmos, 1980.

Leuenberger, M. "'Dein Gnade ist besser als Leben' (Ps 63:4): Ausformungen der Grundkonstellation von Leben und Tod im alten Israel." *Bib* 86 (2005) 343–68.

Lohfink, N. "Enthielten die im Alten Testament bezeugten Klageriten eine Phase des Schweigens?" *VT* 12 (1962) 260–77.

———. "Ich bin Jahwe, dein Arzt' (Ex 15,26): Gott, Gesellschaft und menschliche Gesundheit in einer nachexilischen Pentateuchbearbeitung (Ex 15:25b.26)." In *Studien zum Pentateuch*, edited by N. Lohfink, 91–155. SBAB 4. Stuttgart: Katholisches Bibelwerk, 1988.

Maul, S. M. "Die 'Lösung von Bann': Überlegungen zu altorientalischen Konzeptionen von Krankheit und Heilkunst." In *Magic and Rationality in Ancient Near Eastern and Graeco-Roman Medicine*, edited by H. F. J. Horstmanshoff and M. Stol, 79–95. Studies in Ancient Medicine 27. Leiden: Brill, 2004.

Niehr, H. "JHWH als Arzt, Herkunft und Geschichte einer alttestamentlichen Gottesprädikation." *BZ* 35 (1991) 3–17.

Oeming, M. *Das Buch der Psalmen: Psalm 1–41*. NSK.AT 13/1. Stuttgart: Kohlhammer, 2000.

———. "'Mein Herz ist durchbohrt in meinem Innern' (Ps 109,22): Krankheit und Leid in alttestamentlicher Sicht." In *Krankheit und Leid in der Sicht der Religionen*, edited by M. Oeming, 5–28. Osnabrück: Universität Osnabrück, 1994.

Otto, E. "Magie—Dämonen—göttliche Kräfte. Krankheit und Heilung im Alten Orient und im Alten Testament." In *Heilung—Energie—Geist: Heilung zwischen Wissenschaft, Religion und Geschäft*, edited by W. H. Ritter and B. Wolf, 208–25. Göttingen: Vandenhoeck & Ruprecht, 2005.

Otzen, B. "bᵉlijjaʽal." In *ThWAT* 1 (1973) 654–65.

Pezzoli-Olgiati, D. "Die Gegenwelt des Todes in Bild und Text: Ein religionswissenschaftlicher Blick auf mesopotamische Beispiele." In *Bilder als Quellen (FS O. Keel)*, edited by S. Bickel et al., 379–401. OBO Sonderband. Göttingen: Vandenhoeck & Ruprecht, 2007.

Rothschuh, K. E. "Krankheit." *HWP* 4 (1976) 1184–90.

Ruwe, A., and D. Starnitzke. "Krankheit / Heilung." In *Sozialgeschichtliches Wörterbuch zur Bibel*, edited by F. Crüsemann et al. 315–20. Gütersloh: Gütersloher, 2009.

Scharbert, J. "Krankheit II." In *TRE* 19 (1990) 680–83.

Schramme, Th., ed. *Krankheitstheorien*. stw 2011. Frankfurt: Suhrkamp, 2012.

Seybold, K. *Das Gebet des Kranken im Alten Testament: Untersuchung zur Bestimmung und Zuordnung der Krankheits- und Heilungspsalmen*. BWANT 99. Stuttgart: Kohlhammer, 1973.

———. *Die Psalmen*. HAT 1/15. Tübingen: Mohr/Siebeck, 1996.

Seybold, K., and U. Müller. *Krankheit und Heilung*. Biblische Konfrontationen. Stuttgart: Kohlhammer Taschenbücher, 1978.

Soosten, J. von. "Die 'Erfindung' der Sünde: Soziologische und semantische Aspekte zu der Rede von der Sünde im alttestamentlichen Sprachgebrauch." *JBTh* 9 (1994) 87–110.

Staubli, Th. "Warum man Hühner aß, aber keine Schweine: Biblische Speisetabus und ihre Folgen." In *Im Schatten deiner Flügel': Tiere in der Bibel und im Alten Orient,"* edited by O. Keel and Th. Staubli, 46–57. Freiburg: Freiburg Universitätsverlag, 2001.

Sticher, C. *Die Rettung der Guten durch Gott und die Selbstzerstörung der Bösen: Ein theologisches Denkmuster im Psalter*. BBB 137. Berlin: Philo, 2002.

Wolff, H. W. *Anthropologie des Alten Testaments: Mit zwei Anhängen neu herausgegeben von B. Janowski*. Gütersloh: Gütersloher, 2010.

Zernecke, A. E. *Gott und Mensch in Klagegebeten aus Israel und Mesopotamien: Die Handerhebungsgebete Ištar 10 und Ištar 2 und die Klagepsalmen Ps 38 und Ps 22 im Vergleich*. AOAT 387. Münster: Ugarit Verlag, 2011.

10

"Let This House Be Healed" (Psalm 51)
—Robert B. Coote

ILLNESS: INDIVIDUAL AND CORPORATE

As is well known, in the Bible illness frequently takes on religious meaning through prayer for healing or restoration, based on confession of sin or, more often, protestation of innocence. Illness lies in the hands of God and hence can be addressed by appealing to God, with repentance as far as the illness is regarded as deserved, with complaint as far as undeserved.

Though even today a mainstay of common piety, the connection between sickness and sin is far from obvious to modern liberal intellectual and therapeutic communities and educated religious leaders and counselors, who may be more likely to regard it as an obstacle to accurate diagnosis and effective treatment. Informed observers, however, have supported both sides of this issue; and the potential therapeutic value of confession and complaint at least complicates the judgment. The critique of the common religious connection between sickness and sin depends on among other things a thoroughgoing understanding of its historical roots. It is hoped that this interpretation of Psalm 51 might contribute to such an understanding.

A somewhat less often observed but equally significant dimension of the relationship between religion and therapy in the Bible is this: not only the individual body but also the social body can fall ill. We are liable to perceive the extension of the meaning of illness to social or political disorder, reversible by the same repentance or protest, as metaphorical—a perception that may be one of several reasons behind the demise of national repentance in the much of the West. But in the ancient world the semantic range of words related to "illness" covered a wider area. This wider meaning lay deep in ancient Near Eastern understanding, and it is not uncommon in the Bible. Much of the book of Hosea, for example, is governed by the homology of individual and corporate illness.[1] Most of Psalms consists of prayers of complaint or repentance by the afflicted. In the rhetoric of these prayers, where assumptions of "deserved" and "undeserved" already presuppose a warrant of justice, either individual or corporate, the suppliant's precise ailment is often unclear. The language of illness blends inseparably with the language of social justice and of battle, and all three spheres can be either individual or collective.

As the prayer book, and later hymnbook, of the Temple, the Psalms were always of social significance, even when, as in the First-Temple period, their speaking subject was the individual, normally David or his heir. Early in the history of the Psalter, the relationship between the afflicted monarch and the body politic tended to be merely implicit. Following the fall of Jerusalem and the ruin of the Temple, after the Temple's restoration the body politic frequently replaced the king as subject, and the prayers added to the Psalter consisted mainly of corporate—the "we" of the political nation—complaint over the injustice of the Babylonian devastation of Jerusalem. Of corporate repentance the enlarged Psalter still said practically nothing explicit. However corporate repentance, which played a very significant and distinctive role in the Persian-period corpus of the Prophets[2] and several of the Writings, as well as Jewish practice, was not at all abandoned in the Psalter.[3] The prayers of the king, which continued to preponderate in the Psalter assemblage, readily took on an enhanced corporate significance in their new textual and liturgical context, particularly once the Jerusalem cult lost its reigning Davidic monarch, in the early fifth century BCE. This was especially so, given the interpretation of the Exile developed in the restored Temple's corpus of Prophets, of the king's prayers of repentance: the king, as the embodiment of the indicted, condemned, and sickened political nation, i.e. the disenfranchised and exiled ruling elite, had much to repent. More-

---

1. Hong, *The Metaphor of Illness and Healing in Hosea*.
2. For this essay, "Prophets" with capital "P" designates the texts of the canonical corpus of Prophets; "prophets" with lowercase "p" designates the individual prophets featured in or posited by the Prophets.
3. Among recent treatments: Newman, *Praying by the Book*; Bautch, *Developments in Genre*; Seitz, *The Place of the Reader in Jeremiah*, 67–75; Lambert, *Topics in the History of Repentance*; Boda, Falkand Werline, eds., *Seeking the Favor of God*.

over the Prophets played a further, more particular role in the reinterpretation of Psalm 51, arguably the most ardent, scrupulous prayer of repentance in the Bible.

In this one vital instance of Psalm 51, the most acutely repentant of all the psalms, this corporate significance is made virtually explicit, through reinterpretation, revision, and positioning. The *tertium quid* underlying this transformation was none other than the Temple itself. In Psalm 51 the primary calamity, in conceptual and rhetorical terms at least, is unambiguously an individual person's illness. What made it possible to construe Psalm 51 corporately in terms of the Temple and its wrecked sacrificial cult, i.e. as a plea for the healing of a social illness with supreme collective religious significance, was that the illness referred to was not just of a person, but also of a house: the psalmist likened himself, as will be explained, to a sick house. In the momentous post-Exilic reinterpretation of Psalm 51, the homology of individual and body politic brought into play two related correspondences, both again well rooted in ancient Near Eastern conceptuality: between person and house and between house and Temple.

THE PENITENT AS DISEASED HOUSE

Psalm 51, whose salient lines are as familiar as any in the Psalter, is the most popular penitential psalm in the church today. The text of the psalm known by people today embodies, like much of the Bible, several layers of meaning. These layers reflect different stages in a history of composition and therefore different settings of repentance. Each layer is related to other passages in the Bible, in what scholars now term intertextuality. There are at least four such layers in Psalm 51. In this section, we will look mainly at the first layer, with a glance at the second. In the next section we will look at layer three, which correlates the individual and the Temple, and, briefly, layer four, which reinforces the same correlation.

Psalm 51 seems originally to have had three equal parts or stanzas, here separated by dotted lines.[4]

---

4. In this psalm adjacent lines tied by similarities mark the boundaries between stanzas, as occurs occasionally in the Psalter. Lines of Hebrew poetry typically come in pairs (bicola). I surmise that in Psalm 51 each stanza consisted of six such pairs, here numbered. The translation reflects further conjectures, of the sort that are inevitable when dealing with the ubiquitous obscurities of biblical poetry. The bicolon in brackets is regarded as secondary, since it would fit the first stanza better than the second. Lines of Hebrew poetry are typically only so long; consistent with this constraint, in the third stanza several phrases appear in brackets to indicate that they are probably secondary expansions. The third stanza seems to lack its original final bicolon; perhaps

(1) Have mercy on me, God, in line with your constancy;
   in line with your abundant compassion wipe out my transgressions.
(2) Wash me thoroughly from my iniquity,
   and purify me from my sin;
(3) For I know my transgressions,
   and my sin is ever before me.
(4) Against you, against you only, have I sinned,
   and done what you see as evil,
(5) So that you are justified in your sentence,
   and accurate in your judgment.
(6) Indeed in inquity I was brought forth,
   and in sin my mother conceived me.
——- ——— ——- ——- - ———— ——- ——-

(1) Indeed you desire surety in the **daubed parts**,
   and in the **plugged section** you make me know prudence.
(2) **With hyssop confirm the removal of my sin**, that I might be **pure**;
   wash me, that I might be **whiter** than snow.
(3) Let me hear joy and gladness;
   let the bones you have crushed rejoice.
[Hide your face from my sins,
   and blot out all my iniquities.]
(4) Create for me a pure heart, God,
   and a firm wind renew within me.
(5) **Do not throw me away** from your presence,
   and your sacred wind do not withhold from me.
(6) Return to me the joy of your salvation,
   and with a free/ready wind sustain me.
——- ——— ——— ——— ——— ——-

(1) Let me teach transgressors your ways,
   that sinners might return to you.
(2) Deliver me from (my?) murder, God [my saving God],
   that my tongue may shout aloud your justice.
(3) My lord, may you open my lips,
   that my mouth may proclaim your praise.
(4) For you do not desire sacrifice,
   and [were I to offer it] a burnt offering you do not find
      pleasing.
(5) The sacrifices for God are a broken wind;
   a [broken and] crushed heart you, God, do not despise.

---

it was replaced by the lines added later, as indicated. The translation of many phrases is uncertain: this is particularly true of first stanza (5), second stanza (1) (however not the phrases in bold) and third stanza (2). All phrases in bold echo Leviticus 13–14.

(6?) . . . .

. . . .

____. ____ ____ ____ ____. ____

(Added) Be pleased to bring good to Zion;
    may you rebuild the walls of Jerusalem—
Then you will desire just sacrifices [whole burnt and whole offerings];
    then bulls may be offered on your altar.[5]

The three stanzas can be reduced to these themes: (1) Have mercy, I have sinned; (2) renew my "heart" (i.e. in Hebrew the mind, will, or intent) and especially my wind (i.e. breath); (3) so that in lieu of a thank-offering I can instruct others in your ways and praise—i.e. with thanksgiving, cf. Ps 50:14–15, 23. (Psalm 51 ends on an ironic note: God is pleased with a broken wind and crushed heart, the same wind and heart by which the psalmist, once properly humbled, can appeal for the restoration of heart and wind.) Or most succinctly: (1) I have sinned, but (2) renew my breath (3) to tell others of your mercy.

The psalmist appears to suffer from an illness, as implied in several places in the middle stanza, and on the basis of the ironic pair of lines "purge (as usually translated) me with hyssop . . . that I may be white" the comparison with the "leper," or sufferer from "scale disease," whose treatment is detailed in Leviticus 13 has often been made.[6] This is only partly correct. The middle stanza of Psalm 51 emphasizes inward elements, particularly the "heart" as usual in complaint psalms where a blameless will is essential for a plea of innocence or mercy, and "wind." This emphasis is introduced by two terms in the opening line of the middle stanza that have hitherto not, to my knowledge, been correctly understood, namely *ṭûḥôt* and *sātūm* (51:6 [Heb. v. 8]). The failure to understand these terms goes back at least as far as the Hellenistic period, when the line was translated into Greek, "For

    5. The verb may be either Qal ("bulls may ascend as sacrifices") or Hiphil ("they may offer bull sacrifices"); for this discussion the difference does not matter.

    6. The exact meaning of Hebrew *ṣara'at* has long been a mystery: "the symptoms described in Leviticus 13 do not correspond to any known skin disease" (Milgrom, *Leviticus*, 127). And of course there is no one ailment with a single name in English that afflicts people, clothing, and houses as in Leviticus 13–14. For this reason Milgrom translates *ṣara'at* with the vague phrase "scale disease." It is quite possible that *ṣara'at* is a cover term for various real ailments. At the same time the vagueness of the description of a skin ailment is in line with P's propensity for theory with little basis in empirical reality. The significance of the disease is however quite clear: again in Milgrom's analysis, it signifies what it has in common with the two other sources of impurity dealt with in adjacent laws, corpse/carcass and genital discharges, namely death, an interpretation confirmed by the symbolic value of the ritual devices of blood and additional red items, fresh (Hebrew "living") water, and free-flying bird: Milgrom, *Leviticus*, 12, 128–29, 134.

behold, you love truth: you have made evident to me the secret and hidden things of your wisdom." Since then the terms have been construed virtually universally as abstractions for "inward being," "secret heart" (both NRSV), "hidden self," and the like. The terms are, however, as nearly always in Hebrew poetic speech, graphic and vivid rather than abstract. Furthermore they are grammatically exactly what they appear to be, the feminine plural passive participle of the root *ṭwḥ*, entities that are "plastered, whitewashed, bedaubed," and the masculine singular passive participle of the root *stm*, an entity that is "plugged, stopped up." The reference is not to the "scale-diseased" person in Leviticus 13, but to the "scale-diseased" *wall* of a house in Leviticus 14:33–53 and the rites by which the wall ends up either "healed" or dismantled. The "plastered" entities are the replacement stones (fem. pl.) of the wall, and the "plugged" entity is the place in a wall where the replacement stones are inserted before being replastered.

The ritual prescription is as follows:

> Yahweh said to Moses and Aaron: When you come into the land of Canaan . . . and I put a blight of scale disease in a house, . . . the owner of the house shall come and tell the priest, "There seems to me to be some sort of blight in my house."

The priest shall give orders to clear out the house before the priest goes in to inspect the blight, or all that is in the house will become taboo; and afterward the priest shall go in to inspect the house. He shall inspect the blight. If a blight of green or red spots has formed on the walls of the house, and they appear to be deeper than the surface, the priest shall go outside to the door of the house and place the house under quarantine for seven days. On the seventh day, the priest shall come again, and if on inspection the blight has spread on the walls of the house, the priest shall give orders to pull out the stones with the blight on them and toss them outside the settlement, at a taboo location. He shall have the entire inside of the house scraped, and the mud plaster that is scraped off shall be dumped outside the settlement, at a taboo location. Then they shall take other stones and put them in the place of the stones tossed out, and take other plaster and daub the house.

If the blight breaks out again in the house, after he has had the stones pulled out, the house scraped, and the walls redaubed, the priest shall enter and inspect the house and confirm that the blight has spread, and if it still looks like a blight of scale diseases in the house, then the house is taboo. The house shall be torn down—stones, timber, plaster, and all—and carried outside the settlement, at a taboo location. Anyone who has entered the house while it was under quarantine shall be taboo until evening [i.e. the next day]; all who slept in the house shall wash their clothes, and all who ate in the house shall wash their clothes.

If the priest comes and inspects the house and the blight has not spread in the house after the house was redaubed, the priest shall declare the house pure, since the blight has healed. For de-tabooing the house, he shall take two birds, a piece of cedar, crimson yarn, and hyssop. He shall slaughter one of the birds over an earthen vessel containing fresh water. Then he shall take the piece of cedar, the hyssop, the crimson yarn, and the live bird and dip them in the blood of the slaughtered bird and the fresh water, and sprinkle the house seven times. Having thus confirmed the removal of sin with the blood of the bird, the fresh water, the live bird, the piece of cedar, the hyssop, and the crimson yarn, he shall release the live bird outside the settlement, in the open field. He shall have covered/expiated for the house and declared it pure (Lev 14:33–53).

The disease having been discovered, after a seven-day quarantine the priest returns to find that it has spread. The infected stones are removed, tossed away, and replaced, and the new stones are redaubed or whitewashed. Then comes the wait, the crisis: will the disease disappear or reappear? This is the moment of Psalm 51. If the scaly blotches erupt again, the house is demolished and the stones thrown away ("do not throw me away from your presence"). If they do not reappear, the wall is certified as "healed" and a rite is performed, involving sprinkling blood with hyssop, which "confirms the removal of the sin" (*hiṭṭē'*), after which the wall is "pure." (With respect to Leviticus, the rite does not "purge," the usual translation.) Thus in Psalm 51 the suppliant sees himself as afflicted with "scale disease" as both person and house. "You desire surety beneath the redaubed stones," the psalmist prays, referring to God's hoped-for preservation of the cleansed wall. "In the plugged up section of the wall you would have me know prudence (*hokmâ*)," he adds: in the wake of radical dismantling and reconstruction, the inner integrity of the rebuilt wall signifies "wisdom," i.e. a commitment to just and prudent behavior rooted in fear of God.

The participle *ṭūhôt* occurs in only one other place in the Bible, Job 38:36, a passage that in the history of interpretation has perplexed scholars as much as Ps 51:6. Understandably the usual approach has been to eschew the interpretation of one obscurity by another. But the two passages do in fact go a long way toward explaining each other. The subject of Job 38:34–38 is the rain-producing clouds—how do they do it? "Do you know how to make the clouds produce rain?" God asks Job. Here *ṭūhôt* must refer to the gray expanse of clouds against the sky: "Who [but God] has put *hokmâ* in the *ṭūhôt*," i.e. who but God has the knowledge and skill to put the necessary rain-making devices behind the veil of clouds? The picture of a painted gray surface concealing *hokmâ* is virtually identical to that of Ps 51:6.

Nor is the verb "daub" common in the Hebrew Bible, but Ezekiel 13 should be compared, where daub is said to cover falsehood contained in the "heart" (13:2) and "wind" (13:3). Ezekiel 13:1–16 condemns the prophets for not repairing the wall of the "house of Israel": they have daubed ("whitewashed") the wall to cover up their lies. And for general comparison of the image of Psalm 51 perhaps the most telling passage is Nehemiah 4:7 (Hebrew 4:1), which refers to the repair of Jerusalem's walls by the closing up (*sātam*) of gaps as a "healing" (*'arûkâ*) of the walls. "Nowhere is it stated or even intimated that the infection [of person or house] comes as a punishment for sin . . . Whereas calamitous events are elsewhere in Scripture ascribed to human disobedience of divine law, in this case there is no such attribution . . . Although God is clearly the author of the fungi ['scale disease' v. 34], nowhere is it intimated that they are a punishment for sin."[7] The "sin" or wrong lies in the house by God's act; it is removed, if at all, by God's act; and the removal is certified. The ritual, which in some earlier guise might have entailed a purgation, is "transformed into a symbolic purification; it becomes a religious, not a therapeutic, act."[8] This insight neither obviates nor contradicts the manifest theme of the psalm, the repentance of a remorseful sinner. The analogy is not between the psalmist and the owner or occupant of the house, sinner or not, but between the psalmist and the house itself, which for whatever reason has been afflicted, like the psalmist, by God. As such, the psalmist as much as the house is in need of ritual confirmation of his "de-sinning" (*haṭṭē'*). Nor, however, does this insight preclude the possibility that originally Psalm 51 referred not to precisely the purification rite described in Leviticus 14, but to a purgation rite on which the latter might be modeled.

So far we have dealt with Psalm 51 in its first or original stage, as an individual prayer of a common type. We look briefly now at a second stage of interpretation, which places the psalm together with other psalms of the same type. Psalm 51 is one of the traditional seven penitential psalms of the church, Psalms 6, 32, 38, 51, 102, 130, and 143. Most of the psalms "of David" do not express repentance, as pointed out above. But there are further penitential psalms among the psalms of David in addition to the traditional seven. Psalms 38, 39, 40, and 41 are all penitential; indeed they form a group, of which Psalm 51 was at one time likely to have been a part, as will become clear in a moment. (Psalm 25 is also a penitential psalm, as

---

7. Milgrom, *Leviticus*, 138–39.
8. Ibid., 133.

is Psalm 69 in part, which is similar to both Psalm 25 and Psalm 51.) This group of five penitential prayers—Psalms 38–41, 51—occurs about two-thirds of the way through a collection of "Davidic" psalms consisting mainly of the more usual protestations of innocence and incorporated into Psalms 2–89. This concentrated moment of self-mortification by the king in the royal chapel prayer service brings to mind the annual ritual humiliation of the king in the Babylonian *akitu* rite; it is not unique to the Bible. Whatever the reason for the creation and placement of this uncharacteristic moment in the Psalter, it attracted the attention of later Persian-period editors of the Psalter looking for places in the Temple scriptures where they could expand on the importance of corporate repentance.

THE HOUSE AS TEMPLE

We turn now to the further gradual reinterpretation of the Psalter over time—a thousand years, in my view, from as early as David to Herod and later. The focus will lie on the Persian-period composition of the Psalter in the section of the Psalter that includes Psalm 51 (Psalms 2–89).

The third stage of our treatment of Psalm 51 comes after the Babylonian exile, when the ruling house of David was deported to Babylon and placed at first under house arrest, to be kept in reserve until the right moment for redeployment by the Babylonian regime. The Babylonians never got around to sending the house of David back to Jerusalem. But the Persian conquerors of Babylon did. The Bible makes much of the role of Cyrus the Persian and his successors in sanctioning the restoration of the house of David and its temple in Jerusalem. Unfortunately the Bible is sketchy on the history of the restoration. At least the following is likely. Some of the second and third generations of exiles returned to Jerusalem—how many is not known. Within about 25 years the Temple ("house") was rebuilt, in 520–515 BCE on sparse biblical evidence. The house (dynasty) of David was involved in the rebuilding, as indicated by Haggai and Zechariah. But the house of David did not survive for long thereafter. The dynastic succession listed in Chronicles soon peters out, and Ezra and Nehemiah make no mention of the house of David at all. Thus by the middle of the fifth century, less than a hundred years after the Persian conquest, the house of David had disappeared from the picture altogether.

The failure and termination of the house of David represented a major crisis for the leaders of Jerusalem, especially the priesthood(s) of the Temple, which continued in operation despite the demise of the founding monarchic house. Normally, if a ruling house failed, its city failed with it—a frequent pattern throughout the pre-industrial history of the Middle East and Eastern Mediterranean. By all rights Jerusalem, the city of David, should have fallen into ruins along with the failed Davidic dynasty. The Persian-period compositions of the Hebrew Scriptures show a concerted effort to forestall such a development, and the third stage of the interpretation of Psalm 51 lies at the heart of that effort.

Like Jerusalem and the Temple, the Temple scriptures also survived, under the guardianship of the ruling priesthood. These scriptures included the corpus of the Prophets, whose denunciation of the house of David made all too clear why it had not survived. The corpus also included denunciations of the Davidic temple's cult, including its central element, animal sacrifice. These denunciations appear prominently at critical junctures in several of the prophetic books. The earliest of these is voiced by Samuel in 1 Sam 15:22–23, to justify the Davidic usurpation: "Has the Lord as great delight in burnt offerings and sacrifices as in obeying the voice of the Lord? Surely to obey is better than sacrifice, and to heed than the fat of rams. . . . Because you [Saul] have rejected the word of the Lord, he also has rejected you from being king." The same occurs in Amos 5:21–24: "I hate, I despise your festivals, and I take no delight in your assemblies. Though you offer me your burnt offerings and grain offerings, I will not accept them; and the *šelem*-offerings of your fatted animals I will not look upon . . . but let justice roll like the waters, and justice like a wadi that keeps flowing through the dry season" (NRSV "and righteousness like an everflowing stream"). And Hos 6:6: "For I desire loyalty and not sacrifice, acknowledging God rather than burnt offerings." And more of the same, especially in the great works of Isaiah and Jeremiah. These denunciations are an integral part of the indictment of the Temple that led, in the view of surviving generations, to the Temple's destruction.

In the face of such pronouncements against the Temple's rites, what could justify their restoration and continuance? This question was answered in a number of significant ways in the Temple scriptures themselves, in the process of becoming the Hebrew Scriptures. The use of Psalm 51 was one such way, and an extremely important one.

We will look at this use through two linked features of the psalm. The first is the addition of its last two verses (51:18–19 [Heb. 20–21]). The second is its juxtaposition with Psalm 50.[9] This second feature includes the relationship between Psalm 51 and an entire group of psalms added to the original Davidic prayer collection, which we will call the Levitical collection. We will look at that in a moment. Again bear in mind that the Hebrew

---

9. Cf. Zimmerli, "Zwillingspsalmen"; Gillingham, *Poems and Psalms*, 235.

word "house" can mean several things: not just a physical building, like a house whose walls can become infected with mildew or mold, but also a temple or the Temple in particular ("house" is the usual word for "temple"), a family, a household, an extended household/family, a ruling household or dynasty, the proprietary sovereignty of a household, a monarchy, or "state," and its economy.

Let us deal with these two features of Psalm 51 in order, first the addition to its end, then its placement next to Psalm 50.

The last two verses are widely viewed as an add-on: "Be pleased to bring good to Zion;/ may you rebuild the walls of Jerusalem—/ Then you will desire just sacrifices [whole burnt and *šelem*-offerings];/ then they may offer bulls on your altar." It is not unusual for extra lines to have been added to a psalm. Sometimes these additions are certain; other times they are only likely. One set of add-ons all scholars agree on: the doxologies that conclude each "book" of the Psalter (the final verses of Psalms 41, 72, 89, and 106, and the whole of Psalm 150 to cap the Psalter). The division of the Psalter into five "books" is a very late development, possibly the latest in the formation of the Psalter as we have it. Other examples are equally certain or nearly so: Psalm 25:22, since it lies outside an acrostic pattern; Psalm 34:23 for the same reason; Psalm 53:7, with its surprise reference to Zion, the same as in Psalm 14; and Psalm 69:34-36 [Hebrew 35-37], also with its sudden reference to Zion, in a psalm whose rhetoric has several points of contact with Psalm 51 (cf. 69:9, 30-31); thus probably Ps 3:8 [Heb. 9], and other passages. Why was Psalm 51 secondarily expanded in this way? Usually the reason is not known, but in the case of Psalm 51 the answer seems clear.

Probably this addition was made at the same time Psalm 51 was positioned immediately following Psalm 50. Now Psalm 50 is a very distinctive psalm, and among the psalms unique in its distinctiveness: it expresses the same idea that the Prophets do repeatedly, criticizing the sacrificial cult and asserting that God does not need burnt offerings to make him happy; what God wants is obedience to God's covenant, for people to walk in God's ways. In Psalm 50, God manifests himself at shining Zion as a devouring fire and proclaims, "Not for your sacrifices do I rebuke you; your burnt offerings are continually before me. But I will not accept a bull from your house, or goats from your folds." "I will not accept a bull from your house"—this is the line, as a number of commentators have recognized, to which the addition to Psalm 51 makes a direct response at the very end: "Then they may offer bulls on your altar." When? Following the repentance expressed and thanksgiving vowed in Psalm 51. If I want something to eat, God says, I don't need your help. "Every animal in the forest is mine, the cattle on a thousand hills. I know all the birds of the air, and all that moves in the field is mine. If I were hungry, I would not tell you, for the world and all that is in it is mine. Do I eat the flesh of bulls, or drink the blood of goats? Make thanksgiving your sacrifice to God, and pay your vows to the Most High" (50:10–14). The conclusion of Psalm 50 reiterates the point, anticipating Psalm 51: "Those who bring thanksgiving as their sacrifice honor me."

Clearly the whole of Psalm 51, with its new ending, responds to the challenge of Psalm 50: God says he will reject bull offerings, to which Psalm 51 responds that in the wake of repentance and public thanksgiving one can now expect that God will accept the Temple's offerings. And that to accommodate the restored altar cult God will rebuild the walls of the destroyed house—Temple, Temple precinct, and Temple city—in answer to the repentant prayer for integrity within the walls of the stricken house.

How did the juxtaposition of Psalm 50 and Psalm 51 come about? It came about with the enlargement of the collection of the Temple prayers of the house of David in the priestly Temple in Jerusalem in the Persian period. (The Psalms are often referred to as the "hymnbook of the Second Temple," and while that is far from true of the Psalter as a whole, it does apply to this and subsequent stages in the development of the Psalter.)

The gradual composition of the Psalter can be outlined in five relatively definable stages, not including the oral speech lying behind most of the psalms as prayer or hymn types.[10] Each successive stage incorporated the preceding stage(s). The stages are:

1. *David's prayer service*: songs of complaint and the plaintiff's confidence. Most of Psalms 3–71 with heading "for David," possibly Psalm 86 and others in Psalms 90–150 with "for David." The idea that a significant number of psalms could come from the time of David himself is not a widely held view; obviously this discussion does not depend on its validity.

2. The *prayer book of the Davidic/Solomonic Temple*: Psalms 2–72, Psalm 2 representing "David" and Psalm 72 "Solomon" (note the addition, Ps 72:20: "The prayers of David the son of Jesse are complete "), and possibly others in Psalms 91–150.

3. The *prayer book of the Persian-period Temple*: Psalms 2–89, beginning and concluding with references to the messianic promise of the house of David. We will elaborate on this stage below.

---

10. Of course not every psalm in a given grouping will be accurately represented by such an approximate scheme. To give just one example of an exception, it is very likely that Psalm 19 was introduced quite late into the earliest group of Davidic psalms.

4. The *hymnbook of the* (Hasmonean and) *Herodian Temple*: Psalms 2–150. Note the division between Books III and IV: Books I-III are clearly constructed; 11QPs, the great Roman-period Psalms scroll from Qumran, has only psalms from Books IV and V. The emphasis in Books IV and V on hymnic praise instead of complaint reflects the new splendor of the Herodian Temple. More importantly, Psalms 90–150 lack the promise to the house of David featured in Psalms 2–89 (even though it continues to contain many psalms attributed to David): this suggests the possibility that 11QPs might be an alternative Hasmonean or Herodian collection.[11]

5. The *psalmic torah*, a collection of prayers and hymns *for speculative ethical reflection*: Psalms 1–150, cf. Acts 13:32 "Western" text (D), in which Psalm 2 is identified as the "first" psalm. Here or in the preceding stage the division into Books I-V through use of appended doxologies.

Our interest now is in the *third* of these five stages, Psalms 2–89. Here the Davidic psalms appear divided into two sets, Psalms 2–41 and 51–72. The second set is framed within a set of "Levitical" psalms, Psalms 42–50 and 73–89. This Levitical framework is composed of three overlapping nests corresponding to the three branches of Levites. These three nests of psalms are attributed respectively to three musicians named in the services of the Temple in 1 Chronicles 1–15: Asaph, descendant of Gershom, the oldest son of Levi (1 Chr 6:39); Qorah, descendant of Qehat, the next son of Levi in order of age (6:22, 37); and Ethan, descendant of Merari, the youngest son of Levi (6:44). The nest of Asaph psalms comprises Psalms 50 and 73–83; the Qorah nest Psalms 42–49 and 84–88 (except, for some reason, Psalm 86, labeled a psalm of David); and the Ethan nest by Psalm 89 alone. (This Ethan is equated with Ethan in 1 Kgs 4:31 rather than the expected son of Merari, a change made later, when the pattern just described was not recognized.)

The main subjects of this Levitical framework are the complaint over the destruction of the Temple—to be sung in the Persian-period restored "Davidic" Temple as prayers that manifestly God has favorably answered—and the celebration of the restored Temple cult. In the Psalter, the "communal complaints," i.e. over the Temple, appear almost entirely in the Asaph collection: Psalms 74, 77, 79, 80, 82 (some), and 83. The other notable complaint is Qorahite: Psalm 44.

---

11. David is not mentioned in Books IV and V: the royal psalms 110 and 132 fail to identify the "anointed" of Yahweh with the *melek*, "part of a systematic avoidance of the term *melek* in relation to the Davidic dynasty in the whole of the last two books of the Psalter" (Wilson, online *Review of Biblical Literature* rev. of Haney, *Text and Concept Analysis in Royal Psalms*).

Now an all-important point: the Levitical framework could have enveloped the entire Davidic collection, since the usual approach to recomposition of this kind was to add a new beginning and a new ending. Instead the composer chose to use the Levitical framework to break into the Davidic collection and frame part of it. The composer was then free to insert the front or back end of the framework at any point. The choice must be revealing. An insertion of the front was chosen, and the point of insertion chosen was between Psalm 41 and 51, at the time adjacent to each other (recall the grouping of penitential psalms). Moreover, *just one* Asaph psalm was selected to form the front of the Asaph nest. The underscoring of the juxtaposition of Psalm 50 and Psalm 51 and its argument regarding the Temple's sacrifices could hardly have been more prominent: the most wrenching of David's prayers of repentance preceded by the sole front-end prayer of the singer representing the oldest of the three sons of Levi.

This juxtaposition was obviously extremely important: in terms of structure, it forms the central node, the heart, the nucleus of the Persian-period Psalter, Psalms 2–89. The addition to the end of Psalm 51 makes use of its original metaphor of a scale-diseased "house," now interpreted not figuratively of the dynastic founder David, but concretely of the personified Temple or its priestly officials representing the political nation. The addition to Psalm 51 and its juxtaposition with Psalm 50 enabled the composer of the collection Psalms 2–89 to address this basic issue of the restored cult: what makes the sacrifices of the Temple cult legitimate in the face of the critique of sacrifices in the Temple's Prophetic scriptures? This was a central issue involving the intersection of Temple cult and Temple scriptures, as well as Torah and Prophets, and here it is addressed at the exact structural center of the new Temple prayer/hymn book (Psalms 2–89). Psalm 51 as repentance thus neutralized the critique represented by Psalm 50, redeeming the Torah's central rite of sacrifice from the Prophetic critique of the Temple.[12] Again, for another psalm addition in similar terms, and composed probably around the same time, see Psalm 69:34–36 (or 35–36), in response to 69:30–31.

The centrality of repentance was reinforced and emphasized in the fourth and last development of Psalm 51, the addition of the heading that makes a connection with the Davidic narrative in 1 and 2 Samuel, one of thirteen such midrashic, or interpretive, headings, which are widely regarded as coming late in the development of the Psalter. The narrative heading to Psalm 51 says, "when the prophet Nathan came into him after

---

12. This maneuver can be seen in continuity with the prophetic tradition embodied in the Asaph collection; cf. Weber, "Gottesrede in 'Asaph-Texten.'"

he had gone into Bathsheba." This heading links Psalm 51 to 2 Sam 12:13, in midrashic style, especially through the correspondence of the phrase "against you only have I sinned." The allusion is to more than the story of David and Bathsheba, however. The birth of Solomon that followed David's repentance and the death of Bathsheba's first son by David was a fulfillment of God's promise to build David a "house," i.e. "dynasty," and the means by which the first "house" of the Lord, the Temple, came to be. At the time of the restoration of this Temple in the Persian period, the existence of the "house" or dynasty of David came under acute threat—indeed before long it was defunct—and Psalm 51 was read as a reiteration of David's original "house"-saving repentance.[13]

REPENTANCE AND THE SICKNESS OF THE BODY POLITIC

The third and fourth stages in the development of Psalm 51, based on the "national," or corporate, use of repentance, direct our attention back to the question of corporate repentance in the Bible, and national repentance in the modern world, and its potential role in healing the sickness of the body politic.

Whether in telling a story, making a case, or expressing godliness, the Bible presumes a great repentance. Since the Bible tells the story of a sociopolitical collective as well as individual stories, makes a case for that collective, and expresses the godliness of that collective, it presumes a collective repentance as well as an individual repentance.[14]

In the Hebrew Scriptures, repentance typically represents a great turning point. Corporate and individual repentance tend to become one. The extended story that forms the foundation of the Pentateuch, called J by scholars, makes one of its two or three greatest turns on Judah's repentant appeal to Joseph to let him become Joseph's slave in place of Benjamin: at

---

13. A grand correspondence has been posited between Psalms 51–72 and the narrative of Solomon's succession in 2 Samuel-1 Kings: Goulder, *The Prayers of David*. Goulder argues that this correspondence goes back to David himself (including Ps 51:18–19, pp. 67–68). The argument is unlikely; if the correspondence is valid, it more likely represents an elaboration of the fourth, midrashic stage of the reinterpretation of the psalm. Alternatively, and perhaps more plausibly, Barbiero, "Un cuore spezzato," relates the whole of the psalm to the whole of history of Israel. Attard, "Establishing Connections," shows the added importance of the juxtaposition of Psalms 49 and 50 within the Asaph collection as it may relate to Psalm 51.

14. It goes without saying that a diachronic analysis such as proposed does not preclude a cogent structuring of an eventual result; cf. Auffret, "Étude structurelle du Psaume 51."

this moment Joseph is overcome with grief and joy and the estranged brothers are reconciled, to face the world's great power and receive God's grace and salvation. The great sacrificial rites that form the centerpiece of the Pentateuch place repentance at their core. David's repentance for adultery and murder marks the turning point in the establishment of the Davidic dynasty, whose story makes up the Former Prophets. The Latter Prophets repeatedly call for collective repentance, often enough in the face of what is described as social illness, and the implied repentance of the Prophets themselves forms the basis for the fulfillment of God's deliverance. As for the Writings, as we have just seen, the Psalms as a whole turn on the repentance of David—in Psalms 38–41 and especially Psalm 51—a repentance that is made the focal point of the Leviticalized collection that determines the basic shape of the pre-Hasmonean segment of the Psalter. (The church tradition of "the seven penitential psalms" obscures this feature of Psalms.) Proverbs as a book calls for repentance, and the poetic narrative of Job concludes, apparently, with Job's repentance.

Equally significant is the biblical characterization of repentance as at the same time capricious, fickle, or cynical—as though the penitent delude themselves that their illness is alleviated or dispelled. The theme of repentance is most thoroughly developed in the Prophets, and there the moment never arrives when God stops being suspicious of his people's repentance. It occasions no surprise, therefore, that those who shaped the Persian-period Psalter, the voice of founder David and his Temple heirs, to create the fundamental juxtaposition of Psalms 50 and 51 did not make Psalm 51, Scripture's most profound repentance, the last word.

BIBLIOGRAPHY

Attard, S. "Establishing Connections between Pss 49 and 50 within the Context of Pss 49–52. A Synchronic Analysis." In *The Composition of the Book of Psalms*, edited by E. Zenger, 413–24. BETL 238. Leuven: Peeters, 2010.
Auffret, P. "Étude structurelle du Psaume 51." *Revue biblique* 54 (2006) 5–28.
Barbiero, G. "'Un cuore spezzato e affranto tu, o Dio, no lo disprezzi': Peccato dell'uomo e giustizia di Dion el Sal 51." *Ricerche Storico Bibliche* 19 (2007) 157–76.
Bautch, R. J. *Developments in Genre between Post-Exilic Penitential Prayers and the Psalms of Communal Lament*. Academia Biblica 7. Atlanta: Society of Biblical Literature, 2003.
Boda, M. J., D. K. Falk, and R. A. Werline, eds. *Seeking the Favor of God*. Early Judaism and Its Literature 21. Leiden: Brill, 2006.
Gillingham, S. E. *The Poems and Psalms of the Hebrew Bible*. Oxford: Oxford University Press, 1994.

Goulder, M. D. *The Prayers of David: Psalms 51–72: Studies in the Psalter, II.* JSOTSup 102. Sheffield: JSOT Press, 1990.

Hong, S.-H. *The Metaphor of Illness and Healing in Hosea and Its Significance in the Socio-Economic Context of Eighth-Century Israel and Judah.* Studies in Biblical Literature 95. New York: Lang, 2006.

Lambert, D. A. "Topics in the History of Repentance from the Hebrew Bible to Early Judaism and Christianity." Ph.D. diss., Harvard University, 2004.

Milgrom, J. *Leviticus: A Book of Ritual and Ethics.* Continental Commentaries. Minneapolis: Fortress, 2004.

Newman, J. H., *Praying by the Book: The Scripturalization of Prayer in Second Temple Judaism.* Early Judaism and Its Literature 14. Atlanta: Society of Biblical Literature, 1999.

Seitz, C. R. "The Place of the Reader in Jeremiah." In *Reading the Book of Jeremiah: A Search for Coherence*, edited by M. Kessler, 67–75. Winona Lake, IN: Eisenbrauns, 2004.

Weber, B. "Gottesrede in 'Asaph-Texten." *Old Testament Essays* 25 (2012) 737–60.

Wilson, G. H. Review of Randy G. Haney, *Text and Concept Analysis in Royal Psalms. Review of Biblical Literature* online review, August 2004.

Zimmerli, W. "Zwillingspsalmen." In *Wort, Lied und Gottesspruch II: Beiträge zu Psalmen und Propheten. Festschrift für Joseph Ziegler*, edited by J. Schreiner, 105–13. Würzburg: Echter, 1972.

11

The Medical Interpretation of Jewish Religious Rites in the Nineteenth Century

—Klaus Hödl

In 2002, a regional Austrian animal protection society published in its periodical an article on Jewish slaughter or *shehita*. Its chairman was impassioned in his critique of the Austrian law that permitted Jewish slaughter of animals. In his view, it was one of "*the* most brutal kinds of killing." If it had been permitted for reasons of tradition, he wrote, then by that very same rationale, polygamy could also be introduced, "since it also has a tradition going back thousands of years."[1]

In February 2008, that same animal protection society organized a public discussion event dealing with *shehita*. Representatives of the Muslim faith, Jews, the president of the Islamic Center in Graz, and a klezmer musician and itinerant shepherd, who was a convert to Judaism, were invited to the discussion. As might be expected, the shepherd defended the practice of *shehita*, although not with religious arguments. Rather, he stressed the "'humanity' and absence of pain in this type of slaughter."[2] The medical personnel present disagreed, emphasizing that retention of Jewish slaughter

---

1. Tierschutz-Nachrichten, *Aktiver Tierschutz Steiermark* 4 (2002), 11.
2. Tierschutz-Nachrichten, *Aktiver Tierschutz Steiermark* 3 (2008), 9.

could only be defended if "available scientific and practical knowledge is combined with the existing traditions for the animals' welfare."[3]

These two references to an animal protection society in Styria provide an exemplary window through which to look at the contemporary debate on *shehita*. They make clear various lines of argumentation that structure and mark the current dispute on the topic. The opponents of Jewish ritual slaughter proceed from a dualism between religious tradition in which *shehita* is embedded, and progress, customarily associated with a scientific approach. The champions of kosher slaughter generally reject the accusations against *shehita*, arguing that on the contrary, methods of Jewish ritual butchering are more in keeping with scientific standards than other methods of slaughter, while guaranteeing maintenance of animal protection, and even contributing to the concrete realization of ethical concepts.

The noteworthy aspect of this controversy is that it reflects a discourse[4] that had developed using largely the same arguments already back in the 19th century. For example, the anti-Jewish slant in argumentation as expressed in the position of the animal protection society's chairman cited above was formulated in a lecture delivered in August 1881 before the Society of Palatinate Veterinarians in Neustadt an der Haardt. On this occasion, the speaker stressed that Jewish ritual slaughter was a form of cruelty to animals. He described the method of *shehita* as a traditional procedure that "thousands of years ago, was without dispute probably in relative terms the best ... one that, in the absence of a better method, had also managed to effectively compete with all other methods, well on down into the present century." Yet he stressed that now, *shehita* was no longer in harmony with the contemporary world and had to be replaced by another method of slaughter.[5]

The claim by the Jewish side, in part also advanced by non-Jews, namely that *shehita* was more in keeping with animal protection than the customary method of slaughter, is likewise an argument that was part of the corresponding discourse back in the 19th century. Thus, the Russian-Jewish doctor Isaac Dembo wrote:

> in Jewish ritual slaughter, the animal loses consciousness in a very short time, at the latest three to four seconds after the procedure has begun. This also suggests that the duration of the

---

3. Ibid.

4. The concept of discourse has many diverse meanings, and in the present article is meant to signify a debate on some issue.

5. Bauwerker, "Das rituelle Schächten der Israeliten im Lichte der Wissenschaft," 20–21.

> agonies of death for the animal is infinitesimal... consequently, we who are in favor of shehita wish to point to the first and principal advantage of shehita in comparison with other methods of animal slaughter, namely the relatively painless death that the animal suffers, and thus the substantial adherence to the precept of animal protection.[6]

The analogies in the argument for and against Jewish slaughter put forward and formulated in the nineteenth century, and in our own, suggest a hardening in the patterns of argumentation. Since their original contextual nexus no longer exists, occasionally the reasons put forward for or against *shehita* no longer appear readily comprehensible. Thus the positive or negative connection (depending on point of view) between *shehita* and humaneness appears today hard to grasp, although this was not the case in the nineteenth century. This connection was constructed in the 1860s and 1870s in the context of significant changes in culture and mentality, when everyday violence was seen as a pressing social problem. Contemporaries also proceeded on the assumption that brutal behavior by butchers with cattle to be slaughtered influenced the butchers' attitudes toward the weaker members of society, particularly women and children.[7] The view spread that to give the animal an anesthetic before slaughter was a measure that would serve to decrease the degree of brutalization among butchers, while also protecting the animals from excessive pain and suffering. However, Jewish ritual slaughter laws specified that animals could be slaughtered only if fully conscious. Consequently, anesthesia could not be applied in the context of *shehita*. Subsequently, this was stylized into an exemplary manifestation of the supposedly brutal and violent Jewish character.

Jews tried to refute the accusation that *shehita* was a form of cruelty to animals by projecting the nexus between brutality and slaughter as something solely characteristic of butchers in non-Jewish society. This view is reflected paradigmatically in an 1899 article in a Jewish journal, the *Oesterreichische Wochenschrift*:

> The murder of a prostitute on a country road, the violation and murder of a child in the Salzburg cemetery and the killing of a government official... in all three cases the culprit was a butcher by profession... Powerful passion and brutality are common characteristics among most butchers... But why is it that the Jewish slaughterer... has a very different character?[8]

6. Dembo, *Methoden des Viehschlachtens*, 32–34.
7. Judd, *Contested Rituals*, 63–64.
8. *Oesterreichische Wochenschrift* 20 (1899), 388–89.

The asserted link between *shehita* and humaneness as formulated in the above-mentioned discussion organized in February 2008 in Styria is thus explainable by a discourse on violence in society in the nineteenth century. By the same token, the chairman's statement that permission for kosher butchering could, by the same argumentation, also open wide the door to polygamy, marriage to several wives, is more than just momentary polemics. It can also be shown to derive from discourses in the 19th century, in the framework of which an associative bond was constructed between *shehita* and an excessively high level of sexuality, supposedly characteristic of Jews.[9]

THE PURPORTED DIMENSION OF HEALTH IN CONNECTION WITH JEWISH RITUAL SLAUGHTER

An argument that was central to debate in the nineteenth and early twentieth century but no longer plays a role in contemporary discussion is the medical argument for kosher butchering. It was seen as a method of slaughter that was able, to a significant degree, to protect the consumers of kosher meat from certain diseases. The underlying cause for this was seen to lie in the common practice of careful inspection of the animal (*bedikah*), a core element in *shehita*, which functioned to reduce the consumption of sick animals.[10] An article published in 1911 in the Jewish weekly *Oesterreichische Wochenschrift* stated: "there is a danger of infection by eating the flesh of a tubercular animal ... Only recently has it been established that tuberculosis is a contagious disease ... —and behold, the regulations of Jewish law, anterior by millennia to modern science, contains these prophylactic measures against tuberculosis."[11] This strand of argumentation was bolstered by statistical data. A number of studies on the rates of illness and mortality among Jews indicated a lower degree of mortality due to tuberculosis when compared with the non-Jewish population. One of the first references to this appeared in the American journal *Medical and Surgical Reporter*, where doctor Madison Marsh claimed he had never encountered a Jewish patient ill with TB. To further substantiate his claim, he mentioned correspondence with "several of the most learned and distinguished Jews in the United States," who had also maintained that tuberculosis was indeed very rare among Jews.[12] A discourse subsequently developed stressing that Jews, especially because of the established prophylactic practice of careful

---

9. Judd, *Contested Rituals*, 114.
10. Lauff, *Schechitah und Bedikah*, 24.
11. Funke, "Kommunal-Hygiene des Talmuds," 191–92.
12. Marsh, "Jews and Christians," 343.

animal inspection before slaughter, were largely spared from falling ill with tuberculosis.[13]

In contrast with other previously mentioned arguments in favor of kosher butchering, the reference to its capacity to prevent disease did not constitute a reversal of the arguments brought against Jewish ritual slaughter. The opponents of *shehita* only rarely formulated any association with illness, and that association scarcely played any role in the overall discourse. This notwithstanding, a certain segment of the Jewish community frequently had recourse to the medical argument in a bid to defend kosher butchering against critics, especially the demand that it be banned. The reason for putting emphasis on the aspect of health sprang from efforts to bring the ritual practice into harmony with contemporary social standards and thus gain societal acceptance for *shehita*. Since health represented a central value and medicine had considerable influence in society,[14] it seemed only obvious to describe Jewish butchering as an effective means to prevent sickness. This strategy was in fact also utilized when it came to ritual circumcision, the ritual bath (*mikveh*), and also in regard to keeping the Sabbath. All these spheres were medicalized. In this context, observance of religiously prescribed rites could mean endorsing a healthy way of life. Seen from this vantage, Judaism increasingly forfeited its religiously grounded particularity, by which individuals often explained the performance of the ritual activities. To profess Judaism could now be conceived as advocacy of a healthful style of living—one that could also prove attractive to non-Jews, and was open to them.[15]

The following remarks center on the medical interpretation of Jewish religious practices. I intend here not just to describe that interpretation but to explain it from a historical perspective. The main focus is an attempt to explain the fact that in a specific period in the past—principally although not exclusively in the late nineteenth and early twentieth century—religious ceremonies were viewed as salubrious for the enhancement of health.

---

13. See, e.g., Behrend, "Diseases Caught from Butcher's Meat," 409–22; Drysdale, "Tuberculosis and Meat," 815; Fishberg, "The Relative Infrequency of Tuberculosis among the Jews," 695–99.

14. Frevert, *Krankheit als politisches Problem 1770–1880*.

15. Hödl, *Wiener Juden—jüdische Wiener*, 139. For example, we should also understand calls for the circumcision of all German male neonates, Jewish and non-Jewish, in this context (see *Allgemeine Zeitung des Judentums* 17 [1878] 259–60).

PREREQUISITES FOR THE MEDICALIZING OF RITUAL AND RITE

The beginning of developments through which a growing number of Jews came to view their religious rites not just as religious acts but increasingly also as effective measures to prevent illness can be traced back to the last quarter of the eighteenth century. Social and political upheavals demanded redefining the relation of Jews to the society in which they lived, both individually and as a collective. In this context, a Jewish religious life and its conduct were no longer deemed subject to the sole responsibility of Jews alone. Jewish religious life now was to be brought into harmony with values considered normative for the broader community as a whole. Of central importance in this connection were medical standards. Physicians increasingly provided guidelines for a mode of behavior designed to reduce the risk of disease and thus thought to be relevant for the broader society. The local rulers believed they could only secure the ability of their principality to defend itself militarily if healthy citizens were available for military conscription, as they also sought to prevent the sick from becoming a burden for society.[16]

Until the late eighteenth century, Central European Jews enjoyed an extensive degree of autonomy. Their everyday life was regulated in the main by their communal authorities, who based their administration and dispensation of justice on religious texts. To be a Jew meant to live in accordance with religious laws. However, the special legal position of the Jews was incompatible with the increased strengthening of neo-absolutist practices of rule. At the same time, the economic system of mercantilism, oriented to rendering individuals useful for society as a whole, clashed with the presence of a largely independent group within the society, oriented to its own particular compass and paths to well-being.[17] In this context, the status of the Jews had to be redefined, and a first attempt was the Edict of Tolerance in 1782. The regulations issued by Emperor Joseph II guaranteed Jews their right to view themselves as permanent citizens of their country of domicile.[18] They were granted new freedoms but simultaneously were subjected to new constraints that would act to render a traditional religious existence more difficult.[19]

---

16. Hödl, *Die Pathologisierung des jüdischen Körpers*, 54.
17. Risse, "Medicine in the Age of Enlightenment," 149–95.
18. Wistrich, *The Jews of Vienna in the Age of Franz Joseph*, 20.
19. Häusler, "Toleranz, Emanzipation und Antisemitismus," 83–89.

During this period, the first texts also came into being that suggested how Jews could gain a place in society from which they might better contribute to the common good.[20] These treatises, among which the famous text by the Prussian state chancellor Christian Wilhelm Dohm deserves special mention,[21] generally posit a nexus between the civil equality of the Jews anchored in law and their social utility. They thus presumed that the Jews were injurious to society, and this could only be remedied by instituting legal measures.[22]

Against the backdrop of an intensifying social medicalization—that is, an assessment of social phenomena as healthy or pathological from a medical perspective—Jewish autonomy was also described in terms of pathology.[23] As a result, political initiatives to restrict the special legal position of the Jews acquired a heightened new urgency. It was due to their social isolation, as the military physician Le Jau thought he observed, that Jews suffered from melancholy and depression.[24] Some illnesses, which Jews appeared to be especially susceptible to, were attributed to their practice of certain rites and rituals, and these deleterious rites were to be regulated anew. Jews in turn sought to respond to and counter interference by the ruling authorities in their ceremonies by asserting that Judaism was compatible with the contemporary values of the society, and most particularly with the standards of medicine. For this reason, it was argued, no modifications in their religious practice were necessary. Rather, these commentators contended, Judaism demonstrated how a healthy way of life could be promoted and was therefore of great social relevance.[25]

One example that can serve to present and illuminate the argumentation put forward by Jews concerns the debate on early burial in the late eighteenth century. It formed the point of departure for the controversies sketched below over Jewish rites that took place in the nineteenth and early twentieth century. As mentioned earlier, looking at the discourse on burial, we can trace for the first time the patterns of argumentation that would be utilized in later decades and even on into our own century.

---

20. Sorkin, *The Transformation of German Jewry 1780–1840*.

21 Dohm, *Über die bürgerliche Verbesserung der Juden I & II*.

22. See Michael, "Die antijüdische Tendenz in C. W. Dohms Buch 'Über die bürgerliche Verbesserung der Juden,'" 11–48.

23. See especially Grégoire, *Essai sur la Régénération physique, morale et politique des Juifs*, 57–64.

24. Kottek, "Sozio-politische Bestrebungen zur Hygiene der Juden im 18, Jahrhundert," 15.

25. See Efron, *Medicine and the German Jews*.

EARLY BURIAL AMONG THE JEWS

The beginning of the affair can be dated to 1772, when Duke Frederick of Mecklenburg was informed by a specialist on Oriental cultures that Jews bury their dead immediately after death; and as a result, the erroneous burying of those still alive but thought dead could not be ruled out. In response, the Duke then issued a decree stipulating that Jews in Schwerin were to wait for a period of three days between the occurrence of death and subsequent burial.[26]

The Jews in Schwerin regarded this as direct interference in their autonomy and were unwilling to accept such a move. The Duke's argument that early burial was not based on any biblical passage became the point of departure for their efforts to convince the prince to revoke his decree. They asked two prominent Jewish scholars, including Moses Mendelssohn, for expert opinions on the matter in dispute, and these were to be sent directly to the Duke. In his letter to Duke Frederick of Mecklenburg, Mendelssohn endorsed the position of the Schwerin Jews, stating that rapid burial was required by religious law. Subsequently, the decree was actually altered in such a way that even before the end of the stipulated three days of waiting, a corpse could be buried if a physician established and confirmed that the person was indeed clinically deceased.[27] However, in a separate letter to the Schwerin Jews, Mendelssohn expressed a different viewpoint. He stressed that the supreme commandment in Judaism was the preservation of human life, and this could not be rescinded by force of any customs. He argued that since there was a certain risk inherent in early burial, namely that an individual only apparently dead could be buried, it was actually binding on Jews to obey the orders of the Duke.[28]

The second letter of Mendelssohn became a matter of public knowledge after some time and was an important impetus for continuation of the debate. However, the debate was marked by a new direction in argumentation. Now the focus was not so much on the question of whether the state could legitimately interfere in Jewish religious customs and usage. Instead the discussion centered on whether and to what extent Jewish religious laws were compatible with social norms of health. An affirmative answer would help to facilitate the implementation of Jewish civil equality.

Two statements of opinion expressing the new rationale are of particular importance. The first was written by the Jewish physician Marcus Herz.

---

26. Heinrich, "Akkulturation und Reform," 140.
27. Silberstein, "Mendelssohn und Mecklenburg," 238.
28. Krochmalnik, "Scheintod und Emanzipation," 129.

He agreed with the Duke of Mecklenburg that nowhere in the Bible is there any support for early burial as a requirement. Instead, Herz contended, this goes back to a Talmudic precept. But that, Herz reasoned, did not mean that this regulation was totally irrelevant and should be ignored. However, in his view it could not claim an absolute validity beyond question. Since its establishment as a practice by the Talmudic sages, the conditions that earlier had prevailed and made rapid burial appear desirable had now changed. Herz wrote that the Talmudists must "have had their special reasons dictated then by the conditions of the time and place, but these conditions are unknown to us." He added that they "perhaps no longer fit in with our situation today."[29] Accordingly, Herz adopted a historicizing perspective, suggesting the possibility of changing individual religious regulations—although without at the same time having to reject the entire tradition. The historicizing line of argument, which in the late 18th century was still a very unaccustomed and novel way for Jews to look at their practice of religion, became in the 19th century a central vehicle for approaching their rites from a scientific (medical) vantage.

The second opinion relevant for the debate over burial stemmed from David Friedländer, a prominent *maskil* (advocate of Jewish Enlightenment). It was published in 1787 in the *Berlinische Monatsschrift*. There he criticized a ban on early burial that had been sent to the state rabbi in Prague. But Friedländer did not question its rationale because he supported as rapid a burial as possible. Rather, he was critical because he advocated an approach based on persuasion, changing people's minds, instead of imposing legal measures. On the whole, however, he considered a ban on rapid burial justified because such hasty burial was a "prejudice of such a perverse nature ... that it specifically serves to undermine human bliss and security."[30] Like Herz, he also thought that a postponement of burial was in keeping with *halakha* (the Jewish religious laws and precepts), and that changes in the rites of burial—that is, an adaptation to social and medical rules and regulations—did not constitute or forebode a departure from the pathway of Judaism.

In sum, the positions voiced by Mendelssohn in his letter to the Jewish Community in Schwerin, and by Herz and Friedländer, reflect a readiness to accept the idea of certain modifications in the Jewish ritual of burial. The authors supported their views by arguing that, in this way, the practice would fulfill the criteria of humanity and the standards of contemporary medicine, yet without having to depart in some way from (biblical) religious

29. Herz, *Über die frühe Beerdigung der Juden*, 25.
30. Friedländer, "Ueber die frühe Beerdigung der Juden," 318–19.

regulations. As long as there was a danger that an individual only apparently dead might be buried while still alive, the possibility of such a murder (as non-Jewish opponents contended) could not be excluded.[31] They argued that by means of a postponement of burial or the examination of the deceased by doctors called in to determine clinical death, this criticism could be countered and rendered invalid.

At least for those Jews who were willing to accept (and perhaps also welcome) a role for medicine in the question of burial, secular medical science and religion no longer constituted fundamental, irreconcilable opposites. Physicians joined with the rabbis and expressed their views on the rite with recognized authority. Here lay a central point of departure for a further medicalization of Judaism that would reach its zenith in the early twentieth century.

RITUAL CIRCUMCISION IN THE CONTEXT OF MEDICINE

The stir over interference by princely rulers in the rite of burial had scarcely faded when ritual circumcision emerged at the center of a heated dispute. Unlike in the case of early burial, the polemic against circumcision had a long tradition. Already in antiquity, it had been considered controversial,[32] and since the Middle Ages circumcision had repeatedly nourished anti-Jewish imaginings.[33] The discourse on circumcision in the 19th century was also more complex than the preceding debate on burial, and the makeup of the opponents of circumcision was more heterogeneous.

The first medical statements of opinion on circumcision that were not just sporadic, and thus can be viewed as part of an ongoing debate, were formulated in the early nineteenth century.[34] However, from the 1840s to the 1870s, medical judgments on the value or disadvantages of circumcision were overshadowed by an internal Jewish controversy over Jewish identity.[35] This involved the question of whether *brit milah*, the religious rite of circumcision, was necessary for membership in the Jewish Community, or whether birth from a Jewish mother was sufficient.[36] This discussion should

31. See Büsching, "Ueber die frühe Beerdigung der Juden," 112.
32. Levin, "Brit Milah: Ritual Circumcision," 1125–27.
33. Po-Chia Hsia, *The Myth of Ritual Murder*, 29–30.
34. Hödl, "Die deutschsprachige Beschneidungsdebatte im 19, Jahrhundert," 189–209.
35. See Meyer, "Berit Mila and the Origin of Reform Judaism," 143.
36. Hoffman, *Covenant of Blood*, 5–9; Gotzmann, *Jüdisches Recht im kulturellen*

be viewed against the backdrop of anti-Jewish polemics contending that circumcision was an identifying feature of Jewish particularity, and thus clashed with civil equality for the Jews.[37] In this sense, to a far greater extent than the controversy over burial, the debate surrounding *brit milah* was bound up with the dispute over the legal status of the Jews.[38] Despite the differences between the two controversies, there was a close link between the discourse on burial and circumcision, in that all the arguments of the first debate can also be found once again in the dispute over circumcision. In the following, I address only the aspect of health in the debate on circumcision.

THE SUPPOSEDLY PATHOLOGICAL EFFECT OF *BRIT MILAH*

In the early nineteenth century, one of the first texts focusing on the rite of circumcision from a medical perspective was by the physician Johann Nepomuk Rust (1775–1840), written in 1811. There he reported on cases of syphilis among circumcised boys in Galicia, which he attributed to the practice of *mezizah*, the sucking out of the circumcision wound as part of the Jewish ritual. Rust writes:

> Five years ago in the Krakow Jewish ghetto, there were several newborn infants with ulcerations on their male member; I was called in for consultation ... I carefully examined the mothers, wet-nurses and other household members, but was unable to find a satisfactory explanation for this phenomenon; the disease continued to spread, almost every newborn Jewish infant developed syphilitic chancres, and several who did not seek medical aid developed syphilis ... so it was that I demanded to be directly present during the next circumcision procedure; I now saw that after the procedure was completed, a man sucked out the blood by applying his lips to the wound; I examined the said individual immediately and discovered that the entire interior cavity of his mouth was covered with venereal ulcerations, and

---

Prozeß, 251–302.

37. Gilman, *The Jew's Body*, 91.

38. Thus, Immanuel Kant had already asserted that as long as Jews allowed circumcision to be performed, they could never be of utility to bourgeois society (Brumlik, *Deutscher Geist und Judenhaß*, 35). His statement reflected the view prevalent among a large majority of the Enlighteners, who in many respects regarded Judaism as an antiquated religion that should best be discarded.

that in this way he was infecting the newly circumcised babes with the syphilitic contagion.[39]

With his publication, Rust provided an impetus for a more intensive look by physicians at circumcision. Texts subsequently appeared on similar cases resulting from the practice of *mezizah*, particularly in Warsaw, Vilna and Lvov/Lemberg.[40] In this connection, other sicknesses along with syphilis, such as diphtheria and erysipelas, were mentioned as a consequence of the traditional mode of *brit milah*.[41]

Reference to illnesses was only one among a number of medical aspects raised as criticism against the procedure of traditional Jewish circumcision. Further misgivings involved the largely deficient medical knowledge of the circumcisers (*mohelim*), a deficiency that repeatedly led to injuries among the newly born infant boys. Philipp Wolfers, for example, stated that due to the insufficient medical knowledge of the *mohel*, at times not only the foreskin but a portion of the glans was also removed. He contended that the subsequent treatment of the wound was carried out unprofessionally as well, by pulling so forcefully on the penis that as a result, infections and contusions appeared that could even lead to the death of the neonate.[42] A further consequence of the lack of proper medical knowledge among the *mohelim* was injury to the blood vessels of the infant, which could result in a fatal hemorrhage. In this context, the *mohel*'s ignorance of hygienic standards was also criticized, manifested by a practice of sometimes attempting to stop the bleeding by application of eggshells and horse manure to the wound.[43] Finally, the practice of *priah*, cutting open the inner lamella of the foreskin, was condemned, because it was usually done using sharply pointed fingernails, often dirty, and these contaminated the circumcision wound, causing infection.[44]

---

39. Quoted in Friedreich, "Ueber die juedische Beschneidung aus sanitätspolizeilicher Beziehung," 684.

40. Jaffe, *Die rituelle Circumcision im Lichte der antiseptischen Chirurgie*, 31.

41. Neumann, "Zur Uebertragung der Tuberculose durch die rituelle Circumcision," 569.

42. Wolfers, "Über das Beschneiden des Judenkindes."

43. Goldmann, "Ueber Verblutung bei der Beschneidung von Judenkindern," 204ff.

44. Mombert, "Die Beschneidung israelitischer Knaben," 281; Löw, "Ueber das Beschneiden der Israeliten," 781.

REACTIONS TO MEDICAL CRITICISM OF *BRIT MILAH*

It was not only non-Jewish physicians who criticized the consequences of ritual circumcision that were deleterious to health. Jewish medical doctors also voiced their disapproval. If there was a difference between these two groups, it lay in the conclusions drawn from the critique. While non-Jewish doctors demanded that *brit milah* be abolished because it posed a danger to health, Jewish medical doctors tended only to recommend modifications in the rite of traditional circumcision designed to improve a procedure viewed as problematic.[45] In this sense, the religious rite was to conform to medical requirements but not eliminated.

The decision recommending the abandonment of the practice of *mezizah* by the strictly observant Pressburg (Bratislava) scholar, Rabbi Moses Schreiber (Moses Sofer), a highly respected authority among contemporary Orthodox Jews, was a paradigmatic proof of the need to adapt *brit milah* to scientific standards. Sofer had founded the famous" Pressburg yeshiva (rabbinical academy) in 1806. This was his recommendation in reaction to a letter from Rabbi Eleasar Horowitz in Vienna in 1837, in which Horowitz reported on the deaths of infants from syphilis in Vienna due to sucking out the circumcision wound.[46] Sofer's decision did not do away with the entire ritual but only recommended eliminating a previously constitutive feature of its performance. The intention was to continue with *brit milah*, with a small change, so as to avoid the charge that it was potentially injurious to health. In his decision, Moses Sofer, a leading Orthodox rabbi, endorsed the need to adapt circumcision to prevailing (secular) medical standards.

The Frankfurt rabbi Salomon Abraham Trier, likewise Orthodox and chief rabbi in Frankfurt from 1817 to 1844, similarly advocated for an increasing readiness to adapt elements in Jewish religious practice to the tenets of secular medical science. In a casebook on circumcision published in 1844, Rabbi Trier indicated his acceptance of the regulation introduced by the Frankfurt Medical Office to place circumcision under the supervision of existing "medical policing," i.e. enforcement of public health policy.[47] In this decision, he implied that ceremonies should not violate specific, concrete medical-secular norms, and that broader public interest in safeguarding health among the Jews was justified.

These references to Sofer and Trier should not be viewed as indications of a linear development leading toward a medicalization of religious rites.

---

45. Arnhold, *Die Beschneidung und ihre Reform*, 14ff.
46. Homa, *Mezizah*, 8; Schiffer, *Die Ausübung der Mezizah*, 4.
47. Trier, *Rabbinische Gutachten über die Beschneidung*, IX.

Only a small number of Jewish Communities abandoned the practice of *mezizah* by mouth due to medical misgivings about the traditional practice, and supervision of *brit milah* by a government office was neither planned everywhere nor did all Jews understand and accept such developments. For this reason, the critique of ritual circumcision continued to occupy the attention of a large proportion of Jews in Central Europe. In this connection, other paths were found to adapt *brit milah* to medical requirements. Among such alternatives was the use of some auxiliary device, such as a thin glass pipette, in performing *mezizah*, so as to avoid direct contact between the mouth of the *mohel* and the circumcision wound, or employment of scissors instead of fingernails for carrying out the *priah*.[48]

A new development can be discerned in the last third of the 19th century. It led to an additional impetus toward rationalization and thus a further reinterpretation of the rite. Here not only was an attempt made to change or eliminate individual practices that were deemed in violation of specific social and medical norms. Rather the *brit milah* itself was increasingly viewed as a medical procedure that contributed to better health. In this connection, for example, it was maintained that one effect of removing the foreskin was to harden the glans of the penis, and that this reduced the inclination to masturbate.[49] Since masturbation was believed to be the cause of a series of different ailments, it was possible to view this observation regarding the effects of circumcision as a salient measure in disease prevention.[50]

THE NEW MEANING OF THE SABBATH

In connection with the Jewish Sabbath even more clearly than in the case of circumcision, we can see the development of moves to legitimate religious ceremonies by reference to their medical value. Like circumcision, non-Jews also saw the Sabbath as a characteristic feature of Judaism that furthered Jewish independent existence as a community, but as a concomitant consequence, it also served to impede their interaction with the surrounding social environment and thus rendered Jews identifiable as "others." And in a way comparable with disputes over other rites, Jews also sought in regard to the Sabbath to present and describe its maintenance as being in conformity with the norms of the majority society.

---

48. Löw, "Ueber das Beschneiden der Israeliten," 785.
49. Wallerstein, "Circumcision," 123.
50. Nossig, *Einführung in das Studium der sozialen Hygiene*, 51.

A central strategy pursued since the second third of the nineteenth century was to divest the Sabbath of its religious dimensions and to reshape it into a metaphor for the Jewish sense and spirit of the family. In the context of secularization, Jews in mounting numbers ceased to attend religious services in the synagogue on the Sabbath. However, they did not always see this tendency as negative or a sign of growing indifference toward religious Judaism. Rather, they viewed this as increased leisure time that they could best spend with the family.[51] Since the institution of the family enjoyed a huge positive value in general society, Jews expected that, by stressing the association between the Sabbath and family life, Judaism would be accorded more respect.

Jews indeed had a certain success in that expectation. Increasingly, non-Jews came to see the Sabbath as an exemplary expression of the Jewish sense of family. This is evident in various descriptions of Sabbath celebrations in the popular middle-class magazine *Die Gartenlaube*, as evidenced by the following exemplary description:

> The darkness that had in the meantime arrived permitted us to glance into the interior of the room; it evinced a painstaking cleanliness, and was furnished in a comfortable almost elegant manner. A small chandelier was lit on the ceiling, supplemented by two silver candelabras on the table, covered in white, around which sat a large family at dinner adorned in festive attire, indeed a lovely picture of quiet contentment and domestic satisfaction.[52]

The association with family life was not the only non-religious interpretation of the Sabbath. There were also efforts to push on with its medicalization, in accordance with its double dimension as both a day of rest and a day for and with family. The nexus with family life served, for example, to substantiate the statistically established longevity of the Jews.[53] From this vantage, Jewish family life represented a social-hygienic bond, one that protected individuals against illness and the early mortality associated with it. Joseph Jacobs, a Jewish anthropologist born in Australia and working in Great Britain, put this in a memorable nutshell when he observed that the greater longevity among Jews could be attributed to "the tranquilising effects of Jewish family life . . . on the Sabbath and other festivals."[54]

In addition, the Sabbath as a day without work was interpreted along medical lines. The observance of the Sabbath was seen as a salubrious

51. Kaplan, The Making of the Jewish Middle Class, 69–70.
52. F., "Im Frieden des Sabbathlichtes," 315.
53. See Rosenfeld, "Die Sterblichkeit der Juden," 47–62.
54. Jacobs, *Studies in Jewish Statistics*, vii.

measure that could serve to cure Jews of their supposed special proclivity for mental afflictions. There was a widespread notion, considered substantiated by numerous studies, that in comparison with non-Jews, Jews possessed an above-average susceptibility to hysteria, neurasthenia, nervousness and other maladies.[55] An important explanation for this nosological peculiarity was that the special "hustle and bustle" Jews were purportedly prone to the lack of rest and relaxation, constituted a heavy strain on their nerves. It was in this sense that the Frankfurt physician Max Sichel wrote: "the numerous nervous disturbances of the Jews, in particular conditions of nervous exhaustion ... can be attributed to life in the metropolis, with its eternal haste and scurry, and its more burdensome conditions of existence."[56] And the commandment to rest and to desist from work on the Sabbath appeared to be a precise remedy against this.[57]

The Sabbath increasingly became the veritable quintessence of Judaism. In its observance, Jews sought to demonstrate that their Jewishness was fully compatible with so-called middle-class "bourgeois" social values. An exemplary expression of the prominent importance of the Sabbath was manifested in the Jewish Museum founded in 1896 in Vienna, where the motive underlying its establishment was in significant measure the desire to show to the non-Jewish world a positive side of Judaism. This was highlighted in particular by an exhibit featuring the *Gute Stube* or parlor, a room set aside especially for celebrating the Sabbath.[58]

After several years, the *Gute Stube* exhibit was sent on to Dresden, where it served as the showpiece in the Jewish pavilion in the International Hygiene Exhibition in 1911. An article on the exhibition published in the periodical of the State Association for the Internal Mission of the Lutheran Church in the Kingdom of Saxony stated that the Sabbath parlor was the greatest hygienic blessing ever accorded the human race.[59] In this context, the Sabbath was seen as an institution that prevented disease, its medical versatility far outweighing its religious dimension.

---

55. Weldler, "Die Geisteskrankheiten," 61; Hofer, "Aspekte zum Bild der Juden," 60–61.

56. Sichel, "Die Paralyse der Juden," 98–99.

57. See Hart, *Social Science and the Politics*, 146.

58. Hödl, *Wiener Juden*, 97; for photos of the *Gute Stube*, Old Jewish Museum Vienna, see http://www.jmw.at/de/die-sammlung-ikg.

59. Grunwald, *Bericht über die Gruppe "Hygiene der Juden,"* 22.

CONCLUSION

The present paper has explored the question why, in the late nineteenth and early twentieth century, Jews in Central Europe sought to legitimize their religious rites by medicalizing them. It was stressed that in doing so, they sought to forestall and prevent attacks on Judaism and its rituals. There was at least a tendency among a growing number of Jews to abandon the religious interpretation of Jewish ceremonies in favor of their medical interpretation. From this perspective, Judaism appeared to be in keeping with central social values in the broader society. It was thus possible to convey an image of Judaism to non-Jews that they perceived as positive. For a certain period, it seemed as though Judaism was viewed in a positive light among broad segments of the society. However, in historical retrospect, it is necessary to note that this development did not have a long-term impact.

BIBLIOGRAPHY

Allgemeine Zeitung des Judentums 17 (1878) 259–60.
Arnhold, A. *Die Beschneidung und ihre Reform, mit besonderer Berücksichtigung auf die Verhandlungen der dritten Rabbiner-Versammlung*. Leipzig: Hunger, 1847.
Bauwerker, C. "Das rituelle Schächten der Israeliten im Lichte der Wissenschaft. Ein Vortrag gehalten im wissenschaftlich-literarischen Verein zu Kaiserslautern am 5. Dezember 1881, Kaiserslautern: Gotthold, 1882.
Behrend, H. "Diseases Caught from Butcher's Meat." *Nineteenth Century* 26 (1889).
Brumlik, M. *Deutscher Geist und Judenhaß: Das Verhältnis des philosophischen Idealismus zum Judentum*. Munich: Luchterhand, 2000.
Büsching, A. F. "Ueber die frühe Beerdigung der Juden." *Berlinische Monatsschrift* (1785).
Dembo, I. A. *Anatomisch-physiologische Grundlagen der verschiedenen Methoden des Viehschlachtens*Leipzig: Verlag der Slavischen Buchhandlung, 1894.
Dohm, Ch.W. *Über die bürgerliche Verbesserung der Juden I & II*. Berlin: Nicolai, 1781, 1783.
Drysdale, Charles Robert. "Tuberculosis and Meat." *British Medical Journal* (1889) 815.
Efron, J. M. *Medicine and the German Jews: A History*. New Haven: Yale University Press, 2001.
F., A. "Im Frieden des Sabbathlichtes: Aus den vier Wänden des jüdischen Familienlebens." In *Die Gartenlaube*. 1867.
Fishberg, M. "The Relative Infrequency of Tuberculosis among the Jews." *American Medicine* 2 (November 1901) 695–99.
Frevert, U. *Krankheit als politisches Problem 1770–1880*. Göttingen: Vandenhoeck & Ruprecht, 1984.
Friedländer, D. "Ueber die frühe Beerdigung der Juden." *Berlinische Monatsschrift* 9 (1787).
Friedrich, J. B. "Ueber die juedische Beschneidung aus sanitätspolizeilicher Beziehung." *Centralarchiv für die gesamte Staatsarzneikunde* 5 (1846).

Funke, S. "Kommunal-Hygiene des Talmuds." *Oesterreichische Wochenschrift* 9 (1911).
Gilman, S. L. *The Jew's Body*. New York: Routledge, 1991.
Goldmann, "Ueber Verblutung bei der Beschneidung von Judenkindern," in: *Journal der Chirurgie und Augen-Heilkunde* 13 (1829) 201–10.
Gotzmann, A. *Jüdisches Recht im kulturellen Prozeß*, 251–302. Schriftenreihe wissenschaftlicher Abhandlungen des Leo Baeck Instituts 35. Tübingen: Mohr/Siebeck, 1997.
Grégoire, A. *Essai sur la Régénération physique, morale et politique des Juifs*. 1789. Reprinted, Paris: Boucher, 2002.
Grunwald, M. *Bericht über die Gruppe 'Hygiene der Juden' in der Internationalen Hygiene-Ausstellung Dresden, 1911*. N.p.: n.d.
Hart, M. B. *Social Science and the Politics of Modern Jewish Identity*. Stanford: Stanford University Press, 2000.
Häusler, W. "Toleranz, Emanzipation und Antisemitismus: Das österreichische Judentum des bürgerlichen Zeitalters (1782–1918)." In *Das österreichische Judentum: Voraussetzungen und Geschichte*, edited by A. M. Drabek et al., 83–89. Vienna: Jugend & Volk, 1982.
Heinrich, G. "Akkulturation und Reform: Die Debatte um die frühe Beerdigung der Juden zwischen 1785 und 1800." *Zeitschrift für Religions- und Geistesgeschichte* 50 (1998) 137–55.
Herz, M. *Über die frühe Beerdigung der Juden: An die Herausgeber des hebräschen Sammlers*. 2nd ed. Berlin: Voss und Sohn, 1788.
Hödl, K. "Die deutschsprachige Beschneidungsdebatte im 19. Jahrhundert." *Aschkenas* 13 (2003) 189–209.
———. *Die Pathologisierung des jüdischen Körpers: Antisemitismus, Geschlecht und Medizin im Fin de Siècle*. Vienna: Picus, 1997.
———. *Wiener Juden—jüdische Wiener: Identität, Gedächtnis und Performanz im 19. Jahrhundert*. Innsbruck: Studienverlag, 2006.
Hofer, H.-G. "Aspekte zum Bild der Juden in der medizinischen Literatur der Jahrhundertwende." Diploma thesis, Graz University, 1995.
Hoffman, L. A. *Covenant of Blood: Circumcision and Gender in Rabbinic Judaism*. Chicago: Chicago University Press, 1996.
Homa, B. *Metzitzah*. London: n.p., 1960.
Hsia, R. Po-Chia. *The Myth of Ritual Murder: Jews and Magic in Reformation Germany*. New Haven: Yale University Press, 1988.
Jacobs, J. *Studies in Jewish Statistics: Social, Vital and Anthropometric*. London: Nutt, 1891.
Jaffe, J. *Die rituelle Circumcision im Lichte der antiseptischen Chirurgie mit Berücksichtigung der religiösen Vorschriften*. Leipzig: Fock, 1886.
Judd, R. *Contested Rituals: Circumcision, Kosher Butchering, and Jewish Political Life in Germany, 1843–1933*. Ithaca, NY: Cornell University Press, 2007.
Kaplan, M. E. *The Making of the Jewish Middle Class: Women, Family and Identity in Imperial Germany*. Studies in Jewish History. Oxford: Oxford University Press, 1991.
Kottek, S. S. "Sozio-politische Bestrebungen zur Hygiene der Juden im 18 Jahrhundert." In *Sozialpolitik und Judentum*. Edited by Albrecht Scholz and Caris-Petra Heidel. Dresden: Union Druckerei, 2000.

Krochmalnik, D. "Scheintod und Emanzipation: Der Beerdigungsstreit in seinem historischen Kontext." *Trumah* 6 (1997) 107–49.

Lauff, B. *Schechitah und Bedikah (Rituelle Schlachtung und innere Untersuchung): Auf Grund alttestamentlichen, talmudischen und neuhebräischen Quellenstudiums im Lichte der modernen Hygiene und Fleischbeschaugesetzgebung.* Berlin: Tierärztliche Hochschule, 1922.

Levin, S. "Brit Milah: Ritual Circumcision." *South African Medical Journal* 39 (1965) 1125–27.

Löw, H. "Ueber das Beschneiden der Israeliten und über die Möglichkeit der Anwendung nöthiger Vorsichtsmassregeln, um die Lebensgefährlichkeit dieser Operation zu mildern." *Oesterreichische Zeitschrift für Practische Heilkunde* 47 (1859) 781.

Marsh, M. "Jews and Christians." *Medical and Surgical Reporter* 30 (1874) 342–44.

Meyer, M. M. "Berit Mila and the Origin of Reform Judaism." In *Berit Mila in the Reform Context*. Edited by Lewis M. Barth. Cincinnati: Experimental, 1990.

Michael, R. "Die antijüdische Tendenz in C.W. Dohms Buch, 'Über die bürgerliche Verbesserung der Juden.'" *Bulletin Leo Baeck Institute* 77 (1987) 11–48.

Mombert, M. "Die Beschneidung israelitischer Knaben, ein Gegenstand medizinisch-polizeilicher Ueberwachung." *Zeitschrift für die Staatsarzneikunde* 29 (1849) 267–84.

Neumann, "Zur Uebertragung der Tuberculose durch die rituelle Circumcision." *Wiener Medizinische Presse* 13 (1900) 569–73.

Nossig, A. *Einführung in das Studium der sozialen Hygiene: Geschichtliche Entwicklung und Bedeutung der öffentlichen Gesundheitspflege.* Stuttgart: Deutsche Verlags-Anstalt, 1894).

Oesterreichische Wochenschrift 20 (1899).

Risse, G. B. "Medicine in the Age of Enlightenment." In *Medicine in Society: Historical Essays*, edited by Andrew Wear, 149–95. Cambridge: Cambridge University Press, 1992.

Rosenfeld, S. "Die Sterblichkeit der Juden in Wien und die Ursachen der jüdischen Mindersterblichkeit." *Archiv für Rassen- und Gesellschafts- Biologie* 4 (1907) 47–62.

Schiffer, S. *Die Ausübung der Mezizoh.* Frankfurt: Golde, 1906.

Sichel, M. "Die Paralyse der Juden in sexuologischer Bedeutung." *Zeitschrift für Sexualwissenschaft* 6 (1919–1920) 98–99.

Silberstein, S. "Mendelssohn und Mecklenburg." *Zeitschrift für die Geschichte der Juden in Deutschland* 1 (1929).

Sorkin, D. *The Transformation of German Jewry 1780–1840.* Oxford: Oxford University Press, 1978.

Tierschutz-Nachrichten. *Aktiver Tierschutz Steiermark* 4 (2002).

Tierschutz-Nachrichten. *Aktiver Tierschutz Steiermark* 3 (2008).

Trier, S. *Rabbinische Gutachten über die Beschneidung.* Frankfurt: Bach, 1844.

Wistrich, R. S. *The Jews of Vienna in the Age of Franz Joseph.* Oxford: Littman Library of Jewish Civilization, 1990.

Wallerstein, E. "Circumcision: The Uniquely American Medical Enigma." *Urologic Clinics of North America* 12 (1985) 123–32.

Weldler, N. "Die Geisteskrankheiten unter den Juden Österreichs in den Jahren 1882–1902." *Zeitschrift für Demographie und Statistik der Juden* 4 (1908) 61–63.

Wolfers, P. "Über das Beschneiden des Judenkindes." *Zeitschrift für Staatsarzneikunde* 9 (1825) 205–6.

12

"Whoever Saves a Soul Saves an Entire World"

Pikuah Nefesh in Rabbinic Literature[1]

—Lieve Teugels

Inspired by the rabbinic saying that was chosen as the title of the conference in which it was originally presented: "Whoever saves a soul saves an entire world," I set out to investigate the original context of this saying and see how it functions in the rabbinic discussion of end-of-life ethics. With "rabbinic" I refer to the classical rabbinic period, which is the foundational period of Judaism in approximately the first seven centuries CE. The main literary products of the Rabbis or Sages, as the rabbinic authorities from that period are called, are the Mishnah (third cent. CE), and the Jerusalemite (fourth-fifth cent. CE) and Babylonian (sixth cent. CE) Talmuds.[2]

---

1. I presented a shorter version of this paper at the International Academic Expert Seminar "'Whoever saves a soul saves an entire world': Jewish Perspectives on End-of-Life Ethics" which was held at the Faculty of Theology of the K.U. Leuven in Belgium on 22–24 November 2010.

2. For a general introduction to rabbinic literature, see, e.g., Stemberger, *Introduction*. When treated as a group, or when referring to a majority opinion, the authorities named in rabbinic literature will be called "Sages," or "Rabbis" (capitalised), following standard usage as in, e.g., the translated title of the Hebrew standard work *The Sages*, by Ephraim Urbach. When referring to an individual rabbi, "sage" or "rabbi" (lower case) is used.

The interesting results of my first quick query were, first, that this expression is not often used; on the contrary it occurs exactly once, in Mishnah Sanhedrin 4:5; and, second, that this saying *does* occur in a context that deals, albeit in an unexpected way, with an end-of-life situation. It is found in a legal, judiciary text in which it features in the discussion of capital punishment, i.e. the death penalty.

Apart from this text about capital punishment I will treat a second, longer, text that deals with the preservation of life in cases where that interferes with specific negative Jewish commandments, such as the prohibition of working on the Sabbath or eating on Yom Kippur, the Day of Atonement. Like the first text, the second text features the word "soul," *nefesh* in Hebrew, and specifically the expression *pikuach nefesh*. This is the standard usage in Jewish ethical and halakhic (i.e. legal) texts for stating that the preservation of human life overrides virtually any other religious consideration. In this text, several cases of medically dangerous situations, such as fasting by pregnant women or sick people, are treated.

In dealing with some foundational texts of Jewish thought, this paper explores the religious-anthropological background of Jewish thinking about the value of human life. This is the ideological background behind later, even contemporary, Jewish decision-making on specific medical end-of-life issues, such as organ donation, abortion, and euthanasia.

WITNESSES IN CAPITAL CASES: WHOEVER SAVES A SINGLE SOUL SAVES AN ENTIRE WORLD

> How were the witnesses inspired with awe? Witnesses in capital charges [*nefashot*] were brought in and intimidated [thus]: Perhaps what ye say is based only on conjecture, or hearsay, or is evidence from the mouth of another witness, or even from the mouth of a trustworthy person: Perhaps ye are unaware that ultimately we shall scrutinize your evidence by cross examination and inquiry? Know then that capital cases are not like monetary cases. In civil suits, one can make monetary restitution and thereby effect his atonement; but in capital cases he is held responsible for his blood [sc. the accused's] and the blood of his [potential] descendants until the end of time, for thus we find in the case of Cain, who killed his brother, that it is written: *the bloods of thy brother cry unto me* (Genesis 4:10): Not the blood of thy brother, but the bloods of thy brother, is said—i.e. his blood and the blood of his [potential] descendants. For this reason was man [*adam*] created alone, to teach thee that

whosoever destroys a single soul {of Israel} [Scripture] imputes [guilt] to him as though he had destroyed a complete world; and whosoever preserves a single soul {of Israel}, Scripture ascribes [merit] to him as though he had preserved a complete world.[3]

This mishnah[4] deals with the preparation of witnesses in capital cases in the ancient Jewish court, the Sanhedrin. Some preliminary information about the literary co-text of this passage is due. First of all it should be noted that the Tractate Sanhedrin describes an institution, the constitution, power and jurisdiction of which changed with the shifting political situations in antiquity.[5] The Sanhedrin lost the judicial power to execute the death penalty after the destruction of the Temple in the year 70, if not before. The Mishnah, composed in the third century, however, preserved many Second Temple traditions and presents them as if they still exist and function. Many of the practical and ethical insights about the functioning of the institutions related to the Temple were preserved for various reasons. One of these must have been that they contain fundamental Jewish values and views that transcend the immediate context of the Second Temple situation in which they originated. Such must have been the case with our text too.

In the tractate Sanhedrin a crucial distinction is made between capital cases, in which the accused may be sentenced to death if found guilty, and non-capital cases, in which a monetary fine or another punishment was imposed. Throughout the tractate the distinction between the two is stressed and all sorts of stricter conditions for capital cases are laid out. The purpose of all of these conditions is to provide safety nets to prevent imposition of the death penalty when that could be avoided. These are just a few examples from the immediate context of our passage:

---

3. Mishnah Sanhedrin 4:5 = BT Sanhedrin 37a; braces around "of Israel" added by me. Quotes from the Babylonian Talmud in this paper are from the translation in the Soncino edition. Quotations from the Mishnah in the Talmud are rendered in small capitals; quotations from the Bible are in italics. Explanatory additions between square brackets are already present in the Soncino edition, except from some transcribed Hebrew words, which are added by me.

4. The Mishnah is divided in six parts, called *sedarim*, which are in turn divided in tractates, 63 in total. These tractates consist of chapters, which are sub-divided in smaller units that are each called "a mishnah" (plural: *mishnayot*). A reference to a unit in the Mishnah mentions the tractate, chapter and mishnah, e.g., Yoma 8:5.

5. There are many differences of opinion about the history, composition, function and jurisdiction of the Sanhedrin, mostly due to the discrepancies between what the historical sources (Hellenistic, Roman, Jewish, Early Christian) relate about this institution. What is clear is that the Sanhedrin underwent many changes with the shifting of the political powers, including, but not restricted to the fall of the Temple and Jerusalem after 70 CE. For an overview see, e.g., Mantel, "Sanhedrin."

- Non-capital cases are decided by three judges, whereas capital cases are decided by 23 judges. (1:1)
- In non-capital cases a judge who had argued in favour of acquittal may afterwards argue in favour of conviction and vice versa, but in capital cases one that argued in favour of acquittal may not afterwards argue in favour of conviction. (4:1)
- In non-capital cases a verdict may be reached the same day, but in capital cases it may not be reached until the following day. (4:1)
- If they have found someone innocent in a capital case, they set him free the same day, but if no verdict is reached the judges retire together in pairs, and they eat a little and debate the whole night, but are not allowed to drink wine. If they want to convict someone there needs to be a majority of at least two, and if that is not the case they need to bring in more judges until there is a majority of at least two, up to a maximum of 71 judges. And if then there is a majority of 36 against 35 they have to debate until one judge that favoured conviction approves of acquittal. (5:5)

Returning to Mishnah 4:5 quoted above, the idea expressed here is that a witness or a judge who argues in favour of conviction without absolute proof that the accused is guilty will be held responsible for killing the convict and his or her possible descendants. The inclusion of the descendants is derived by means of a midrash[6] of Gen 4:10, where the Hebrew text reads *demei achikha*, in plural, literally "the bloods of your brother." From here, the Rabbis derive that not only the brother's blood, but more "bloods," namely of his descendants, are meant. Additional biblical proof is adduced by means of a reference to the creation of Adam, the first human being. Since he was created alone, and the whole human world depends on his existence, we can deduce that the whole world depends on the existence of each and every human being who in Hebrew is called *ben adam*—literally: descendant of Adam. Whoever destroys a human being is held responsible for the destruction of a complete world, and whoever saves a human being, conversely, has the merit of preserving an entire world. Thus, the witness is himself put to trial, not before the court, but before Scripture, which in the rabbinic mind is the same as before God himself. This is the context for the adage "whoever saves a single soul saves an entire world." It is a legal, judiciary context, not a medical one.

---

6. Much could be said about the genre, definition, and characteristics of midrash (see, e.g., Stemberger, *Introduction*, 233–40), but for this purpose it should suffice to know that midrash is the rabbinic way of interpreting the Hebrew Bible.

An attentive reader will have noticed that there is ambiguity as to the universality of the claim. In the text quoted above I have put "of Israel" between braces. The textual witnesses of this passage vary in this respect. One manuscript version of the Mishnah (Ms. Munich), and the Jerusalem Talmud (the *Yerushalmi*) read "a single soul," without "of Israel. " The version that includes "of Israel" was included in the Babylonian Talmud (or *Bavli*), which is generally seen as the most authoritative rabbinic work. Because the Yerushalmi is older, it is likely that the more universalist version is the original one. This version also makes more sense because of the reference to Adam, whom the Bible presents as the first human being, not the first Jew. The version of the text in the Babylonian Talmud is a stumbling block for interpreters, not in the least Jews who want to use this text to underscore the positive Jewish attitude to life in general. This has, for example, been an issue with the film *Schindler's List*, for which the quotation "whoever saves a single soul saves an entire world" appeared as a motto on posters and other advertising material. One quick Google search shows that this generated a lot of commotion when people, notably critical Jews, discovered that the "real" version of the text was different. Compared to the Bavli, the Yerushalmi has long been the lesser-known work. Only specialists in rabbinic texts would know that there are two versions, the more universalist probably being the original one. This does not take away from the fact that in the Babylonian academies around the sixth century CE, at the height of Jewish intellectual creativity, a narrow particularist view prevailed, and that students of Judaism, historians and ethicists alike will have to come to terms with that.

In conclusion, what is remarkable is that in this discussion about the death penalty, *not* having to execute it was the main concern. This is in line with the general attitude towards the value of human life in rabbinic literature. An expression often used in this context is *pikuach nefesh*. This concept and its halakhic and ethical consequences are the topic of the remainder of this paper.

SAVING OF LIFE (*PIKUACH NEFESH*) SUSPENDS BIBLICAL LAWS

The passage that gave its name to the expression *pikuach nefesh* is found in Mishnah Yoma 8:7, and its elaboration (*gemara*) in the Babylonian Talmud Yoma 84b.[7] The expression *pikuach nefesh* specifically refers to opening

---

7. The Jerusalem and Babylonian Talmuds follow the same division in six *sedarim* as the Mishnah (see n. 3 above). Each discussion in these *talmudim* typically includes

up (*pakach*) a heap of rubble to rescue a person (*nefesh*, lit. "soul") buried underneath on the Sabbath when all work, including digging, is otherwise forbidden. By *pars pro toto*, *pikuach nefesh* came to refer to the obligation to save endangered life, including one's own life, in all circumstances where Jewish law needs to be transgressed to do so. Together with the two previous *mishnayot*, a thematic unit (Mishnah Yoma 8:5–7) can be distinguished that deals with several cases of *pikuach nefesh*.

Tractate Yoma (literally "the day") deals with the observance of Yom Kippur, a day of repentance and complete fasting that is considered the holiest day of the Jewish year. Moreover, all the restrictions about working on the Sabbath also apply to Yom Kippur, which the Bible dubs a *shabbat shabbaton*—a Sabbath of Sabbaths, a day of complete rest (Leviticus 16:31 and 23:32). Therefore the discussion in our passage, in typical rabbinic style, side-tracks into Sabbath observance, whether or not coinciding with Yom Kippur. Moreover it also touches upon the eating of non-kosher food. All three: Yom Kippur, Sabbath, and the dietary laws are *biblical* commandments, which puts them in the most serious category of Jewish laws that under no condition can be abrogated, *except*, as we will see, when a human life is at stake.

This is the relevant passage in Mishnah Yoma 8:5–7.

> (5) If a woman with child smells [and craves food], she must be given to eat until she feels restored. A sick person is fed at the word of experts. And if no experts are there, one feeds him at his own wish until he says: enough.
>
> If one is seized by a ravenous hunger, he may be given to eat even unclean things until his eyes are enlightened. If one was bitten by a mad dog, he may not give him to eat the lobe of its liver, but R. Matthia b. Heresh permits it.
>
> (6) Furthermore did R. Matthia b. Heresh say: if one has pain in his throat, he may pour medicine into his mouth on the Sabbath, because it is a possibility of danger to human life [*safek nefashot*] and every danger to human life suspends the [laws of the] Sabbath.
>
> (7) If debris falls on someone, and it is doubtful whether or not he is there, or whether he is alive or dead, or whether he be an Israelite or a heathen, one should open [*mefakchin*] [even on

---

the text of a unit of the Mishnah, followed by some commentary/elaboration called *gemara*. Not all sections of the Mishnah have corresponding *gemara* in either or both Talmuds (for more details I refer to the work mentioned in n. 1). A reference to the Babylonian Talmud includes the name of the tractate, and the folio on which the text is found in the standard editions, preceded by BT, e.g., BT Yoma 84b.

Sabbath] the heap of debris for his sake. If one finds him alive one should remove the debris, and if he be dead one should leave him there [until the Sabbath day is over].

I will now discuss the various cases mentioned in this mishnaic unit as well as its *gemara* in the BT Yoma 82a–85b.

The Pregnant Woman

It is assumed in *mishnah* 5 that we are dealing with Yom Kippur when no Jewish adult should eat or drink. However, there are some exceptions to this rule: A pregnant woman and a sick person are allowed to eat, the unstated reason being that their life or the life of the unborn baby might be endangered if they fast. The *gemara* on this passage reads as follows:

> Our Rabbis taught: If a woman with child smells [and craves] the flesh of holy flesh, or of pork, we put for her a reed into the juice and place it upon her mouth. If thereupon she feels that her craving has been satisfied, it is well. If not, one feeds her with the juice itself. If thereupon her craving is satisfied it is well; if not one feeds her with the fat meat itself, for there is nothing that can stand before [the duty of] saving life [pikuach nefesh], with the exception of idolatry, incest and bloodshed [which are prohibited in all situations]. (BT Yoma 82a)

Here we have the main rule of *pikuach nefesh*. The duty of saving life suspends most other commandments: If for some reason a person needs even pork, the quintessential non-kosher food, they should give it to her. As in other rulings that we will encounter below, one should start with the "lesser transgression": if a little taste of meat juice is sufficient to satisfy the woman's craving, this should be enough. However if she can only be satisfied with the real thing, even fat (pig) meat should be given to her.

There are, however, three exceptions to the rule of *pikuach nefesh*: one should never commit the three cardinal sins of murder, idolatry and illicit sexual relations. The *gemara* goes on with some examples of cases where it is preferred to shed blood instead of letting a crime happen, for example in the case of a betrothed girl that is about to be raped (one should kill the rapist) or in the case where one is forced to rape or murder someone (one should rather be killed or kill oneself). The latter case is an example of martyrdom for the "sanctification of the name" (*kiddush ha-shem*).[8]

---

8. Since early rabbinic times, *kiddush ha-shem* and martyrdom have become practically synonyms. A well-known example is Rabbi Akiva who died a martyr's death in the

What we can learn from these three exceptions to *pikuach nefesh* is that, contrary to what is often claimed, Judaism does not uphold the absolute "sanctity of life"; rather, it believes in the great value of preserving human life. Baruch Brody summarizes his discussion of the casuistry of suicide and euthanasia in Jewish rabbinic and halakhic sources as follows:[9]

> I now want to return to the question raised at the beginning of this essay, viz., whether traditional Judaism is committed to the doctrine of the sanctity of human life. I think that it is evident from what we have seen that it is not. No doctrine of the sanctity of human life could justify penitential acts of suicide. No doctrine of the sanctity of human life could justify killing oneself to avoid sinning under coercion. No doctrine of the sanctity of human life could justify killing oneself to avoid a mocking and cruel death at the hands of one's enemy. No doctrine of the sanctity of human life could justify withholding care that would keep a dying person alive but in pain. No doctrine of the sanctity of human life could justify risking a loss of life to avoid pain. Major traditional Jewish authorities have justified all of the above. None of them could have been committed to a belief in the sanctity of human life. What then is the traditional Judaic opinion? I think that it is comprised of several major elements: (a) a belief in the great value of preserving human life and in the corresponding obligation to come to the aid of those whose life is threatened . . .

The above *gemara* is just one example of how traditional Jewish texts and values, in this case the exception of the "big three" transgressions for which one should rather give up a life than commit them, can shed light on contemporary situations in which difficult ethical choices are made from a Jewish perspective.

---

hand of the Romans because he refused to stop teaching Torah when this was forbidden. Older famous examples are Eleazar, and Hannah and her seven sons who refused to eat pork when forced to do so by the Seleucid oppressor, known from 2 Maccabees 6 and 7. See Hillel Ben-Sasson, "Kiddush ha-shem and Hillul ha-shem"; Cohen, "Hannah and Her Seven Sons."

9. Brody, "A Historical Introduction to Jewish Casuistry on Suicide and Euthanasia," 74.

The Sick Person

A sick person is fed at the word of experts. And if no experts are there, one feeds him at his own wish until he says: enough.[10]

R. Jannai said: If the patient says, I need [food], whilst the physician says: He does not need it, we hearken to the patient. What is the reason? *The heart knoweth its own bitterness* (Proverbs 14:10). But that is self-evident? You might have said: The physician's knowledge is more established; therefore the information [that we prefer the patient's opinion]. If the physician says: He needs it, whilst the patient says that he does not need it, we listen to the physician. Why? Stupor seized him.

We learned: a sick person is fed at the word of experts. [That implies]: Only upon the order of experts, but not upon his own order? [Further it implies]: Only upon the order of "experts", but not upon the order of a single expert? — This refers to the case that he says: I do not need it. But should one feed him upon the order of one expert? — This refers to the case when someone else is present who agrees that he does not need it. [If so, wherefore state that he] is fed at the word of experts. Surely that is self-evident, for it is a possibility of danger to human life and "in the case of the possibility of danger to human life we take a more lenient view"! — It refers to a case in which two more people are present who say that he does not need it. And although R. Safra said that "Two are as a hundred and a hundred are as two" applies only to witnesses, but with regard to opinion we go according to the number of opinions, all that applies only to opinions concerning money matters, but here it is a case where there is a possibility of danger to human life. But since in the second part [of the Mishnah] it states: and if no experts are there, one feeds him at his own wish, is it to be inferred that in the first part we deal with the case that he said he needed it? There is something missing [in the Mishnah] and this is how it reads: These things are said only for the case that he says: I do not need it; but if he says: I need it, then if two experts are not there, but one who says: He does not need it, then one feeds him at his own wish.

Mar son of R. Ashi said: Whenever he says. "I need [food]", even if there be a hundred who say, "He does not need it", we accept his statement, as it is said: *The heart knoweth its own bitterness.* We learned in the Mishnah: if no experts are there one feeds him at his own wish. That means only if no experts are there, but not if such experts were there? — This is what is meant:

> These things are said only for the case that he says, "I do not need it", but if he says, "I need it", then there are no experts there at all, [and] one feeds him at his own wish, as it is said: *The heart knoweth its own bitterness.* (BT Yoma 83a)

This long discussion boils down to the idea that one cannot be careful enough: if a patient feels he needs food on a fast day, s/he should be given to eat, whatever the experts say, because "The heart knoweth its own bitterness". This verse from Proverbs envelopes the discussion like a frame. The sages mentioned in the *gemara* agree that the opinion of the experts is only necessary in case the patient refuses food: if one or more experts think s/he needs the food, s/he should be given food. The reason of the patient's refusal might be that s/he is in a stupor.

The various possibilities hinted at in the *gemara* are further spelled out in the later halakhic codes, most notably the Shulchan Arukh. The various cases in which the patient wants food or refuses food and one or several doctors present take the same or different positions are laid out. For example, if one doctor thinks that the law needs to be breached, but the patient and another doctor deem this unnecessary, the law should be upheld, i.e. the patient should not eat. Rabbi Jakobovits, in his standard work on Jewish Medical Ethics, has a chart tabulating the various combinations of a patient and one or more experts having conflicting views as to whether the law of fasting on Yom Kippur needs to be breached or upheld, based on the source in Shulchan Arukh "Orach Chaim," as well as various *responsa* in support of the decisions.[11]

One remaining problem is how a refusing patient will be fed. Can he or she be force-fed? This problem is still very actual in modern medical practice. A person refusing a cure (or food) because this would involve a breach of the law is called a *chasid shoteh*—a pious fool. According to many authorities, such a person should be convinced, if not forced, to eat or take medicine.[12]

---

11. Jacobovits, *Jewish Medical Ethics*, 65; see also Freedman, *Duty and Healing*, 309–13.

12. Jacobovits, *Jewish Medical Ethics*, 52, and see the references in n. 40 there. Rudman, "Fetal Rights and Maternal Obligation," 118, states that a patient can be forced to take medicine or undergo surgery (e.g., amputation) if the psychological damage done hereby is not greater than the physical benefit. He quotes Rabbi Moshe Feinstein in support of this view. In the same article he also mentions convincing/forcing (summarized as "coercing") a sick person or pregnant woman to eat on Yom Kippur if not doing so would clearly bring them or the foetus in danger.

The Bulimia Patient

> If one is seized by a ravenous hunger, he may be given to eat even unclean things until his eyes are enlightened. (Mishnah Yoma 8:5)

The word translated as "ravenous hunger" in the second part of *mishnah 5* reads *bulimia* in Hebrew—a loanword from the Greek. This is considered a disease and a possible life-threatening condition which can be measured from the fading light in the patient's eyes. If no kosher food is available, even feeding the patient non-kosher food will do—and all this on Yom Kippur. The succinct statement of the Mishnah that one who has a bulimia attack should be "given to eat even unclean things until his eyes are enlightened" is elaborated in the *gemara*. It is stated that one should start feeding the patient the less forbidden foods first, i.e. "common food" before food that has not been tithed, or carrion etc. Thereafter the discussion treats one specific food: honey.

> Our Rabbis taught: If one was seized with a ravenous hunger, he is given to eat honey and all kinds of sweet things, for honey and very sweet food enlighten the eyes of man. And although there is no proof for the matter, there is an intimation in this respect: *See, I pray you how mine eyes are brightened. Because I tasted a little of this honey* (1 Samuel 14:29). What does "although there is no proof for the matter" mean? Because in that case no ravenous hunger has seized him. Abaye said: This applies only after a meal, but before the meal, it even increases one's appetite, as it is written: *And they found an Egyptian in the field, and brought him to David, and gave him bread, and he did eat, and they gave him water to drink, and they gave him a piece of cake of figs, and two clusters of raisins, and when he had eaten, his spirit came back to him, for he had eaten no bread, nor drunk any water, three days and three nights* (1 Samuel 30:11, 12).

> R. Nahman said in the name of Samuel: If one was seized by a ravenous hunger, one should give him to eat a tail with honey. R. Huna, the son of R. Joshua said: Also pure flour with honey. R. Papa said: Even barley-flour with honey [is effective] . . . (BT Yoma 83b)

In a modern study in Dutch,[13] Dr. M. Elzas suggests that the disease bulimia mentioned here might refer to cases of spontaneous hypoglycaemia caused

---

13. Elzas, "Geneeskunst in de Babylonische Talmoed: Bulimie," 2300–303. See also

by a tumour in the pancreas called "nesidioblastoma." This is indeed a life-threatening disease. Dr. Elzas finds the prescribed treatment with honey and fine flour particularly interesting as this corresponds to the modern treatment of spontaneous hypoglycaemia. Honey raises the blood sugar quickly, whereas the combination with flour, which has a similar but slower effect, would prolong the effect of the honey. In his opinion the remedy with honey and flour is presented here as the standard rabbinic therapy for hypoglycaemia, particularly when this is caused by a nesidioblastoma, of which he sees the oldest attested case described here. In my view this goes one step too far into historicising a text which is not necessarily meant as such (more on this further). But it does make sense that experience taught the Rabbis that honey has a fast relieving effect on people who feel faint with hunger.

The *gemara* continues with three cases of sages who report how they themselves have been struck by a bulimia attack.

> R. Johanan said: Once I was seized by a ravenous hunger, whereupon I ran to the eastern side of a fig-tree, thus making true in my own case: *Wisdom preserveth the life of him who hath it* (Ecclesiastes 7:12) for R. Joseph learned: One who would taste the [full] taste of a fig, turns to its eastern side, as it is said: *And for the precious things of the fruits of the sun* (Deuteronomy 33:14). R. Judah and R. Jose were walking together when a ravenous hunger seized R. Judah. He seized a shepherd and devoured his bread. R. Jose said to him: You have robbed the shepherd! As they entered the city, a ravenous hunger seized R. Jose. They brought him all sorts of foods and dishes. Whereupon R. Judah said to him: I may have deprived the shepherd, but you have deprived a whole town. (BT Yoma 83b)

Dr. Elzas, questionably treating the talmudic discussion as history, goes even further to suggest that this section of the *gemara* still deals with bulimia caused by a nesidioblastoma and that the three sages who are mentioned here must be related, sharing a gene that causes the growth of the tumour.[14] This would explain why such a rare disease would occur in three talmudic sages, two of them being of the same generation (Jose and Judah). Leaving this far-fetched theory for what it's worth, it is not necessary to see the whole *sugya* (Talmudic discussion of a topic) as a well-knit literary, or even less, an historical unity, to see that "ravenous hunger" was and still could be the

---

Preuss, *Biblisch-Talmudische Medizin*, 209: "Bulimie."

14. In order to state his case he has to demonstrate that the Rabbi Jochanan mentioned here was in fact Jochanan ben Nuri who lived before Rabbi Jose and Rabbi Jehuda, and that he was in fact their grandfather.

indication of a serious life-threatening condition that requires immediate feeding to save the patient's life, putting aside the law of fasting on Yom Kippur.

The Person Bitten by a Mad Dog

> If one has been bitten by a mad dog, he may not give him to eat the lobe of its liver, but R. Matthia b. Heresh permits it. (Mishnah Yoma 8:5)

The issue of the lobe of the dog's liver—which is of course non-kosher food—has to do with the fact that this was considered a kind of homeopathic medicine against rabies. The therapeutic use of parts of the rabid animal, particularly the liver, for individuals bitten by such an animal, was recommended by many ancient physicians including Dioscorides, Galen and others. Also Pliny describes the use of this remedy in his Natural History.[15] Rabbi Matthia ben Heresh too believed that it worked; however, he seems to have been an exception among the Rabbis. Whether or not the Sages allow this exception to the dietary laws and the laws of fasting on Yom Kippur, depends on whether or not they believe in the effectiveness of the remedy. Administering an effective remedy for such a fatal disease on a fast day- because it was clear that rabies was fatal—would constitute *pikuach nefesh* and therefore be allowed. However, the general opinion of the Sages, and thus the halakhah, is that this remedy is not effective and therefore affords no reason to transgress biblical law.

One reason for the Sages' scepticism could be that Rabbi Jehuda haNasi, the final editor of the Mishnah, had a negative experience with this remedy. The Jerusalem Talmud (JT Yoma 8:5, 45b) relates that a German servant of Rabbi Judah haNasi who was bitten by a mad dog was given of its liver to eat. However the effort was futile and the patient died, from which the Jerushalmi concludes that "let no man tell you that he was bitten by a mad dog and lived."

Although feeding a rabies patient a piece of the mad dog's liver was not allowed on Yom Kippur because it was not deemed effective, nevertheless a bite from a rabid dog *was* considered particularly life threatening and thus enough reason to transgress biblical law. This is confirmed in the Babylonian Talmud Shabbath 121b:

---

15. For references, see Preuss, *Talmudische Medizin*, 224–25, esp. n. 7. Rosner, "Rabies in the Talmud," 198–200; Rosner, *Medicine in the Bible and the Talmud*, 50–53.

> Rabbi Joshua ben Levi said: All animals that cause injury [i.e. kill] may be killed [even] on the Sabbath. Rabbi Joseph objected. Five may be killed on the Sabbath, and these are they: the Egyptian fly, the hornet of Nineweh, the scorpion of Adiabene, the snake in Palestine, and a mad dog anywhere.

This ruling of *pikuach nefesh* was also codified by Maimonides and Joseph Karo.[16]

The Throat Ache

Mishnah Yoma 8:6 continues with more medical advice by Rabbi Matthia.

> Furthermore did R. Matthia b. Heresh say: if one has pain in his throat, he may pour medicine into his mouth on the Sabbath, because it is a possibility of danger to human life (*safek nefashot*) and every danger to human life suspends the [laws of the] Sabbath.

The sage's name must have been the main reason for the editor of the text to include this material here, as the issue is no longer eating on Yom Kippur. Such clustering of related traditions by a named sage is not uncommon in rabbinic literature. The fact that "on the Sabbath" is mentioned, indicates that a digression into Sabbath laws starts here: the administration of medicine is considered "work" because making medicine usually involves grinding, which is one of the 39 kinds of work forbidden on the Sabbath.[17]

Rabbi Matthia endorses an exception to the Sabbath laws in case of a throat ache, as he considers it a condition that might develop into a more serious, life-threatening disease. The Mishnah does not discuss this issue further and leaves it open whether the Sages in general think along the same lines as Rabbi Matthia. The *gemara* in the Babylonian Talmud picks up this question and records a discussion among various sages about scurvy, one of

---

16. Maimonides, *Mishneh Torah*, Laws of the Sabbath, Chapter 11, paragraph 4; Karo, *Shulchan Aruch*, Orach Chayim, Chapter 316, paragraph 10. See also Meir ha-Kohen, *Mishna Berura*, 246: "One may kill any animal or creeping creature on Shabbos whose bite is definitely fatal even if it is not running after him." The example of a mad dog is given in the note there.

17. Cf. Jacobovits, *Jewish Medical Ethic*, 74: "The sabbatical ban on medicines, introduced to guard against the possibility of pounding spices on the Sabbath, is of Talmudic origin." See also the references to the *Shulchan Arukh* and the Talmud mentioned there. The 39 forbidden categories of work, including grinding, are listed in Mishnah Shabbat 7:2.

the symptoms of which is bleeding gums and possibly pain in the throat.[18] Thus the topic has shifted from a throat ache in general to a more specific dangerous disease that involves oral problems. Following a story in which Rabbi Johanan receives a remedy for scurvy from a matron and wonders whether he can also use this on the Sabbath, and some sidetracks into various other remedies for scurvy, the *gemara* (BT Yoma 84a) continues with the Sabbath issue:

> When R. Johanan suffered from scurvy, he applied this [remedy] on the Sabbath and was healed. How could R. Johanan do that?—R. Nahman b. Isaac said: It is different with scurvy, because whereas it starts in the mouth, it ends in the intestines. R. Hiyya b. Abba said to R. Johanan: According to whom is it? According to R. Matthia b. Heresh who said that if one has pains in his throat one may pour medicine into his mouth on the Sabbath?—I say: In this case, but in no other.

The sages mentioned here debate whether scurvy is a serious enough disease to allow the administration of medicine on Shabbat—in other words: is this a case of *pikuach nefesh* or not? R. Nachman ben Isaac admits that scurvy is different (from a common throat ache?) because it can turn into a dangerous intestinal disease. R. Hiyya b. Abba, however, mockingly wonders if this is yet another of the disputed R. Matthia b. Heresh's remedies. He concludes (I say) that in this case, i.e. in the case of scurvy, he agrees with him, as the condition may be life threatening, but not for just any throat ache.

In the following, some other of R. Matthia's reputed remedies are discussed, partly repeating the cases already mentioned in the Mishnah, i.e. the bite of the mad dog and the throat ache. In two *baraitot*[19] two other cases related to R. Matthia are added: jaundice[20] and asphyxia.

---

18. On scurvy in the Talmud, see Rosner, *Medicine*, 55–60.

19. A *baraita* is a tannaitic source that does not occur in the Mishnah. "Tannaitic" refers to the teachings of the Tannaim, the oldest rabbinic sages (roughly before 200 CE) that are mentioned in the Mishnah, the Tosefta, and other texts from that period. The sages from the period thereafter, mentioned in the Talmuds, are called "Amoraim." Often *baraitot* are recognizable by characteristic introductions that mark them as tannaitic, such as *tanya* (for it was taught) used in the second passage. Apart from the version in the Mishnah, alternative lists of remedies advocated by R. Matthia seem to have circulated.

20. Heb.: *yerakon*. This disease is not listed among the conditions for which R. Matthia ben Heresh has a remedy in the Mishnah. On *yerakon*, see Preuss, *Talmudische Medizin*, 187–90, esp. 190, where he mentions R. Matthia's remedy of donkey flesh. Dioscurides recommended the urine from a donkey. This latter remedy is forbidden in the BT Bechorot 7b because of its origin from an unkosher animal: "The question, however, arose concerning [the urine of an ass] which people drink and is good for

> Shall we say that the following [teaching] supports his view? If one is attacked by jaundice [*yerakon*] one may give him to eat the flesh of a donkey; if one was bitten by a mad dog, one may give him to eat the lobe of its liver; and to one who has pains in his mouth may be given medicine on the Sabbath—this is the view of R. Matthia b. Heresh; but the Sages say: These are not considered cures—Now what does "these" mean to exclude? Won't you say it is meant to exclude medicine? No, it is meant to exclude blood-letting in case of asphyxia. Thus also does it seem logical. For it was taught: R. Ishmael son of R. Jose reported three things in the name of R. Matthia b. Heresh: One may let blood in the case of asphyxia on the Sabbath, and one whom a mad dog has bitten may be given to eat the lobe of its liver, and one who has pains in his mouth may be given medicine on the Sabbath, whereas the Sages hold: These are not considered cures. Now what does "these" exclude? Would you not say "these" excludes the two latter ones, and not the first one?—No, it means to exclude the first two ones, and not the last one.

The talmudic Amoraim debate the meaning of the two different *baraitot* reporting the teachings of R. Matthia and the opinion of the Tannaim about these.[21] In the first version "these are not considered cures" is meant to refer to the treatment of jaundice by donkey meat and the treatment of rabies by the dog's liver. Since they are not cures, they are also not allowed on Sabbath. Letting blood in case of asphyxia, however, was considered an effective cure and therefore allowed on Sabbath in a case of *pikuach nefesh*. In the second version, blood letting and feeding the dog's liver are considered effective cures, whereas giving medicine for a throat ache is not considered effective and therefore not allowed on the Sabbath.

To refute the above conclusion, yet another tannaitic tradition related to R. Matthia b. Heresh is quoted, which is in conflict with the conclusion that was just made[22] (BT Yoma 84b).

> Come and hear: For Rabbah b. Samuel learned: If a woman with child has smelled [food], one feeds her until she is restored; and one who was bitten by a mad dog is given to eat from the lobe of its liver, and one who has pains in his mouth may be given jaundice. What is the ruling?—R. Shesheth replied to this. We have learnt this in the Mishnah: that which goes forth from the unclean is unclean, and that which goes forth from the clean is clean, and this [urine] also comes from an unclean animal." See also Rosner, *Medicine*, 70–74.

21. For the distinction between Tannaim and Amoraim, see n. 18.
22. This is indicated by the formula *ta shma* (Come and hear).

> medicine on the Sabbath—these are the words of R. Eleazar b. Jose in the name of R. Matthia b. Heresh. But the Sages say: In this case, but not in another. Now what does "in this case" refer to? Would you say to the woman with child? That is self-evident; for is there anyone to say that in the case of a woman with child it would not be permitted?—Hence it must refer to the medicine. This is conclusive.

In this *baraita* the version of the Mishnah is repeated but followed by the Sages' remark "in this case but not in another". Since this cannot refer to the pregnant woman (the case of the dog's liver seems to be forgotten), it cannot but refer to the throat medicine: in this case (in case of scurvy?), administering throat medicine on Sabbath is allowed, but in no other cases.

Even though the argument is already marked as "concluded,"[23] one final remark is added. R. Ashi quotes the Mishnah as we know it ("our Mishnah") to prove that the latter conclusion is correct: since the tannaitic sages separated R. Matthia's remedy of the mad dog's liver, which they don't allow on Shabbat, from the remark about the throat ache, which they do not comment upon, by inserting the word "furthermore," it must follow that they agreed with his idea that throat medicine can be given on the Shabbat. If not, they would have quoted both remedies together and afterwards have stated that they do not permit either of them.

> R. Ashi said: Our Mishnah too justifies this inference. R . Matthia B. Heresh said furthermore: if one has pains in his mouth one may give him medicine on the sabbath. And herein the Rabbis do not dispute him. For if it were that the Rabbis dispute him, he should teach these together, and afterwards mention that the Rabbis dispute it. This is conclusive evidence. (BT Yoma 84b)

"BECAUSE IT IS A POSSIBILITY OF DANGER TO HUMAN LIFE AND WHEREVER THERE IS DANGER TO HUMAN LIFE, THE LAWS OF THE SABBATH ARE SUSPENDED"

This saying concludes the opinion of R. Matthia ben Heresh in *mishnah* 6. The formulation in the Mishnah (because it is . . .) connects this remark directly with Rabbi Matthia's opinion about the necessity of the administration of throat medicine on the Sabbath. This confirms the conclusion of the *gemara* that a throat ache might be life threatening. The idea that the threat

---

23. By means of the formula *shema mina* (This is conclusive).

might not be immediate but that a sore throat could turn into something worse if not treated, is furthered in the following discussion in the Talmud.

> Because it is a possibility of danger to human life. Why was it necessary to add and wherever there is danger to human life, the laws of the sabbath are suspended?—Rab Judah in the name of Rab said: Not only in the case of a danger [to human life] on this Sabbath, but even in the case of a danger on the following Sabbath. How is that? If e.g. the [diagnosis] estimates an eight-day [crisis] the first day of which falls on the Sabbath. You might have said, let them wait until the evening, so that the Sabbaths may not be profaned because of him, therefore he informs us [that we do not consider that]. Thus also was it taught: One may warm water for a sick person on the Sabbath, both for the purpose of giving him a drink or of refreshing him, and not only for [this] one Sabbath did they rule thus, but also for the following one. Nor do we say: Let us wait, because perchance he will get well, but we warm the water for him immediately, because the possibility of danger to human life renders inoperative the laws of the Sabbath, not only in case of such possibility on this one Sabbath, but also in case of such possibility on another Sabbath. Nor are these things to be done by Gentiles or minors, but by Jewish adults. Nor do we say in this connection: We do not rely in such matters on the opinions of women, or of Samaritans, but we join their opinion to that of others. (BT Yoma 84b)

In the above *gemara* the discussion takes on a broader scope and goes beyond the case of the throat medicine. At stake is the reach of the word "Sabbath": are we only dealing with danger on the present Sabbath or do we need to treat on this Sabbath so as to prevent the danger from extending to the next Sabbath?[24] A *baraita* ("Thus also it was taught") is quoted which teaches that it is permitted to warm water for a patient on the Sabbath, even if the actual danger would only occur on the next Sabbath. Moreover the *baraita* states that a Jewish adult male himself should warm the water instead of having this done by a *"shabbes goy"* or a child (who would not be liable if working on the Sabbath). In other words: it is a *mitsvah*, a religious duty, to break the Sabbath if there is even a remote chance that a life might be in danger. Moreover the laws as to the majority of opinions are also stretched

    24. The reasoning seems a bit forced as it should not really matter whether the danger extends to the next Sabbath or to another day. I think an exegetical problem is being solved here. The words "danger to human life" (*safek nefashot*) are repeated in the Mishnah while this is not really necessary to make the point. The Rabbis, in typical midrashic style, "read" this repetition as indicating that also the Sabbath on which the person is in danger might be repeated.

for such a case: the opinion of a woman or of a Samaritan would, exceptionally, count if in this way a majority would obtained who believes that this is a case of *pikuach nefesh* for which the Sabbath laws should be set aside.

Pikuach Nefesh: A Person Covered by Debris

Mishnah 7 continues the deviation from the Yom Kippur laws into the discussion of breaking the Sabbath laws when a person is in danger. A new case is broached here: a person trapped under a collapsed structure. As has already been said, the case treated here, opening up a pile of debris on the Sabbath to save a life has given the name to the expression *pikuach nefesh*, as a form of the verb *pakach* (*mefakchin*) is used here for "opening up."

> If debris fall on someone, and it is doubtful whether or not he is there, or whether he is alive or dead, or whether he be an Israelite or a heathen, one should open (*mefakchin*) [even on Sabbath] the heap of debris for his sake. If one finds him alive one should remove the debris, and if he be dead one should leave him there [until the Sabbath day is over]. (Mishnah Yoma 8:7)

On the Sabbath, when such work as digging or removing rubble is normally forbidden,[25] a Jew is obliged to dig somebody out of the rubble. The Mishnah mentions several conditions where there is some doubt: even if one is not sure a person is underneath, he should dig; even if one is not sure whether the victim still lives, he should dig. When one is sure the victim is dead, one should not dig until the Sabbath is over, because there is no longer a condition of *pikuach nefesh*. I will momentarily get to the last condition as to "whether he be an Israelite or a heathen".

In the *gemara*, the issue of "digging" a person out of rubble is extended into other situations where "work" needs to be done in order to save a life.

> Our Rabbis taught: One must remove debris to save a life on the Sabbath, and the more eager one is, the more praiseworthy is one; and one need not obtain permission from the Beth Din. How so? If one saw a child falling into the sea, he spreads a net and brings it up—the faster the better, and he need not obtain permission from the Beth Din though he thereby catches fish [in his net]. If he saw a child fall into a pit, he breaks loose one

---

25. There are some differences of opinion as to which of the 39 categories of work forbidden on the Sabbath "digging" belongs (see note 16). Some commentators see this as a variation of *soter*, i.e. demolishing; others see it as a form of *bone*, i.e. building. The problem may also be the "carrying" of digging equipment. See Evers, *Op het leven!*, 133 n. 1 for references.

> segment [of the entrenchment] and pulls it up—the faster the better; and he need not obtain permission of the Beth Din, even though he is thereby making a step [stairs]. If he saw a door closing upon an infant, he may break it, so as to get the child out — the faster the better; and he need not obtain permission from the Beth Din, though he thereby consciously makes chips of wood. One may extinguish and isolate [the fire] in the case of a conflagration — the sooner the better, and he need not obtain permission from the Beth Din, even though he subdues the flames. Now all these cases must be mentioned separately ... (BT Yoma 84b)

All these cases need to be mentioned separately because different forms of work are involved.[26] The Beth Din is a Jewish court: in cases of immediate danger each Jew can judge for him or herself whether the situation could possibly be fatal, such as in the case of a child falling in water or an infant staying alone in a room.

The last condition mentioned in the Mishnah, "whether he be an Israelite or a heathen", is the hardest to evaluate. Some of the sages quoted in the *gemara* in BT Yoma 84b-85a seem to be of the opinion that it is not deemed necessary to save a gentile's life on the Sabbath. There are a few passages that suggest this is the case, the clearest of which being the following:

> If debris had fallen upon someone [etc.]. What does he teach herewith? — It states a case of "not only". Not only must one remove the debris in the case of doubt as to whether he is there or not, as long as one knows that he is alive if he is there; but, even though it be doubtful whether he is alive or not he must be freed from the debris. Also, not only if it is doubtful whether he be alive or dead, as long as it is definite that he is an Israelite; but even if it is doubtful whether he is an Israelite or a heathen, one must, for his sake, remove the debris. (BT Yoma 85a)

The duty of *pikuach nefesh* is often based on the biblical injunction in Leviticus 19:16 "You shall not stand upon/profit by the blood of your neighbour."[27] In the Talmud it is debated whether "your" or "his neighbour" (*re'ekha/ re'ehu*), which occur frequently in biblical law, refer to Israelites only or also to non-Israelites, whether "strangers," "temporary residents," or other categories. More often than not, the Talmud excludes non-Jews from the

---

26. See n. 16.

27. Eisenstein, "Pikku'aḥ Nefesh," 152–53. Leviticus 19:16 is given here as the main argument for *pikuach nefesh*. The problem of the saving of non-Jews on the Sabbath or holidays is not mentioned.

category "neighbour."[28] Hence the law of *pikuach nefesh*, if based solely on Lev 19:16, would not be applicable to non-Jews according to most Talmudic texts.

Yet the view that the law should not be broken to save a non-Jew's life has been nuanced and debated by many Jewish authorities after the Talmud. These authorities base the duty to preserve the life of "strangers" as well as Jews on Lev 25:35.[29]

> If one of your countrymen becomes poor and is unable to support himself among you, help him as you would a stranger or a temporary resident, so he can continue to live among you.

Hence it is derived that a "stranger" should be supported too. Maimonides and others define a "stranger" as any non-Jew who observes the seven Noachide commandments, i.e. not a complete heathen who does not uphold any moral standards.[30] Maimonides, Nachmanides and other halakhic authorities plainly hold that non-Jews as well as Jews should be helped "once they accepted the basic laws of humanity."[31] The issue, however, remained problematic, as the *Shulchan Arukh*, the main code of Jewish law, in principle upheld the talmudic view that the law should only be breached for Jews.[32] In the seventeenth century, when the question became rather acute since there were more and more Jewish doctors working in non-Jewish en-

---

28. E.g., BT Baba Kama 38a, dealing with Exod 21:35; Baba Metsia 87b, dealing with Deut 23:25; and Baba Metsia 101b, quoting Lev 19:13. Steven Fraade, in an illuminating study on the matter, explains how biblical *nomos* was not intended to include non-Jews and how the Rabbis had to come to terms with this when facing legal issues involving non-Jews. His study focuses upon Baba Kama 38a which treats the case of a gentile's ox goring a Jew's ox and vice versa (cf. Exod 21:35: "when a man's ox injures his neighbour's ox"). In this source the Sages debate whether "neighbor" includes non-Jews. This case can shed a light on the issue of *pikuach nefesh* when this is solely based on Lev 19:16, because in both biblical texts the word "neighbor" is used. Cf. Fraade, "Navigating the Anomalous," 145–65. See also Sperber, "Gentile," 485–86.

29. For a discussion of this problem, including references, see I. Jacobovits, *Jewish Medical Ethics*, 62–63.

30. On the Noachide commandments see, e.g., Berman, "Noachide Laws." The Noachide laws include the prohibition of idolatry, blasphemy, bloodshed, sexual sins, theft, eating from a living animal, and the injunction to establish a legal system.

31. Jacobovits, *Jewish Medical Ethics*, 62, see also nn. 43 and 44 there.

32. Interestingly many authors seem to ignore this issue completely. See, e.g., Evers, *Op het leven!*, 121–36: "Patientenselectie" (Selection of Patients), who even quotes Mishnah Yoma 8:7 but avoids the discussion of this serious problem. The author seems to imply that there is no difference between Jewish and non-Jewish patients in this regard, as he discusses the Dutch situation in which Jewish patients would form a minority of the patients of Jewish doctors. But he does not explicitly touch upon the halakhic problem initiated by the Talmud.

vironments, many *responsa*[33] were devoted to it. Often the rabbis advised doctors to stay away from such situations by avoiding professional calls on the Sabbath or telling the patients to do what was necessary themselves.[34] As to non-observant Jews, a similar problem arose, as the argument that one Sabbath should be breached so as to allow the patient to observe many more Sabbaths in the future—a major biblical support for the case as will be seen in the next paragraph—does not apply to them either.

Biblical Proof: The Sabbath Is to Live by, not to Die By

The talmudic treatment of the duty to save life (on Yom Kippur and) on the Sabbath ends with some discussions by rabbinic sages who want to adduce biblical proof for the proposition that saving life is more important than the Sabbath. First, a story is told of three famous rabbis taking a stroll while discussing the matter.

> R. Ishmael, R. Akiba and R. Eleazar b. Azariah were once on a journey, with Levi ha-Saddar and R. Ishmael son of R. Eleazar b. Azariah following them. Then this question was asked of them: Whence do we know that in the case of danger to human life (pikuach nefesh) the laws of the Sabbath are suspended?— R. Ishmael answered and said: *If a thief be found breaking in* (Exodus 22:1). Now if in the case of this one it is doubtful whether he has come to take money or life; and although the shedding of blood pollutes the land, so that the Shechinah departs from Israel, yet it is lawful to save oneself at the cost of his life—how much more may one suspend the laws of the Sabbath to save human life! R. Akiba answered and said: *If a man come presumptuously upon his neighbour etc. thou shalt take him from My altar, that he may die.* (Exodus 21:14) ... Now if in the case of this one, where it is doubtful whether there is any substance in his words or not, yet [he interrupts] the service in the Temple [which is important enough to] suspend the Sabbath, how much more should the saving of human life suspend the Sabbath laws! R. Eleazar answered and said: If circumcision, which attaches to one only of the two hundred and forty-eight members of the human body, suspends the Sabbath, how much more shall [the saving of] the whole body suspend the Sabbath! (BT Yoma 85a–b)

---

33. Responsa (Latin: plural of responsum, "answers") are written decisions and rulings given by halakhic authorities in response to questions addressed to them.

34. Ibid, 63 and n. 47 there.

Rabbi Ishmael compares the situation of *pikuach nefesh* to a biblical law that states that one may kill a burglar in self-defence, even when it is not clear whether he has the intention to kill. Hence, if shedding blood when one's own life might be in danger is allowed in some cases, how much more[35] the breaking of the Sabbath laws, which is a lesser offence, is allowed to save a life.

Rabbi Akiva comes with another biblical text: In Exodus 21 it is stated that anyone who kills a person shall be put to death. However, v. 14 reads that "if someone schemes against another person to kill him, he must be dragged even from my altar and be put to death." Rabbi Akiva derives from this that if even the Temple Service should be interrupted to save the endangered person's life, then all the more can the Sabbath be broken to save a life.

A third proof is adduced by R. Eleazar who compares saving a life to circumcision: if a child can be circumcised on the Sabbath (which is allowed), thus "saving" one of its members, how much more should one suspend the Sabbath rest to save an entire body, i.e. a life.[36] In the Gospel of John this same saying is attributed to Jesus.[37]

Hereafter the context of the "journey" seems to be left, as three other sages adduce more biblical prooftexts to state that saving life is worth more than keeping the Sabbath laws. All three passages are taken from the biblical laws about Sabbath observance.

> R. Jose son of R. Judah said: *Only ye shall keep My Sabbaths* (Exodus 31:13), one might assume under all circumstances, therefore the text reads: "Only" viz. allowing for exceptions. R. Jonathan b. Joseph said: *For it is holy unto you* (Exodus 31:14 cont.). I.e., it [the Sabbath] is committed to your hands, not you to its hands.
>
> R. Simeon b. Menassia said: *And the children of Israel shall keep the Sabbath* (Exodus 31:16). The Torah said: Profane for his sake one Sabbath, so that he may keep many Sabbaths. Rab Judah said in the name of Samuel: If I had been there, I should have told them something better than what they said: [*You shall therefore keep my statutes and my rules; if a person does them,*] *he shall live by them* (Leviticus 18:5), but he shall not die because of them. Raba said: [The exposition] of all of them could

---

35. The rabbinic hermeneutic rule of *kal vachomer* (a minori ad maius) is applied here. On rabbinic hermeneutics, and specifically this rule, see Stemberger, *Introduction*, 15–30, esp. 18.

36. See also the parallels in BT Shabbat 132a; Mekhilta Shabeta on Exod 31:13.

37. John 7:23.

be refuted, except that of Samuel, which cannot be refuted. (BT Yoma 85b)

The first argument, started by R. Jose son of R. Judah and continued by R. Jonathan ben Joseph is a famous midrash on Exod 31:14 which is also known from the NT where it is expressed by Jesus.[38] Rabbi Jose accentuates the word "only", and applies a rabbinic hermeneutic rule to the occurrence of this word: when a conjunctive is found that is not absolutely necessary for the meaning of the text, it carries special meaning;[39] in this case R. Jose reads it as a reducing meaning—which is to say that there are valid exceptions to keeping the Sabbath. Rabbi Jonathan ben Joseph interprets the second half of the verse and focuses on the words "unto you": the Sabbath is for you, meaning, its observance should not bring your life in danger, but it should enhance your life.

The second biblical prooftext brought in by R. Simeon is a famous one, but it is tricky in that it in fact says that the Sabbath is worth more than a human life. It is also a hard explanation to uphold when dealing with non-observant Jews or non-Jews.[40] Rab Judah must have noticed this because he comes with a final biblical argument, which he had heard from the sage Samuel, to prove why the Sabbath is subservient to life:

> You shall therefore keep my statutes and my rules; *if a person does them, he shall live by them* (Lev. 18:5), but he shall not die because of them.

---

38. Mark 2:27.

39. The rabbinic hermeneutic rule (see note 34) of *miut* (reduction) is applied here, because of the occurrence of the word *akh* (only). See Stemberger, *Introduction*, 23.

40. There are still well-informed Jews who are of the opinion that a person's life is subservient to Sabbath and that "Profane for his sake one Sabbath, so that he may keep many Sabbaths" is the main argument for *pikuach nefesh*. See, e.g., the online article of Gil Student, "Shabbat and Gentile Lives," 2001. Writing after the passing of Dr. Israel Shahak, a human-rights activist who claimed that Judaism was racist because it would treat non-Jews with different ethical standards from Jews, and bearing upon the issue of saving a gentile's life on the Shabbat, he concludes: "When Dr. Shahak criticized Judaism of being racist by denying medical treatment to Gentiles on Shabbat, he was wrong on many counts. First, this is not practiced today, as can be evidenced by the treatment of Gentiles by Jewish doctors in Sha'arei Tzedek Hospital in Jerusalem or by Hatzoloh volunteers in New York. Second, the determination is not race-driven. In theory, it applies to both non-religious Jews and Gentiles. It also does not apply to all Gentiles. As we have seen from Ramban, we are allowed to violate Shabbat to save Gentiles who have officially taken it upon themselves to live righteous lives. Third, and perhaps most importantly, the permission, or lack thereof, to violate Shabbat to save someone's life is not in any way a valuation of that person's life because no life, whether Jewish or Gentile, is more important than Shabbat."

"Them" refers to the biblical commandments. A later talmudic authority, Raba, agrees that this is the only valid proof.

Samuel, Rab Judah and Raba believe that observing religious commandments only makes sense when they enhance life, not when they bring it down. This is an idea that underlies most of Jewish thought in general and Jewish medical ethics in particular.

BIBLIOGRAPHY

Brody, Baruch. "Chapter 1: A Historical Introduction to Jewish Casuistry on Suicide and Euthanasia." In *Suicide and Euthanasia: Historical and Contemporary Themes*, edited by Baruch Brody, 39–75. Dordrecht: Kluwer, 1989.

Ben-Sasson, Haim Hillel. "Kiddush ha-shem and Hillul ha-shem." In *Encyclopaedia Judaica*. CD-Rom ed. Judaica Multimedia, 1997.

Berman, Saul. "Noachide Laws." In *Encyclopaedia Judaica*. CD-Rom ed. Judaica Multimedia, 1997.

Cohen, Gerson D. "Hannah and Her Seven Sons." In *Encyclopaedia Judaica*. CD-Rom ed. Judaica Multimedia, 1997.

Dorff, Elliott N., "End-of-life: Jewish Perspectives." *The Lancet* 366 (2005) 862–65.

———. *Matters of Life and Death. A Jewish Approach to Modern Medical Ethic*. New York: Jewish Publication Society, 2004.

Elzas, M. "Geneeskunst in de Babylonische Talmoed: Bulimie." *Nederlands Tijdschrift voor Geneeskunde* 116/51 (1972) 2300–303.

Eisenstein, D. "Pikku'aḥ Nefesh." In *Encyclopaedia Judaica* 16 (20072) 152–53.

Evers, R. *Op het leven! Medische ethiek bezien vanuit joodse optiek*. Kampen: Kok, 1997.

Fraade, Steven. "Navigating the Anomalous." In *The Other in Jewish Thought and History: Constructions of Jewish Culture and Identity*, edited by Laurence Jay Silberstein and Robert L. Cohn, 145–65. New York: NYU Press, 1994.

Freedman, Benjamin. *Duty and Healing: Foundations of a Jewish Bioethic*. New York: Routledge, 1999.

Jacobovits, Immanuel. *Jewish Medical Ethics: A Comparative and Historical Study of the Jewish Religious Attitude to Medicine and its Practice*. New York: Bloch, 1959.

———. "Medical Ethics, Jewish." In *Encyclopaedia Judaica*. CD-Rom ed. Judaica Multimedia, 1997.

Hakohen, Israel Meir. *Mishna Berura: Hebrew-English edition*. vol.3 c: Laws of Shabbos §308–24. New York: Feldheim, 1984.

Mantel, Hugo. "Sanhedrin." In *Encyclopaedia Judaica*. CD-Rom ed. Judaica Multimedia, 1997.

Preuss, Julius. *Biblisch-Talmudische Medizin: Beiträge zur Geschichte der Heilkunde und der Kultur überhaupt*. Berlin: Karger, 1911.

Rosner, Fred, *Medicine in the Bible and the Talmud: Selections from Classical Jewish Sources*. New York: Ktav, 1977.

———. "Rabies in the Talmud." *Medical History* 18 (1974) 198–200.

Rudman, Z. C. "Fetal Rights and Maternal Obligation." *Journal of Halacha and Contemporary Society* 13 (1987) 113–24.

Sperber, D. "Gentile." In *Encyclopedia of Judaism* 7 (1999) 485–86.

Stemberger, Günter. *Introduction to the Talmud and Midrash*. 2nd ed. Edinburgh: T. & T. Clark, 1996.
Student, Gil. "Shabbat and Gentile Lives." 2001. http://www.aishdas.org/student/shabbat.htm.
Urbach, Ephraim U. *The Sages: Their Concepts and Beliefs*. 2 vols. Jerusalem: Magnes, 1987.

Part 4

Religion, Illness, and Care of the Sick in Greco-Roman Antiquity and Christianity

13

Illness and Healing in Christian Traditions

—Gregor Etzelmüller
and Annette Weissenrieder

RECENT ANALYSES OFTEN PROCLAIM a positive connection between religious attitudes and health. After evaluating about 1200 clinical studies on the relationship between religion and mental/physical health, the authors of the *Handbook of Religion and Health* come to the following conclusion: "(R)eligious beliefs and practices rooted within established religious traditions were found to be consistently associated with better health and predicted better health over time."[1] The studies, which mainly focus on Christian believers, seem to suggest an understanding of Christianity as a religion of healing.

Along the same lines, the New Testament scholar and church historian Adolf von Harnack described Christianity as a religion of healing as early as 1892, and explained that its mission had been successful largely because the early church cared for the sick and the needy. "Because [the early church] promised and produced healing and outshone all other religions and cults in this respect, its success was already assured before it won over society completely with its superior philosophy. Christianity not only offered the real Jesus instead of the imaginary Asclepius, but it fashioned itself as a 'religion of healing,' deliberately presenting itself 'as medicine for body and

1. Koenig, *Handbook*, 591, cf. Miller and Thoresen, "Spirituality, Religion, and Health," 24–35.

soul,' and it considered one of its most important duties to be taking care of the physically ill."[2]

Naturally, Christianity's self-commendation as a religion of healing must be read critically in contrast with the factual history of Christianity. Throughout this history, people with handicaps were also always stigmatized and excluded.[3] Well into the second half of the 20th century, for instance, people with mental disabilities were prevented from taking communion in most Protestant congregations. Historically, churches and congregations were not merely inclusive actors, but also effected and supported the exclusion of people with illnesses and disabilities. Even Harnack's commendation of Christianity as a religion of healing must be seen critically given its background, the colonial missionary project. It must at least be admitted that the spread of Western medicine in the context of the Christian mission had negative as well as positive effects.

Harnack's advocacy of current Christianity and his representation of early Christianity as a religion of healing are therefore currently subject to a great deal of criticism. Instead of looking for the social causes of illness and disability, critics say that von Harnack develops an idealized image of a healthy person with which all people are expected to comply as a standard. He is said to support "the hegemony of normalcy within which the different is paternalistically accommodated."[4] Systematic theologian Sharon V. Betcher correctly pointed out that von Harnack's image of Jesus is that of a "vital, pure and busy" Jesus, corresponding more closely to the modern ideal of industriousness and health than to the synoptic texts. Von Harnack, she says, ignores "the biblical interpretation of Jesus with Isa 53, i.e., the Song of the Suffering Servant, one of the most important intertexts for crafting the figure of Jesus in the synoptics. Shaped through Isaianic imagery, Jesus appears grotesque—despised, rejected, a man of suffering, acquainted with infirmity, one from whom others hide their faces (Isaiah 53:3)."[5]

Based on the perception of the sick, rejected and grotesque Jesus, Betcher primarily criticizes the coupling of religion and physical health. Those who preach the miracle stories of the New Testament as accounts of

2. Von Harnack, *Medicinisches*, 96.

3. Cf. Barnes, "A Legacy of Oppression," 3–24; Wienberg, "Inklusion von Menschen mit Behinderungen," 169–82.

4. Betcher, "Disability and the Terror of the Miracle Tradition," 170; cf. Hutchinson, "Disabling Beliefs?," 1–23, 4, with additional literature.

5. Betcher, "Disability and the Terror of the Miracle Tradition," 171. The "metaphorical reconceptualization of Jesus Christ as a 'disabled God'" is a common starting point of different liberation theologies based on the experiences of disabled people (cf. Hutchinson, "Disabling Beliefs?," 5).

healing, she says, marginalize people with disabilities and promote "a 'Pick up your bed and walk' mentality that circulates in Western cultures as the ethos of morality ... and intact economic resources, i.e., labour power."[6] According to Betcher, the miracle stories in the New Testament should not be understood within the context of illness and healing, but rather of slavery and societal liberation: "slavery, not disability as we today construe it, may have been more precisely that which was signified by bodies blind, maimed, lame and deaf."[7] Thus Christianity should not be commended and lived out as a religion of healing, but as a religion of societal liberation.[8]

Betcher's christologically based criticism of von Harnack is not only justified, but also indicates a circumstance that theologians prefer to ignore: the fact that illness is also a societal evil, that societies can make people sick and disabled. At the same time, however, Betcher's criticism also provokes the question of whether illnesses and disabilities only represent a societal evil. Are there not also people—as often seen in the New Testament—who are crippled not just due to slavery and who suffer not just from social marginalization, but who also suffer from natural evils, from the cruelty of natural processes? Consider the woman with the issue of blood (Luke 8:43–48 par., see also pp. 280–282 below). Theology is constantly in danger of ignoring not just the cruelty of the human world, but that of all creation.[9] Heidelberg physician and philosopher Viktor von Weizsäcker, who more than almost anyone was sensitive to the social conditions of illness, once gave a talk in which he asked theologians, "Have you ever seen and experienced the progressive, radical collapse of spiritual, moral and religious life in a cancer patient?"[10] Cruelty comes not just from other human beings, but from creation itself.

Given the complex discussion sketched out here, our goal in the following is not to commend Christianity as a religion of healing. Instead, we want to question the valency of this concept. This will take place from a Protestant perspective, based on connections between New Testament

---

6. Betcher, "Disability and the Terror of the Miracle Tradition," 166; cf. 162; this criticism is more apparent in Swiss Catholic theologian Wilhelm's text, "'Normal' werden—war's das?," 103–5, which criticizes not only a specific use of the biblical healing stories, but the stories themselves.

7. Betcher, "Disability and the Terror of the Miracle Tradition," 173; cf. 175.

8. Ibid., 174. This contemporary recommendation also corresponds to early Christian art, which was also not focused on healing, but on political liberation. "Salvation [in early Christian art] is represented as a deliverance from the power of the Roman emperor." Mathews, *The Clash of Gods*, 76 (cited in Betcher, ibid., 174).

9. Cf. Thomas, *Neue Schöpfung*, 16.

10. Von Weizsäcker, *Grundfragen medizinischer Anthropologie*, 274.

exegesis, systematic theology and practical theological issues. If one is to be able to understand Christianity as a religion of healing, this must first be demonstrated by the biblical texts themselves. However, the biblical texts contradict an understanding of healing solely in the sense of physical recovery. In our opinion, if Christianity is to be claimed as a religion of healing, this must be stated as follows: As a religion of healing, Christianity does not directly aim to create better health, but rather a community that accepts the sick and suffering—one that does everything possible to heal them (including making the necessary societal changes), but also helps people to be sick in a healthy way and allows the sick and suffering to make their own specific contributions to the development of the Christian congregations.[11] In a religion of healing, the sick and suffering are not merely objects of medical and ministerial care; instead, every person contributes in a specific way toward the formation of this healing community.

The following remarks are intended to ask whether such an understanding of Christianity as a religion of healing is plausible with regard to early Christianities and the diversity of Christian denominations. Thus we will begin with the biblical miracle stories and ask what these stories are really about (pp. 264–267). To create a better understanding of the biblical miracle stories, we will then contextualize them within the intersection of ancient rational medicine, healing cults and Old Testament texts (267–283). This will allow us to see differences in early Christianity that persist even today in the various denominations (pp. 284–290). The two final chapters attempt to develop an understanding of Christianity as a religion dedicated to care for the sick that can also stand up to critical questioning from the field of disability studies (pp. 290ff.).

THE FOCUS IS NOT ON THE MIRACLE ONLY

For New Testament miracle stories, form-critical classifications like therapies, exorcisms, gift miracles etc. are still foundational. These classifications distinguish between miracles that are historically plausible and others that should be considered wonders. It is unsettling, however, that form-critical analysis does not include insights on ancient diseases.[12] The focus is on the miracle of healing, while the aspects of the stories relating to the hermeneutics of illness and the living environment are almost completely ignored.

11. Cf. Mieth, "Der behinderte Mensch aus theologisch-ethischer Sicht," 127–30.

12. Bendemann (*Christus der Arzt*) and Weissenrieder (*Images of Illness*) tried in different ways to show that the healing stories include a wide range of aspects, of which healing is only one.

Recently, systematic theologian Betcher has attracted a great deal of attention with her book *Spirit and the Politics of Disablement* and her article "Disability and the Terror of Miracle." Betcher evaluates New Testament miracle stories as "texts of terror" that have only one focus: the *miracle* of healing.[13] Her approach explicitly denounces the religious interpretation of an illness: in a miracle story, illness would be demonized and understood as God's punishment. But to what extent are miraculous aspects really constitutive in the healing stories?

Two points show that it is not as easy to differentiate between the two directions as it might seem at first glance: The New Testament has no single term that is translated "miracle." The English term "miracle" derives from the Latin term *miraculum*. In Greek, terms like δυνάμεις (*dūnameis*) powers, ἔργον (*ergon*) work, σημεῖον (*semeion*) sign, τέρας (*teras*) and θαῦμα (*thauma*) wonder are important terms that signify a miracle story; however, they are not used to refer to a supranatural event. For space reasons we are referring here to θαῦμα (*thauma*) only. New Testament passages refer to θαῦμα *thauma* (marvel or wonder), which is very often understood as puzzlement, perplexity, or curiosity. However, in antiquity wonder is closely connected with the faculty of vision (a wonder to see) and is related to mind and wisdom. In the particular context of the Gospel of Luke, the terms *thauma / thaumazein* refer to the belief and knowledge, especially in the infancy narratives (Luke 1:21, 63; 2:18, 33). Aristotle's understanding of *thauma* is foundational for understanding the ancient concept(s) of "miracle." *Thauma* is not used for things that defy causal explanation, but refers to wonder aroused by unexpected events. Such occurrences described as *alogon* (1460a13.28–9.36), *atopon* (1460a35), and *adūnaton* (1460a27) inspired veneration and typically motivated an inquiry into the causes of the wonder (*Metaph.* 982b12–19). It is a matter of knowing that you don't know, which requires wisdom. Therefore, "wonder" does not necessarily refer to a "supra-natural" domain.[14] The *aporia* for deep insight proceeds from seeing and interpretation. The Gospel of Luke does not operate on the basis of a naïve belief in miracles, but rather makes complex distinctions between miracle, wonder and suspicion, seeing and knowing. Especially for Luke, this means that the focus is not only on the miracle. Instead, he tries to make the miracles plausible within their social context, which includes the ancient understanding of health as well as religious distinctions and political realities. Thus New Testament miracle stories refer to the wonder of

---

13. See Betcher, *Spirit and the Politics of Disablement*, 1–24.

14. Wilson Nightingale, "On Wandering and Wondering," 23–58; Schaeffer, "Wisdom and Wonder in 'Metaphysics' A: 1–2," 641–56.

healing, but with an emphasis on making distinctions between miraculous events. This is especially true if we give credence to the historical, political, and social information included in the healing stories.[15] This factual information makes the miracle understandable in the world of the readers and circumvent the distinction between fact and fiction. This is connected with a second important aspect:

Betcher and many others refer to terms like θεραπεύειν *therapeuein*, which is often translated as "to make healed," "to heal," or "to cure." However, the Greek terms that we translate as "healing," ἰάομαι *iaomai* and *therapeuein*, should not be interpreted in a sense of bodily restitution only. In the LXX, *therapeuein* carries connotations of treatment for illness and more generally service (Tob 12:3 but cf 6:9; 1 Esdras 1:4; Judith 11:17).[16] More often, the terms are used in ancient medicine as "taking care," "looking after the ill person" and "medical treatment."[17] *Iaomai*, on the other hand, was used predominantly in the LXX to refer to divine healing (Tob 12:14; Pss 6:2; 30:2; 41:4, and passim; Wis 16:10; Sir 38:9). It signifies much more the act of a divine person, service or healing, than the sick or healed. It was also the designation given to Asclepius in the *iamata*.[18] However, the language of transformation or therapeutic change—to use the terminology of medical

---

15. For more details see von Bendemann, *Christus medicus*, and Weissenrieder, *Images of Illness*.

16. Wells, *The Greek Language of Healing*, 103–19.

17. We limit ourselves here to a few examples regarding *therapeuein*. See, e.g., CH *Morb* II.3: "If you wish to attend this patient *therapeuein*, treat his head with vapour-baths, and fashion a connection to the external air by incising." In CH *Morb*. II.6, the author is saying: "You must treat *therapeuein* this patient as follows: wash him with hot water two or three times every day . . . the first days clean him downwards, and give him water to drink, for water usually provokes vomiting . . .]" (LCL, Jones, trans.). And Plato says: "[T]he slaves are usually doctored by slaves, who either run round the town or wait in their surgeries; and not one of these doctors either gives or receives any account of the several ailments of the various domestics, but prescribes for each what he deems right from experience, just as though he had exact knowledge, and with the assurance of an autocrat; then up he jumps and off he rushes to another sick domestic, and thus he relieves his master in his attendance on the sick. [720d] But the free-born doctor is mainly engaged in visiting and treating the ailments of free men, and he does so by investigating them from the commencement and according to the course of nature; he talks with the patient himself and with his friends, and thus both learns himself from the sufferers and imparts instruction to them, so far as possible; and he gives no prescription until he has gained the patient's consent, and only then, while securing the patient's continued docility by means of persuasion, [720e] does he attempt to complete the task of restoring him to health." (Plato, *Leg* IV 720d-e, LCL; see also *Georg*. 513). And a translation of Acts 17:24f. also has "to serve" for *therapeuein*: "And he is not served by human hands, as if he needed anything, because he himself gives all men life and breath and everything else."

18. See LiDonnici, *The Epidaurian Miracle Inscriptions*, 84–131.

anthropologist Arthur Kleinman—is not *iaomai* or *therapeuein*. For Mark this is not surprising, in that *therapeuein* is not generally used in Mark; in Matthew, however, it is used several times in summaries (4:23, 24; 8:7, 16; 9:35; 10:1, 8; 12:10, 15, 22; 14:14; 15:30; 17:16.18; 19:2; 21:14); however, the verb is not used to describe a therapeutic change except in Matthew 12:22. The therapeutic change is normally described in terms of reversal, e.g., the leper is cleansed (Matt. 8:3), the fever leaves Peter's mother-in-law (Matt. 8:15), and the daughter of the leader of the synagogue who has just died is resurrected (Matt. 9:25). Matthew 14:36 describes Jesus' healing of many with the word διεσώθησαν, which has a theological meaning—to save—and is also used in the context of the Asclepius tradition. Therefore the term σώζειν (*sozein*, to save) connotes the use of one religious system over another, the Asclepius tradition vs. early Christianities. Thus the terms *therapeuein, iaomai* or *sozein* refer to serving people, which is life-enhancing and changes their life. It may be better to refer to this in terms of a vocabulary of change rather than one of health.[19]

We already indicated that early Christianity must be related to its context, of which ancient medicine and philosophy are an important part. It was therefore of vital importance for early Christianity that *ancient medicine and philosophy* were themselves in a process of differentiation. Christianity had to relate on the one hand to the differentiation of "rational" medicine out of practice-oriented medicine, on the other hand to the differentiation of a scientific-rational medicine out of the healing cults of the time, and finally to the coexistence of rational medicine and philosophy. Early Christianity not only searched for its own point of view in this process of differentiation, but also related the point of view to its theological principles.

ANCIENT "RATIONAL" MEDICINE AND ITS RELATIONSHIP TO ANCIENT HEALING CULTS

"Rational medicine"[20] is widespread, above all, in the *Corpus Hippocraticum* and in later works by medical theorists such as Herophilus and Galen,[21] who brought physical and scientific legality to the fore.

---

19. Kleinman, *Patients and Healers in the Context of Culture*, 303–10.
20. Cf. on the relationship between "rational" medicine and New Testament Weissenrieder, *Images of Illness*, chap. 2. Cf. also Weissenrieder and Etzelmüller, "Christlicher Glaube und Medizin."
21. Cf. also Tieleman, *Galen and Chrysippus on the Soul*; see also his contribution in this volume.

The "birth" of the Greek art of both medicine and medical literature was seen in Hippocrates, and one could say that "rational" medicine originated in Greece in the fifth century BCE, when the first treatises of the Hippocratic Corpus were written.[22] But this is no longer the simple matter of fact it once was. Scholarship is becoming more sensitive not only to eurocentric bias, but also to the notion of "rational." Today it is necessary to specify what the term means with reference to ancient Greek medicine.

The view that rational medicine originated when the Hippocratic Corpus was written is supported by writings such as *De morbo sacro* and the six treatises of *De morbis popularibus*, which at first glance appear to argue against supernatural practices and beliefs. Although ancient physicians such as Hippocrates thoroughly supported this perspective, some caution is advised since it can be all too easy to interpret the writings of the Hippocratic Corpus as a kind of enlightenment movement of antiquity or as a "Greek miracle" leading toward natural science, and therefore to hold them up as a paradigm of rational biomedical science, which, from the point of view of a belief in progress, appears to be an early form of our contemporary bioscientific medicine.[23] In philological and medical-historical exegetical research we read again and again that the Greeks "already knew X," "while Y"—something that seems common knowledge to us now—"they did not yet know."[24] The designation of ancient medicine as "rational medicine" goes hand in hand with a certain late modern attitude of reservation toward the "supernatural" and the "magical," which we bring under critical examination in this volume.[25] Rational is understood here as *logikos* in the sense of theoretically substantiated, indicating a closeness to the natural philosophy of antiquity. The beginning of rational medicine consists therefore most clearly "in the discovery of disease as a *natural process*: a particular type of cause produces *as a rule* a particular type of effect."[26]

This strongly supports the supposition that one cannot assume a religious foundation for medicine. Various methodological approaches such as the doctrine of the microcosm-macrocosm and the doctrine of the bodily

---

22. Herter, "Die kulturhistorische Theorie der hippokratischen Schrift 'Von der alten Medizin,'" 464–83; and Fantuzzi, "De Prisca Medicina pseudoippocartico," 21–26.

23. This is also true for the designation of "superstition," which in New Testament studies is often connected with ancient medicine. See Martin, *Inventing Superstition*.

24. This applies, for example, to the question of whether "circulation of the blood" was already known in antiquity. On this question see Duminil, *Le sang, le vaisseaux, le coeur*, 169–74.

25. In this connection see also Chaniotis's notable essay on the region of Lydia and Phrygia in "Illness and Cures in Greek Propitiatory Inscriptions" 323–44.

26. So Tieleman in his contribution in this volume.

fluids confirm the purely rational background of medicine. There are some possible reasons to reject this one-sided interpretation:

For one, it is striking that in the *Corpus Hippocraticum* an entire treatise is dedicated to the phenomenon of dreaming, which then becomes the reason and preparation for the medical doctor's diagnoses (*De victu* IV): the dreaming soul gives information about the state of the body. Thus the treatise begins as follows: "Anyone who has a correct understanding of the signs that occur in sleep will discover that they have great significance for everything" [CH *De victu* IV 86 (6.640 Littré)]. This statement occurs within the context of the author's explanation that dreams have great significance not just as "signs" and "indicators" of the body, but that they should also be understood and valued as divine prophecies of the future. A belief in the divine origin of dreams and their prophetic power was widespread in antiquity and was common even in intellectual circles.[27] Here, the dividing line between the rational and the irrational is clearly different than our "modern" view would expect. In addition, the *per professionem* "dream interpreter" Artemidorus not only testifies to the god's manifest healing successes in his holy sites, but also rejects the possibility of arbitrariness in interpreting medical dreams (*Onir.* 4,22) when he writes: "You will see that the (divinely ordained) treatment completely follows the rules of medicine and in no way deviates from their rationality." We hear additional reports from the orator Aelius Aristides (around 145 CE), who received instructions from the healing god Asclepius, and who followed these instructions. Aristides writes: "Even when we were stricken in body, we did not come to ignoble supplication of the doctors. But although, to speak by the grace of the gods, we possessed the friendship of the best doctors, we took refuge in it was better to be saved through his agency, and that if it was not possible, it was time to die."[28] Comparable statements come from Galen, though he draws a clear line: dreams should not be the exclusive source of medical findings.[29] Nonetheless, he does not describe the divine works of the healing god Asclepius as "irrational," since even he could only work within the boundaries established by nature (ἀδύνατα φύσει).[30]

In addition, the closeness of Hippocratic medicine to the practice of the healing cults is also testified by the *Hippocratic oath (Ius)*. There it says:[31]

27. See van der Eijk, *Aristoteles. De insomniis*, 102–32.

28. Aristides Orationes 28.132 (translation: Behr). See the contribution of Georgia Petridou in this volume.

29. Galen *MM* 3.2 (X 164 Kühn) and *Introc. S. medic.* 3 Deichgräber (XIV 679 Kühn).

30. Galen *UP* 9.14; 2.159 Helmreich; XIV 615 Kühn.

31. The treatise goes back to the opening of the training center of the Asclepiads for

"I swear by Apollo Physician, by Asclepius, by Health, by Panacea and by all the gods and goddesses, making them my witnesses that I will carry out, according to my ability and judgment, this oath and this indenture" [CH *Iusiurandum* 1 (LCL 1: Jones)]. With this oath, the Hippocratic tradition is aligned with the healing God Apollo who is also named in numerous other sources as the "father" of the Asclepiads.[32]

Notably, Hippocrates swears his oath not only by Apollo, but also by Asclepius, who was known as the healing God.[33] A number of healing temples (*Asklepieia*) are known to us from this time. The healing qualities are reflected by the image constellation. Asclepius' help and healing of human suffering is indicated in several ways: he touches the sick, and conversations are signaled by the attentive posture of his body, which expresses a direct connection to the sick.

Parallel to Asclepius' affirmation of the doctors, we find the question of divine power (*dūnamis*), which comes from the gods. The first-century written treatise *Decorum* assumed that the potency of gods "was interwoven into the mind of medicine." "[M]edicine is found to be held in honor by the gods. And the physicians have yielded to the gods. For in medicine the ruling power *dūnamis* is not unessential. In fact, though the physicians take many things in hand, many [illnesses] are also overcome for them spontaneously" [CH *Decorum* 6 (Translation: LCL with some changes)]. Spontaneous healing was therefore ascribed to the gods.[34] And it is worth noting

---

a broader layer and led to the fact that the medical tradition of Cos could be continued by founding it on a wide base. The social context at the beginning of the oath shows that with this opening, however, the privileges of the family of Asclepiads were also in question. It is a question repeatedly discussed in the literature: whether the oath is really to be attributed to the doctor's school founded by Hippocrates (so Kudlien, *Beginn des medizinischen Denkens*, 19; Deichgräber, *Der hippokratische Eid*, 48–49; Kollesch and Hartwig, "Der hippokratische Eid," 253–326; Schubert, *Der Hippokratische Eid* and Diller, *Hippokrates, Schriften*, 7).

Some remarks refer to possible medical topics in antiquity: thus the ban is meant to ensure societal protection against suicide by poison, which was made possible by pharmacists and doctors who prepared highly efficient poisons (Theophrastus *Historia Plantarum* IX 16,8); on the subject of abortion, there are references calling abortion *uvulae* which are not otherwise mentioned in the *Corpus Hippocraticum*. However, other *abortativa* are mentioned (see *De muliebribus* I 68 and *Superfetatione* 27); the fear of impotence among men is shown by the ban of the stone cut (only at this point are skillful men mentioned in the CH). In addition, the reference to the healing cults points to the question of coupling the healing cult with rational medicine.

32. See Plato *Phaedo* 270 c; CH *Epistulae* 2.17–24 (IX 314.1–8 Littré).

33. Cf. Ovid *Met.* XV, 637–640, 658–662, 669–679, 736–744; Pausanias II,27,2. Regarding the images see Weissenrieder, "He is a God!," 134–56.

34. But it seems to be unclear whether this healing was a deliberate act of God or a natural process, because nature was divine; see therefore Edelstein, *Ancient Medicine*,

that the Hippocratics are mindful of prayers to the gods: "They should have brought them [the patients] to the sanctuaries, with sacrifices and prayers, in supplication to the gods" [CH *De morbo sacro* 4 (VI. 362 Littré)]. In addition, *De natura muliebri* begins with the statement that "the divine is the main cause among human beings ... He who works skillfully must first begin with the things divine."[35] Furthermore, in the Prognostics, the author asks "whether there is something divine in the diseases," and Galen uses the Hippocratic text to focus on studying the prognosis of that which is divine.[36] Stephanus adds, "Such a doctor fully and justly deserves our admiration because the doctor, by using prognosis, is assimilated to God as far as [this is] possible for human beings."[37] In this sense, prognosticating an illness was close to prophesying. Therefore we can say that religious interpretations of illness and scientific-medical knowledge seem not necessarily to have been perceived in antiquity as being in competition. The doctor Herophilus also mentions medicine and drugs as "the hands of the gods," which we have also seen in Plutarch[38] and Galen.[39] This is especially striking because Celsus says (ironically?) that Herophilus, among others, "did not treat any kind of disease without drugs" [Cel. *Medicina* 5, *prooem.* 1 (*CML* 1, 190 Marx)].

Nevertheless, this picture of the coupling of rational medicine with the healing cults of its time requires a correction: the *Corpus Hippocraticum* contains two treatises that touch on the question of whether one should attribute certain illnesses to a divine origin: the treatises *Airs, Waters, Places* and *On Sacred Disease*.[40] Both determine that there is no illness with sacred or even divine origin, because everything is produced according to the laws of nature—or at least according to the law of the illness. Thus the author opens the text *On the Sacred Disease* as follows: "I am about to discuss the disease called 'sacred.' It is not, in my opinion, any more divine or more sacred than

---

216–17.

35. CH *Nat.Mul.* 1 (Littré 7.312). However, it is unclear whether "divine" has the same meaning here as in *Morb.Sacr.*

36. CH *Progn* 1; Galen *In Hippocratis Prognosticum* 1.4: Galen uses τουτέου instead of τούτων.

37. Stephanus *Commentary on the Prognosticon of Hippocrates* 1.18 (Translation: Duffy with some changes).

38. Plut. *Quaestiones symposiacae* 4.1.3 (*Moralia* 663 b–c).

39. Gal. *De Compositione Medicamentorum Secundum Locos* 6.8 (XII 965f. Kühn).

40. CH *De morbo sacro* 1; Littré VI, 356–364. The writing is characterized by an effort to grasp "epileptic phenomena" scientifically. The purpose is to release the illness from its religious connotation. Therefore, the author uses the term "sacred illness" only within a controversial context at the beginning and the end of the text. Instead, the author writes "this illness / suffering" rather than epilepsy. *Epilēpsis* merely means the single attack and is not a name of an illness.

other diseases, but has a natural cause, and its supposed divine origin is due to men's inexperience, and to their wonder at its peculiar character."[41] It is in this context that we also find polemical statements against magicians and charlatans; he argues against understanding the illness as demonic possession or as an unpredictable, sudden and divine effect on a human being, both of which the author challenges because he does not allow for the possibility of divine influence here. In this respect he remains solidly grounded in rational medicine. The divinity alone, not the illness, is surrounded by cleanness and holiness. For this sole reason, a divinity can by no means be the cause of an illness. This evaluation occurs only when there is a lack of interpretation or an absence of meaning: "Being at a loss, and having no treatment that would help, they concealed and sheltered themselves behind the divine and called this disease sacred in order that their utter ignorance might not be manifest" [CH *De morbo sacro* 1 (Littré VI 354.15ff.)]. The lack of interpretation is combined with the second factor, namely the question of guilt. The author writes: "Accordingly I hold that those who attempt in this manner to cure these diseases cannot consider them either sacred or divine; for when they are removed by such purifications and by such treatment as this, there is nothing to prevent the production of attacks in men by devices that are similar. If so, something human is to blame, and not a godhead" [CH *De morbo sacro* 3.1 (Littré VI; Translation: Jones)].

This human guilt is interpreted in the course of the treatise as an inherited illness (CH *De morbo sacro* 5.1.). If the *Corpus Hippocraticum* is taken at face value, it is exclusively the nature of an illness which is examined in order to interpret an illness. The "rational" medicine of antiquity is therefore ambivalent concerning its religious foundation. Its religious self-image is supported by the Hippocratic oath. This religious foundation has its basis in the healing cults of Apollo and Asclepius, for one thing stands out: nowhere are temple medicine and the temple cult of Asclepius called into question. Nevertheless, rational medicine dissociates itself from religious interpretations of illness by rejecting divinity as the cause of illness.[42]

---

41. CH *De morbo sacro* 1.1 (translation: Jones); cf. Grensemann, *Die hippokratische Schrift "Über die heilige Krankheit"*; van der Eijk, "The Theology of the Hippocratic Treatise On the Sacred Disease."

42. Cf. the contribution of Tieleman in this volume.

THE RECEPTION OF "RATIONAL MEDICINE" AND ANCIENT HEALING CULTS IN EARLY CHRISTIANITY

Early Christianity was obliged to relate to the discourse of its context, of which ancient medicine and healing cults are an important part.

A possible conflict with the healing cult of Asclepius might be reflected in John 5:1–18, the healing miracle of the man at the pool at Bethesada. Already in early 19th century archaeological expeditions, archaeologists discovered a large tank situated about 100 feet north-west. Further excavations discovered the remains of Hadrian's Temple of Asclepius and Serapis, as well as smaller healing pools of the Asklepieion, and two other large pools. The discovery shows that John's Gospel may reflect a detailed knowledge of the site, giving the name of the pool as Bethesda, its location near the Sheep Gate and its five porticos with rushing water.

A second example may be reflected in Acts 28, where Paul is, for the only time in Acts, acclaimed a god and savior by the natives (the story is different in Acts 14) after surviving a shipwreck and failing to die from a snake bite.[43] Like Asclepius, Paul must pursue his mission to Rome; he acts as a seer, since he predicts that a shipwreck will endanger the crew, and he also displays his power over the snake, though unlike Asclepius, where the snake is a sign for the healing God, Paul kills it! Just like Asclepius, Paul is associated with political rulers here. Paul meets with "the chief official, the *primus*, of the island of Malta." The use of this title has been confirmed through an inscription from the time of Tiberius.[44] The title was used to designate Publius as a representative of the provincial Roman elite, and it was often associated with special proofs of loyalty to the Roman Empire. Another inscription reads: "He served the God Augustus."[45] In healing Publius, Paul is therefore serving the ideal of well-being represented by the Roman Empire. He is not acting as an independent healer, but as one who is connected with the political leadership of the area. Just as with Asclepius, Paul is thus described as embodying the well-being of the State and is therefore paid with homage, "to be honored with many honors" (*timais timan*). Paul, who arrived as a shipwrecked Jew, leaves the Island as the real benefactor, primus and one of the gods. And like Asclepius, Paul has the ability to heal and lay his hands on an ill person. Yet this healing power does not come from him personally, but is rather experienced through prayer. All of these connections between the Asclepius tradition and the account of Paul's experiences

---

43. See Weissenrieder, "He Is a God!"
44. Cf. Ashby, "Roman Malta," 26.
45. See ibid., 26–27.

on Malta demonstrate the significance of the medical background involved in reading the narrative of Acts 28.

A quotation from the apologist Justin (155 CE) demonstrates that this competition with the Asclepius tradition was intensified in the early church. When explaining the function of Christ for his contemporary pagan world, Justin states, "And in that we say that He made whole the lame, the paralytic, and those born blind, we seem to say what is very similar to deeds said to have been done by Aesculapius" [Justin *Apol.* I,22,6 (Translation: Roberts/Donaldson)]. Both Asclepius and Christ are described as a *Soter*, a savior (Justin *Apol.* I,37,7 and Aelius Aristides *Oratio* 48,40; 39,3.6).[46]

When Paul in Acts 28 is presented in the light of the healing cult of Asclepius, there is of course a fundamental limitation: The cause of the illness, dysentery, is not traced back to a divine power but to the conditions associated with the origins of dysentery, such as rain, wind, age and cold. In so doing, Acts focuses entirely on the medical indications for dysentery.[47] Therefore the author focuses on information that was plausible in the light of the ancient medical science. The text does not distinguish between the natural and supernatural interpretation contexts.

Rational medicine can be seen as the context for some New Testament healing stories. There are numerous references to rational medicine in Luke. In his descriptions, the author of the Gospel of Luke employs constructs of illness that were understandable within the culture of antiquity and that can only be viewed in this context. We can understand the discrepancies from the Gospel of Mark as an intensification of the indicators of illness in the Lucan text.[48] Medical writings of the ancient period confirm this thesis.

Ancient medicine is familiar with two models of epilepsy.[49] Both of these start from the assumption of damage to the brain due to bodily fluids, brought on by the congestion of breath in the arteries. One form manifests itself in conspicuous seizures; the other results in paralysis. Whereas both phenomena are mentioned together in the Gospel of Mark (9:17–18, 20; 9:26)—an impossible scenario in the context of ancient medicine—the author of the Gospel of Luke omits the symptoms describing paralysis in the boy and limits himself to the depiction of a seizure brought on by phlegm, which includes a fit of dramatic physical movement. Jesus is presented here not as an exorcist, but more as physician.

46. See in more detail Dörnemann, *Krankheit und Heilung*.

47. Cf., e.g., CH *De epidemiarum popularibus* I 3.15–17.

48. For more details see Bendemann, *Christus der Arzt* and Weissenrieder, *Images of Illness*; also Popkes, "Die Heilungen Jesu," 186–202.

49. See in detail Weissenrieder, *Images of Illness*, chap. 7.

It is in fact remarkable that Luke, who interprets epilepsy in the context of ancient medicine, still mentions a demon (Luke 9:42). Any interpretation of this text always has to take the ambiguity of the term *pneuma* into consideration: On the one hand the unclean spirit refers to a demonic interpretation of the illness, epilepsy (also mentioned in *De morbo sacro*); on the other hand *pneuma* also refers to unclean *pneuma* inside the human body, which is the cause of the epilepsy. If one follows the interpretation of the unclean spirit as a demon, the question regarding the function of this demon arises.[50]

The author of *De morbo sacro* denies that epilepsy has a divine origin in the sense of something god-sent. He criticizes his opponents for their impiety, *asebeia—apistis*, and for their atheism, *atheos*, which consist of their practicing purificatory rites and incantations as if the sick person were possessed by a demon. Therefore they misunderstand the illness as god-sent and divine. In this sense, the author calls these people *atheos*, because they believe that the gods are responsible for sending illness and can be influenced by sacrifices.

The classicist van der Eijk made a helpful remark in understanding the role of demons. Demons are to be understood as being "beyond human control, for the nature of this illness is sometimes beyond human control, though not divine."[51] This might explain why Jesus has power over this disease while the disciples do not: If Jesus has power over an illness seen as beyond human control, he is divine,[52] and it is indeed interesting that the crowd were astonished at the majesty of God after Jesus rebuked the demon. This reaction is only plausible if Jesus defeats the power that was interpreted as being beyond human control.

A hint is found in the story of the healing of Peter's mother, who was ill with a high fever (Luke 4:39). In addressing the fever, Jesus treats the fever as a demon and thus as a responsive person. Luke distinguishes between the sick person and the disease that invades the patient as an independent force from the outside.[53] Precisely for this reason, the patient is freed of the

---

50. For further details on epilepsy see Wohlers, *Heilige Krankheit*; Temkin, *The Falling Sickness*, and Weissenrieder, *Images of Illness*, chap. 7.

51. Van der Eijk, "The 'Theology' of the Hippocratic Treatise, On the Sacred Disease," 191.

52. We find a similar expression in *Vict* IV.87, where the author writes: "Prayer is a good thing, but while calling on the gods one should also put in effort oneself." (6.642 Littré)

53. Cf. Oeming, "Art. Krankheit," 292: The patient has become the "victim of a demonic attack." "That which disturbs physical or emotional well-being comes from outside."

religious responsibility for her illness. This results in the paradoxical situation that the introduction of a demon is to be interpreted as antidemonic. Accordingly, the mention of the demon in Luke's story of the healing of the epileptic boy demonstrates that the cause of the disease is not to be found in his alleged sins, but is to be understood as being beyond human control.

That Jesus can be experienced as a doctor is clear in Lucan healing stories, which are presented against the background of ancient medicine. Jesus is therefore presented more as a doctor than a healer. Unlike Mark's presentation, which is focused on exorcism, Luke tells a medical healing story. He speaks explicitly of *iaomai* (9:42) which is also used in ancient medical texts and in several healing temples of Asclepius. This is also true for *therapeuein*. In New Testament exegesis it is often wrongly assumed that both terms imply a complete cure. However, both terms have a wide range of meanings, one of which is healing. More often the terms are used in ancient medicine as "taking care," "looking after the ill person" and "medical treatment."[54] In the Hippocratic Corpus, *iaomai* is a characteristic of a good doctor. The term describes the obligation of a doctor, Jesus in the New Testament, to tend an ill person. Terms that have previously been translated and interpreted as healing, like *therapeuein*, should be considered more in the sense of "taking care." The only term known in the New Testament designating full health is *hygiein*, which is found only one time in New Testament (e.g., John 5:9; see p. 273).

Let us summarize: The previously mentioned New Testament texts provide rational interpretations of illness. Regarding their differentiation, these texts take different paths: On the one hand, Mark and Acts in particular were more related to ancient healer and exorcist traditions. Despite a complete replacement of the religious framework, the early Church adopted several aspects of the healing cults and exorcist traditions. The basic healing cult traditions like fasting, temple sleep and repentance with tears therefore became part of Christian rites.[55]

On the other hand, early Christianity was related to the rational medicine of the ancient world. This coupling can especially be seen in the Gospel of Luke, where medical studies were preferred to the religious interpretations of illness. Accordingly, the early church generated a large number of doctors.[56] The independent features of the Christian conception of health and illness in late antiquity can be seen here. The ethos of healing and care

---

54. See above at pp. 264–267.

55. Cf. Zeppezauer, "Krankheitskonzepte in der Hagiographie," 261–73; Markschies, "Gesund werden im Schlaf."

56. Cf. von Harnack, *Medicinisches*, 1–14, 108; see also Brennecke, "Heilen und Heilung in der Alten Kirche."

free of charge, and the creation of diaconal institutions and hospitals, were extensively cultivated. Since the earthly Jesus, as a physician, particularly devoted himself to the poor, Jesus was particularly known, in places where the early church saw him as a physician, as the physician of the poor.[57] Accordingly, the Christian hospitals—unlike the holy sites dedicated to Asclepius, where it was expensive to undergo a cure—took in patients regardless of their class and resources (like many doctors did).[58]

"In order to be healed in the pagan holy sites of Asclepius, a sacrifice was demanded in advance and a payment afterward." By contrast, Christian healers like the brothers Cosmas and Damian as well as Cyrus and John healed people in Menuthis "without money." According to Markschies, the Christian healing practice is distinguished from the ancient healing cults solely by its "particular attention to free healing and its stronger focus on the weak members of society."[59] "You have received healing for free, so you must also freely give healing,"[60] warned the bishop Cyril.

THE RELATIONSHIP OF OLD TESTAMENT TRADITIONS AND RATIONAL MEDICINE IN EARLY CHRISTIANITY

So far we have seen that early Christianity goes hand in hand with ancient medicine. Nevertheless, that view is questioned for illnesses that fall under the category of impurity as these occur in Old Testament, especially in terms of the irregular female issue of blood and leprosy, which are both discussed in Leviticus. These illnesses exclude people from the community of humans and of God. Basically, therefore, the word field *katharizein—hiereus—haptō*—clean, priests and touch—can be found in the texts with varying levels of frequency.

In the New Testament, especially in the Gospel of Luke [leprosy: Luke 4:27, 5:12–16; 7:12; 17:11–19; the woman with the issue of blood: Luke 8:43–48 par], both illnesses appear frequently, which is surprising considering the pagan readers of the Gospel of Luke. In recent exegetical discussion,

---

57. Brennecke, "Heilen und Heilung in der Alten Kirche," 32.

58. Ibid.: "Asclepius, according to Origenes and many after him, only wants to heal the pure from illness; Christ, on the other hand, is the physician of the lost. And drawing on much older educational polemics against Asclepius and his cult, the Christians accuse him of greed (the cures at the holy sites were not cheap!). Christ, by contrast, is the physician of the poor," 43; Kollmann, *Jesus und die Christen als Wundertäter*, 362–63, 367–68.

59. Markschies, "Gesund werden im Schlaf," 208f.

60. Cyr. Al., or. 18,3 (PG 77, 1105 B).

it is often argued that normal or "harmless"[61] bodily functions are identified as unclean—either arbitrarily or with misogynistic intent—and used as an argument for social exclusion. To what extent does this interpretation apply within the sphere of impurity in the New Testament?

The Illness Construct of Leprosy (*lepra*) in the Gospel of Luke

Behind the interpretation as a cleansing story, which is widespread in New Testament exegeses, is the implication that *lepra* is a harmless skin secretion. However, an analysis of the story against the background of Jewish and secular medical texts[62] shows that the etiology of the illness was interpreted in a similar manner both in Jewish texts (see Qumran,[63] and the Jewish medical book *Kitab-al-Tabakh*) and the "secular" medical text: namely as the influence of harmful factors in the environment on the body and an imbalance of bodily fluids. In addition, both secular and Jewish medicine banish the sick persons from the city because of possible contamination. Thus the distinction between a cleansing and a healing story is not obvious. This can also be shown by the text itself: First, it is striking that in Luke 17:12 it is simply left open whether the ten lepers reside outside or inside the city (*eisērchomai*).[64] They seem to move within the vicinity of the border, and it is not clear whether the lepers are identified as sick and unclean, and therefore have to stay outside the town. Luke 17 also has a fragility in terms of its geographical classification, "between Samaria and Galilee." Recent

---

61. Wohlers, "Aussätzige reinigt!"

62. The Hippocratic authors observe a relationship between wind and moisture conditions and the outbreak of *lepra*. The author of *De humoribus* writes, "North and south winds can all be predicted based on illness because for that person who is possessed of good and accurate knowledge, there are clues upon which he can base his considerations; such as, for example, certain types of lepra (skin diseases) and pain in the extremities which bring on itching when rain is approaching, and other such associations." (CH *De humoribus* 17; translation: Jones LCL) In the Hippocratic texts, the influence of environmental factors on the illness *leprosy* is always connected to an imbalance of bodily fluids. See esp. Weissenrieder, "Stories under the Skin."

63. The author puts forward the following explanation, which can be compared to some of the texts of the *Corpus Hippocraticum*: If *ruach*, air, enters a person's arteries, making it impossible for the blood to "rise and fall" regularly, this can have various consequences. If the air supply, and consequently the circulation of the blood are disturbed, this will initially produce a swelling or a light spot. The author of the 4Q fragment then considers this point on the skin to be a dead spot, since ruach and blood no longer "rise and fall." *Ruach* is responsible for obstructing the movement of blood, but it also reestablishes a normal flow of blood. See in detail Weissenrieder, *Images of Illness* and eadem, "Stories Just under the Skin," 73–100.

64. Weissenrieder, *Images of Illness*, chap. VII.

studies have shown that the text probably refers to a region in which Jews and Samaritans lived together, a region in which plural living situations and religious differences ranked among the top concerns.[65] Josephus, at least, reports extensively about this region, without scrimping on examples of bloody incidents.[66] And it is surely worth noting that he describes this conflict as a plague. Thus it makes sense to analyze both aspects—illness and conflict—at the same time.

More than almost any other behavior, violence—with its sense of inevitability and its destructive potential—has been closely associated with the imagery of an infectious illness. Infection creates victims, and violence sets off a chain reaction. Violence and illness can both be identified with impurity in societies, so both are to be counteracted with ritual efforts. Thus violence within the social body becomes the agent of an infectious logic, and it develops a virus-like power that can only be conquered through immunization strategies and by isolating those who are ill. Krämer assumes that the epidemic spread of illness and violence can be disrupted by the rite of sacrifice.[67] In this sense, the sacrificial victim suspends the transmission of illness and violence.

Therefore, the role of the priest is noteworthy. In Old Testament texts, priests define the purity or impurity of the person, and the act of seeing plays a central role, just as it does in Luke 17: Jesus' special act of seeing (v.14)—which the Lucan author conceives as a symbol of divine power analogous to the touching of a "leper" in Luke 5:12–16—corresponds to the act of seeing by one of the "lepers," who sees and confirms the healing of his illness (v.15), thereby apparently taking over a function normally reserved for priests. Once he sees that he is healed, he thus decides against going to the priests for a sacrifice, but instead decides to go home.[68] This special form of seeing provides the cataphoric link to the argument about seeing the Kingdom of God that immediately follows the healing. Thus we can assume that the special form of seeing becomes visible in the healing and is made explicit through the explanation.

This interpretation is further supported by the use of *allogenēs*, which the author uses to describe the one Samaritan who is healed. On a general level, this term emphasizes a person's foreignness or "otherness." In Luke

---

65. Böhm, *Samarien und die Samaritai bei Lukas*; Weissenrieder, "Stories Just under the Skin," 80–100.

66. Josephus *Bell.* 2.466 and 477–480 and *Ant.* 14.205–207.

67. Krämer, *Medium, Bote, Übertragung*, 138–58.

68. See in detail Weissenrieder, "Stories Just under the Skin"; and Weissenrieder, *Images of Illness*.

17:11–19, *allogenēs* indicates a reevaluation of the theme of purity: A pure person is one who sees the Kingdom of God.[69]

The narrative thus does not question the Jewish interpretation of leprosy, but deepens it: not the priest, but each and every patient is able to confirm the healing without sacrifice that is associated with a new interpretation of reality.

The Illness Construct of the Flow of Blood

The woman's illness, described as an issue of blood, is more closely defined by the term ῥύσις αἵματος *rūsis haimatos*, which we also encounter in Leviticus 15. The use of the term "issue of blood" ῥύσις αἵματος (*rūsis haimatos* Mark 5:25; Luke 8:44ff.; see also Lev 15:7, 19, 27) speaks for accepting the text as part of an Israelite discussion on cleanness and uncleanness.[70] Leviticus 15 could therefore function as a reference to Luke 8:43–48. This conclusion is contradicted by the fact that the terminology of cleanness characteristic of Lev 15, *katharsis and akatharsis* (Lev 15:20–27) is missing here. Neither the expiatory sacrifice nor the rules of restriction are themes.[71] For the hemorrhaging woman of Luke 8:43–48, Luke's complete disregard of this semantic frame indicates that purity and uncleanness are not determinative sociocultural categories in the proper historical interpretation of the narrative.

Nevertheless, an analysis of the text against the background of the purity code seems debatable when one considers the use of *haptomai*, which recalls the semantic frame of reference of cleanness and uncleanness. Therefore, Bovon concludes, "Her condition is all the more dramatic because her discharge of blood renders her ritually unclean and thus socially isolated. Contact with her is forbidden by the law. Thus the word ... 'to touch' is the key here."[72] In Luke 8:43–49, however, the touching does not appear within the context of restrictions, nor is there any mention of a priest who points out the woman's cleanness. Rather, a semantic opposition is created between divine reality and human reality. Within human reality, an "issue of blood" is described as a chronic illness, which brings massive economic consequences: the sick woman is impoverished. Although the woman spent all her money to be healed, the consulting physicians were unable to heal her. The divine reality is represented by Jesus' extraordinary power (8:46),

---

69. Weissenrieder, *Images of Illness*.

70. See Weissenrieder, "The Plague of Uncleanness," 207–12; and Weissenrieder, *Images of Illness*.

71. See conversely Kahl, "Jairus und die verlorenen Töchter Israels," 66–67.

72. Bovon, *Das Evangelium nach Lukas. 1,1—9,50*, 337.

which was released with the touching of his garment. The divine power, which brings healing through touch (Luke 5:13) or by word (Luke 5:17, 24), is plausible within the context of Luke's Gospel. Thus the text does not lead us to consider the influence of the purity code on the hemorrhaging woman or on Jesus' being touched by her.

First it is striking that, in contrast to Mark's version, Luke does not include two crucial points that would permit an interpretation in the sense of the purity code. According to Mark 5:29, the woman felt that she was "healed" of her "plague" *mastix*, an expression repeated with emphasis in 5:34. The term is used only once in Luke 7:21, listed along with several other descriptions of illnesses. If one considers the usage of *mastix* in the LXX, Ps 37(38):18 stands out in particular. In verses 4, 6, and 8, various symptoms are listed that are also named in the context of leprosy: no "soundness in my flesh," the "wound stink" and "are corrupt." Verse 12 lists the social consequences of the illness: the people nearest to the sick stand at a distance, which indicates social isolation. Accordingly, the term "plague" *mastix* may be interpreted as terminology that differs from other disease constructs, at least those associated with uncleanness in the purity code. In Leviticus 15, the term is not applied to an irregular "issue of blood," but we are aware of 4Q274, a central text regulating behavior for illnesses identified with uncleanness. The "plague" is explicitly mentioned here in relation to a "woman suffering from her menstruation." Therefore it is possible that the word "plague" was omitted because its use would point to the disease construct for an issue of blood that characterized the purity code and, with it, Leviticus 15.

Our thesis is further supported by a second conspicuous omission: Luke does not mention the source of the issue of blood, which Mark describes as a "fountain of blood." In Lev 12:7 (LXX), this phrase appears as the source of an issue of blood in the context of instructions for women who have given birth and is an equivalent of "uterus." If the author is avoiding this term, which is indigenous to the purity code, then this in turn represents a conscious decision in terms of understanding the illness. The etiology of the issue of blood does not appear to be important to him, otherwise he would have left the gender-specific references in the text or would even have emphasized them. As it is, it is simply clear that blood is flowing.

By neglecting the use of the terms that Mark employs—"plague" and "fountain of her blood"—as well as those indicating cleanness and uncleanness, the author does away with the fundamental references to the purity code of Leviticus 12–15 and concentrates solely on the issue of blood as an indicator of illness and the social consequences that accompany it.

If Luke has made the signs of disease the focal point, the second essential question becomes that of the severity of the illness. In the introduction to his ninth chapter dealing with issue of blood, Caelius Aurelianus descibes the following: "An outflow of blood from a hidden part (of the body) can often lead to an improvement on health, but can just as often be highly dangerous. In some cases, it can lead to immediate death, if the body becomes weakened by an excessive issue (of blood). In other cases, death comes in the final phase (of the illness), when consumption develops or when an internal wound fails to heal." (Cael. Aur. *Tard.Pass.* 2.9.117) This statement is further supported by similar terminology from the physicians of antiquity. A variety of terms are employed interchangeably to describe regular and irregular issues of blood. For example, the Hippocratics mention "female flow" (CH *Aphor.* 173) and "flow," Soranus describes regular and irregular issues of blood with "female flow" (Sor. *Gyn.* 2.41, 43), and Pliny treats the following terms as equivalent: *profluvium* (*Nat.Hist.* 26.160) and, more frequently, *sanguis profluvia* (26.131, 133), *fluctiones mulierum* (21.123) and *profluvia feminarum* (27.103; 29.9). None of these expressions refers to the etiology or pathogenesis of the illness. They simply describe the facts without evaluating them. Therefore, the term *rysis haimatos*—the flow of blood mentioned in Luke 8:43–49—does not indicate an illness. The severity of the disease is not linked to the term "issue of blood"; rather, it is determined by a series of other criteria, e.g., the heaviness of the blood flow or the duration. The duration is reported in Luke 8:43–49, as well as in Mark, to be twelve years. In addition, the texts mention the physicians the woman has consulted and the hopelessness of a cure. If the inclusion of the illness's duration in the text seems unusual to today's readers, the perspective shifts when one considers that, according to the *Corpus Hippocraticum*, an exact record of the length of an illness was of great relevance to the case history: the number of weeks, month or, very occasionally, years—are seen as signs of intensification of the illness and of the imminence of death. If a physician diagnoses a patient as being near death, the therapy is discontinued. The patient is already considered to be dead. Therefore, the interest is in the degree of illness and not—as is often assumed in exegesis—in uncleanness.

A further measure of support for this thanatological reading may be found in the narrative composition. The relevance of the community and the function of the individual within the community form the background: Only the community can guarantee subsistence for the individual, both economically and socially. Both aspects are illustrated by the reference in Luke 8:43 to the unsucessful visits to the physicians, and to the fact that the woman's family relationships are not mentioned (by contrast: Jairus's daughter). Illness can be defined as a loss of function in the social body. However, it would be an oversimplification of this point to infer the woman's exclusion from society on the basis of illness. After all, it is significant that the woman with the issue of blood steps forth out of the crowd and attains healing within the obscurity of the multitude (vv. 45, 47). One should consider the connotation of the crowd in Luke's Gospel: it distinguishes itself in that it can be interpreted as a "summoned gathering of Jesus' close relatives" (Bovon, 2002, 336–37 n31). If the woman with the issue of blood lingers within this group, this could indicate her affiliation with the crowd of believers. The transformation of the bleeding woman and her state of privation, however, is set in motion not by an intermediary, but by the woman herself.

This transformation is particularly made clear through the verbs of movement: while the people are depicted as waiting (v. 40), verbs of movement are repeatedly applied to the woman (come up behind him v. 44; touch v. 44; comes trembling v. 47; falling down v. 47). The verbs are accompanied by details that express a paradox, namely that the woman approached from "behind him" and "hid." One could describe this as a "paradoxical interpretation." The central point is not the exclusion from the community, but the lack of functionality imposed on the woman due to her long-term illness and the absence of hope for her cure. The bleeding woman's lack of function stands out in contrast to Jairus, who, as a ruler of a synagogue and a homeowner (v. 41), represents various acts of belonging. Second, the transformation is also indicated through the speech function as a sign of seclusion of the incident for the people and the disciples (vv. 45–46), and verifies the incident's visibility for Jesus. Afterward the situation changes because not Jesus and the disciples, but the people, are named as the forum for proclaiming the woman's healing (v. 47). The triumph over the presence of death in Luke does not occur by integrating the bleeding woman into the community, when Jesus makes her his daughter (v. 48). Not only is her relationship to Jesus implied. Amid the crowd, the healed woman is given a function as the daughter of Jesus, which amounts to a repeal of her "paradoxical integration."

In summary, the focus on leprosy and the issue of blood is not on Jesus' questioning or even overriding the Israelite law of purity, but on overcoming the dimension of death, which has two consequences: the economic implication (only mentioned with the bleeding woman) and the "paradoxical integration." The etiologies of both illnesses, the issue of blood and leprosy, remain vague when viewed against the background of ancient medicine: (1) Both illnesses can indicate a serious illness that accompanies an injury, a rupture of tissues, etc., and (2) an issue of blood or leprosy can represent a therapeutic evacuation. The implication that either an issue of blood or leprosy should be described as "harmless" is not obvious from ancient medical texts.

RELIGION AND MEDICINE IN REFORMATION CHRISTIANITY AND IN THE PENTECOSTAL MOVEMENT

The various options for relating faith, healing traditions and rational medicine that we can see in early Christianity have shaped Christianity, including Protestantism, to the present day.

The traditional Reformation churches build on the Lucan model here. It is particularly enlightening to look at Calvin and his Geneva reformation.[73] Calvin explicitly denied that the church and its bodies had special healing powers. With regard to his contemporary world, Calvin states in the Institutio that Christ "no longer distributes miracles through the hand of the apostles" (*Inst.* IV, 19, 19), for the "the gift of healing disappeared" (*Inst.* IV, 19, 18).

Naturally Calvin does not dispute that God continues to address the illnesses of the faithful and to heal them—but according to Calvin, this is done in a subtle, hidden way (cf. *Inst.* IV, 19, 19), not least through the healing arts, which Calvin calls a gift from the Holy Spirit (*Inst.* II, 2, 15). For precisely this reason, the Ecclesiastical Ordinances of the Church of Geneva of 1561 requires, that "a doctor and a surgeon [be hired] for the poor in the hospital as well as for the needy in the city."[74]

Of course, Calvin does not simply want to hand over the patients to the physicians; he argues for a close relationship between religion and medicine. For one thing, pastors should regularly "visit the hospital to see whether everything is in order."[75] This interest on the part of religion in providing the best possible patient care ultimately led to the founding of a medical school in Geneva. The historical cultural significance of this step becomes clear when one considers that "modern medicine and natural science mainly emerged after the Reformation, and largely within the Protestant or Protestant-influenced regions."[76]

For another thing, pastors are particularly called to care for the souls of the sick, since they "first and foremost require the services of our spiritual

---

73. Cf. Schreiner, *The Theatre of His Glory*; Smit, "On Illness and Providence."
74. Les Ordonnances ecclésiastiques de 1561, 259, 14–16.
75. Ibid., 259, 12–13.
76. Weizsäcker, "Frage der 'christlichen' Medizin," 226–27.

office."77 With this attention to the sick, their perception changes as well: "They are false interpreters, ... who say that all afflictions, without any distinction, are sent on account of sins; as if the measure of punishments were equal, or as if God looked to nothing else in punishing men than to what every man deserves ... Next, we ought to observe that there are various reasons why he afflicts men ... Hence we infer, that we cannot always put our finger on the causes of the sufferings which men endure."78

A strong charitable commitment, a link with scientific medicine, pastoral attention and breaking away from the religious doctrine of illness as a punishment—these four characteristics shape the Reformed tradition from Calvin on. Two hundred fifty years after Calvin, they are once again clearly visible in the writings of Reformed theologian Friedrich Daniel Ernst Schleiermacher. Even more clearly than Calvin, Schleiermacher states, "on no account must the evils affecting the individual be referred to his sin as their cause."79 Christ himself, he says—Schleiermacher refers to John 9:3 and Luke 13:5—taught "that natural evils ... are assuredly not linked to the sin of the individual—so far as we can isolate it—in such a way as to warrant our measuring his sin by the evil he suffers."80

This clarification has two consequences: because the origin of natural sufferings like illness is now understood as a natural consequence of human mortality, illnesses become the subject of scientific medical research. The experience of illness develops into a constant impulse "to bring these forces more fully under human control."81 As Jesus demonstrates his amazing healing powers in John 9:25, in the story of the man who was blind from birth, so too should humanity increasingly use natural suffering in order to demonstrate its ability to control nature.82

On the other hand, the disconnection between natural suffering and sin sharpens the focus on social evils—disregard for the sick, their disintegration and exclusion. Because illness is never simply a natural form of suffering, but also a societal form, the part of the illness caused by human action must be consistently sought out, and then every effort made

77. Cf. Calvin's letter to Viret, October 1542, OC 11, 457–460, 457.
78. Calvin, *Commentary on John*, 296.
79. Schleiermacher, *The Christian Faith*, 320: summary sentence for §77.
80. Ibid., 321.
81. Ibid., 317.
82. However, Schleiermacher does mention that Christian faith by no means aims to eliminate suffering in and of itself. It does, however, warn against any "activity specially directed towards the cessation of suffering as such" (Schleiermacher, *The Christian Faith*, 324). For this would be a "sensuous" act that "would really be determined by the interests of the lower side of life" (ibid.).

to minimize this.[83] This is precisely why Schleiermacher, even if he was no social pioneer, supported his Lutheran colleague in his fight to improve patient care at the Berlin hospital Charité during his years as a pastor there.[84]

In our opinion, this Reformed tradition, echoing the Lucan model, can be read as linking religion and scientifically based medicine. However, just as the Gospel of Luke is countered by the miraculous traditions described by the Gospel of Mark and Acts in the New Testament canon, today's traditional Reformed churches are challenged by the Pentecostal movement to offer themselves as a source of healing, and to build a network that immunizes them against illness. "Prayer for divine healing is perhaps the most universal characteristic of the many varieties of Pentecostalism and perhaps the main reason for its growth in the developing world."[85]

The question of why religious healing works—one that most ethnologists face in their field research—has still not been satisfactorily answered.[86] The Heidelberg ethnologist William S. Sax primarily relates the healing power of rituals to stress reduction, to working through social conflicts and to building trust.[87] One could argue that the healing rituals change the framework conditions of a system—for instance the family, but also the body[88]—to such an extent that this change also affects the physical level. "Recent research on the physiological effects of meditation, behavior therapies, biofeedback, and placebos suggest a number of different ways by

---

83. With regard to disability studies, it can be said that Schleiermacher belongs to the prehistory of the "social model" of disability. The core theory of this model developed by English social researcher Michael Oliver is that "the level of impairment in the sense of clinically relevant symptoms must be clearly differentiated from disability in the sense of a social impairment. According to the social model of disability, disability is created through systematic exclusion, and is not simply the result of medical pathology" (Waldschmidt, "Warum und wozu brauchen die Disability Studies die Disability History?," 17). In addition, more recent postcolonial disability studies believe more strongly that social processes not only exclude people with impairments, but also generate the seemingly natural evil of impairment. Thus, according to Sharon V. Betcher, Disability, the impairments named in the miracle stories of the New Testament can fundamentally be read as real consequences within the slave economy. In the Roman Empire, the amputation of an ear was a form of punishment for slaves (cf. Betcher, "Disability and the Terror of the Miracle Tradition," 174–75). In terms of Schleiermacher's era, one could also think of unhealthy working conditions as well as the effects of war.

84. Cf. Nowak, *Schleiermacher*, 76–77.

85. Anderson, *Pentecostalism*, 30.

86. See the contribution of Koch and Meissner in this volume.

87. Sax, "Heilen Rituale?," 232.

88. Cf. Sax, "Healing Rituals," 302: "the power of public rituals lies in the fact that they are the chief site where both collective and individual identities are created, reiterated, and transformed."

which indigenous therapies may affect biologically-based diseases. In that the epidemiological web causing and sustaining physiological diseases not infrequently includes major psychosocial factors, indigenous healing may at times work to affect such diseases by altering those factors."[89]

The fact that healings in the Pentecostal movement are long-lasting could be because the healed persons are integrated into a community of mutual support, to which they in turn contribute something unique as sons and daughters of Jesus.[90] At the same time, Max Weber's argument about the rationalization of lifestyle applies here[91]—the faithful give their entire lives over as the price for their healing through Christ, and prioritize the creation of social networks and the building of the community of Christ over personal pleasures.[92]

The tight relationship between religious communication and a praxis of caring and curing that appears in the Pentecostal movement can be read within the resonance field of the New Testament texts. If, following the Gospel of Mark, one sees Jesus as a religious healer or exorcist, the distinction between religion and medicine becomes less convincing.[93] Like the Gospel of Mark, the majority of the world today views healing as being entirely part of religion. "In a situation where secular society provides adequate health care only for those with the means to purchase it, the economically disenfranchised frequently turn to the only available source of healing: the divine."[94]

The differing ways of handling illness, in the Pentecostal movement on the one hand and in the Reformed churches on the other, can be reconstructed as different ways of reading the scripture and thus of understanding Jesus. If healing in the Gospel of Luke does not aim to effect complete healing, but rather describes Jesus' obligation as a physician to the sick, then

---

89. Kleinman and Sung, "Why Do Indigenous Practitioners Successfully Heal?," 24.

90. Cf. Chesnut, *Born again in Brazil*, 92–107.

91. See Cockerham, Abel, and Lüschen, "Max Weber."

92. "In the ideological and comportmental realms, believers further restore and preserve their health through a Manichean worldview and an ascetic moral code . . . Put into practice, Pentecostal dualism becomes a strict moral code that requires converts to renounce their earthly vices. Men in particular must exit the carnal drama of the street and take up roles in the spiritual theaters of home and church. In abjuring vice, men abandon some of the main behavior associated with the male prestige complex" (Chesnut, *Born again in Brazil*, 170; cf. 108–25).

93. As argued, for instance, by Kollmann, who focuses on the shamanic portrayal of Jesus in the Gospel of Mark in his work *Jesus und die Christen als Wundertäter* (cf. 289–90) as evidence of a cautious opening of the Christian religion to magic and shamanism.

94. Chesnut, *Born again in Brazil*, 179.

the Reformed churches take up this version in their charitable work. If the churches want to remain true to this tradition, they cannot remove themselves from hospitals, but must ensure that the chaplains—as is often the case in North American hospitals[95]—become part of the medical team. "A high-level division of labor must be replaced by teamwork between health professionals and religious chaplains in order to avoid losing sight of the patient as an individual."[96]

"Research in the field indicates that spirituality and religion are seen as a core aspect of life, and patients want physicians to address issues of spirituality in the context of medical care. A public survey done in 1996 by *USA Weekend* showed that 63% of patients believe doctors should ask about spirituality issues, but only 10% have actually been asked."[97] When one considers the (quite ambivalent) influence of religious attitudes on recovery processes, doctors should be sensitive to their patients' religious attitudes. However, since they are often not "spiritual specialists," it makes sense for them to work closely with those who are. "In hospital settings, chaplains are a good place to begin. In a community-based setting, the patient's own spiritual leader or, if the patient is not affiliated with any specific group, a spiritual specialist who is willing to work from the patient's perspective is often the most viable option. Support groups, study groups, worship experiences all can be a part of this strategy. The use of literature and tapes, prayer (best done with a religious professional if possible) are relatively easy responses to spiritual distress."[98]

Neurologist Mechthilde Kütemeyer convincingly explains how the presence of a theologian who is integrated into the medical exchange can positively affect and change the clinical processes:

> [The pastor] described to us the distress experienced by patients in hospital rooms, visited without warning by doctors and nurses; the patients' powerlessness while waiting hours for examinations; lying on the uncomfortable stretcher in the lobby of

---

95. Cf. Padilla and Moczynski, "Navigating the Institutional Culture," who note "that any time that a chaplain enters into a health care setting seeking to advocate for a patient, he or she will become immersed in a network of relationships characterized by a medical or care-giving team that is focused on caring for a patient. . . . the chaplain then effectively, or functionally, joins this care-giving team and must pay attention to the implied responsibilities that each of the relationships entered into entails" (35).

96. Körtner, "Für einen mehrdimensionalen Spiritualitätsbegriff," 31; cf. Kliewer, "Allowing spirituality into the healing process," 623; Padilla and Moczynski, "Navigating the Institutional Culture," 48.

97. Kliewer, "Allowing Spirituality into the Healing Process," 616–17.

98. Ibid., 622–23.

the X-ray department, subject to cold, noise, the gazes of people walking around them and the rough voices of doctors who are busy with other patients—the whole range of impositions that patients endure without complaint, their space, time and bodies belonging to the "clinic." The theologian gathered a wealth of experience during her attendance—findings about the condition, fears, desires and needs of the patients and mementos of their lives. If an unconscious patient had to be transferred to the intensive care department, unable to speak, she was able to share details about the person's character and habits as well as his or her desire to live or die with the employees there, so that the caretakers were not treating a "case" but an individual.[99]

During day-to-day clinical work, theology becomes the advocate for a cause that is often linked with non-medical forms of patient treatment, namely the interest in a consistent form of medicine that focuses consistently on the individual.[100] "The modern biomedical enterprise—with its threefold work of knowledge acquisition, technology development, and care delivery—urgently needs the guiding visions and values embodied in the faith traditions. When technological momentum or economic necessity alone guides the health care enterprise, the sustaining impulses of respect, meaning and purpose often fall aside."[101]

The New Testament texts can of course also be used to justify the healing actions of the Pentecostal movement. This could perhaps be described as a form of following Jesus that is foreign to us and must first be approached with a willingness to learn. These types of learning processes can be seen even in the mainline churches today, where anointing and healing services are increasingly being offered.[102]

However, the concept of healing ministry should be seen in light of the above explanations of the ancient and ur-Christian definition of healing. The healing that is requested in such religious services does not need to consist of repairing a physical deficit; instead, people can learn—within a life-affirming environment—how to be sick in a healthy way. The Heidelberg theologian and psychoanalyst Dietrich Ritschl pointed out the various processes that can be described using the term "healing." He distinguishes

---

99. Kütemeyer, "Neurologie und Psychosomatik," 196.

100. Cf. Roser, "Innovation Spiritual Care"; and Bawell Weber, "Erfahrungen mit Spiritual Care in Deutschland und den USA," 208.

101. Marty, "Foreword," viii.

102. See *The Church's Ministry of Healing*; Church of England, *A Time to Heal*; Atkinson, *The Church's Healing Ministry*; Ernsting, *Salbungsgottesdienste in der Volkskirche*, 124–262; Malia, *Healing Touch and Saving Word*.

between healing as (1) self-healing, (2) repair, (3) learning to live with limitations and (4) accepting our mortality.[103] Concentrating solely on the first two dimensions would not do justice to the finite and limited realities of human life.

In addition, services that are explicitly defined as healing services offer the possibility of individual blessings and anointment. Given the isolating power of illness, which often stigmatizes the patient, touch can take away some of this power. This becomes clear when Jesus touches lepers (Mark 1:41), people with a fever (Mark 1:31) and people who are near death (Mark 5:39–41), lets himself be touched by a woman who is considered to be a sinner (Luke 7:39), and finally is touched by all who are sick (Matt 14:35–36).

The anointment is meant to express to the public and to the anointed person that this person is a creature of God, accepted by God and equipped with royal dignity. Anointment can help people with illnesses and disabilities, whose dignity is often denied, experience this dignity in a bodily sense.

With regard to illness as a social evil, such religious services should counteract the exclusion of sick people and break open the loneliness that is experienced during illness.[104] However, in a society whose ideal of health turns members of the society into handicapped persons, such services also play a prophetic function, uncovering the marginalization caused by certain discourses and cultural attitudes. Thereby, it is specifically the memory of the crucified, suffering and disabled Christ which "serves as an effective contrast to the idealized and commercialized images of the body."[105] In this regard, anointing and healing services should simultaneously aim to strengthen individuals while transforming their environment.[106]

CHRISTIANITY AS A RELIGION DEDICATED TO SERVING THE SICK

Even though the interpretation of illness as a punishment from God is fairly uncommon in the New Testament, we still encounter it today in the clinical world. A study on the significance of religiousness in the treatment of breast cancer, performed at a hospital in a small German city demonstrates

---

103. Ritschl, *Zur Theorie und Ethik der Medizin*, 113, 220–22.

104. Cf. Ernsting, *Salbungsgottesdienste*, 249–51.

105. Rappmann, "The Disabled Body of Christ as a Critical Metaphor," 25; cf. Hutchinson, "Disabling beliefs?," 6–8.

106. See Ernsting, *Salbungsgottesdienste*, 69.

that 20% of the patients tortured themselves with questions of guilt and saw their illness as a punishment from God.[107]

> They ask themselves, "Why me?" (Ms. B.; Ms. H., both age 60, Protestant) and search for reasons in their lives that could have caused God to punish them. One patient, for instance, asks herself, "Why are you in particular being punished in this way?" (Ms. C., age 69, Catholic) and then immediately finds a possible answer in her own faulty behavior: "Well, maybe because I'm not so religious. I don't go to church." (Ms. C.). Another patient speculates, "I think that maybe I did some things wrong in my life and so maybe I'm getting 'my punishment' now, you know, like my 'just deserts' from the Lord" (Ms. H.).[108]

Recently, medical studies both in the U.S. and in Germany have shown: "Religious people who become upset by the belief that God has abandoned them . . . may inadvertently subvert the success of their recovery. It is important for future research to examine such health-limiting aspects of religion or spirituality in patients."[109]

If Christianity sees itself as a religion of healing that follows Jesus Christ, then it must first of all counteract this interpretation of illness. If Christ did not talk about guilt to the sick people who asked him for help, instead seeing only their need, then the church should also see and treat people with illnesses as sufferers rather than sinners.

Of course, this insight must be gained over and over again. There have been times in the history of Christianity when the interpretation of illness as punishment for sins was understood to be *the* Christian interpretation. In particular, Early Protestant orthodoxy believed illness to be the result of sin. Accordingly, preachers told sick people to confess their sins and be forgiven before visiting a doctor. For if illness is seen as punishment for sins—as stated by Lutheran orthodox preachers like Johann Sigwart in 1611—"ist es vnmüglich/ daß man derselben vberhaben seye/ oder wider abkomme/ es seye dann/ daß die Sünden erkennet vnd bereuet werden" ("it is impossible / for one to be superior to it / or to escape from it / unless / the sins are recognized and repented of.")[110] Pietism largely took on and popularized

---

107. Cf. Murken and Müller, "Gott hat mich so ausgestattet," 127.
108. Ibid., 125–26.
109. Powell, Shahabi and Thoresen, "Religion and Spirituality," 50; see also Zwingmann et. al "Positive and Negative Religious Coping"; Thomas et. al., "Einfluss verschiedener Formen von Religiosität."
110. Sigwart, Drey Predigten, 95, cited in Holtz, "Unsicherheit des Lebens," 142.

this viewpoint.¹¹¹ In various religious traditions as well as in their secular derivatives, this view continues to have an effect even today.

In this regard, Friedrich Daniel Ernst Schleiermacher once again noted the liberating attitude of Jesus (see p. 285 above). Schleiermacher differentiates between natural and social evils.¹¹² These, he says, are distinguished by their relationship to the sin (§75). While social evils exist only where sin reigns, "death and pain . . . are found where no sin exists" (§76, 319). Death and illness as natural phenomena are not the result of sin, but of the mortality of human beings (cf. §75). For precisely this reason, "natural evils . . . , objectively considered, do not arise from sin" (§75, 319). Theologically speaking, then, interpreting one's own illness as punishment for individual misdeeds, something that clinicians encounter even today, is objectively wrong.

At the same time, Schleiermacher also tells us why this interpretation of illness persists today. Although Schleiermacher reveals the objective error of this religious interpretation of illness, he does not deny its subjective power: since our awareness of and trust in God will always be limited, we must also expect that we will continue to consider our illness as guilt in times of serious sickness. It makes sense to interpret illness as a self-inflicted evil because every patient can find guilty moments in his or her life that can be interpreted as the reason for the illness.¹¹³ The interpretation of one's own illness as punishment is often reinforced by the interpretation of others. Healthy people, reminded by every sick person that they, too, could become ill, protect themselves against this idea by viewing the other's illness as the consequence of a badly lived life.¹¹⁴

In these interpretations, which causally link individual guilt with illness, we can see the power of sin, which shatters trust, sows the seeds of unkindness, and destroys hope.¹¹⁵ By inducing people to see others' illnesses as self-inflicted, sin prevents solidarity with those who are ill. By portraying

111. Ernst, *Krankheit und Heilung*.

112. On the following, cf. Etzelmüller, "Christentum als Religion der Heilung," 451–56.

113. Cf. Morgenstern, "Trauer zwischen Schuld und Scham," 598: "If, despite searching for meaning, no meaning can be found, we look for guilt. And—this is the terrible thing—we feel guilt even when there is no guilt at all."

114. Cf. Schneider-Flume, "Perfektionierte Gesundheit als Heil?," 139 f.: "While as a rule we no longer conclude that certain illnesses were caused by certain moral failings, our esteem for self-responsibility makes it even easier to assign guilt to patients because they presumably did not do enough for their health, for instance by eating unhealthily, etc."

115. On the underlying communication theory-related understanding of sin, cf. Brandt, "Sünde."

God as one who punishes people through illness, sin unsettles the basic confidence of the sick. Instead of awakening hope, religion—under the power of sin—creates a sense of despair that closes people off from life. Accordingly, more recent studies show that negative religious coping is associated with a higher rate of depression.[116] Thus we can conclude that illness is not the result of sin; rather, that we see illness as a self-inflicted punishment demonstrates the power of sin, which conquers us again and again.

A Christianity that sees itself as a religion dedicated to serving the ill not only opposes the vitally harmful view of illness as a punishment from God, but also motivates the followers of Christ to resist illness.

The stories of Jesus healing the sick make it clear: an illness that destroys a person is not the will of God. Karl Barth articulately stated in his Church Dogmatics: "As Jesus acts in His commission and power, it is clear that God does not will that which troubles and torments and disturbs and destroys man. He does not will the entanglement and humiliation and distress and shame that the being of man in the cosmos and as a cosmic being means for man. He does not will the destruction of man."[117] This discovery makes it necessary to let go of the idea of God as an all-determining reality that shaped the theology of the 20th century.[118] In opposition to this idea, Jesus' healings of the sick make it clear that not everything that happens in this world corresponds to the will of God.

Of course, if illness is no longer directly connected to the will of God, we must ask ourselves how to interpret illnesses in terms of creation theology. The increased medical focus within our perception of severe illnesses, and how they are harmful to life, is only compatible with a doctrine of creation that states: God has created a world whom he granted the freedom to develop itself. This is expressed even in the biblical creation stories. By no means does God create everything, but rather empowers his creations to take creative action themselves.[119] The earth brings forth creaturely life.

---

116. Cf. Thomas et.al. "Einfluss verschiedener Formen von Religiosität auf die Schwere und den Verlauf der Depression im Alter," also Zwingmann, "Positive and Negative Religious Coping," 543: "Depressive coping was predicted negatively by positive religious coping and positively by negative religious coping."

117. Barth, Church Dogmatics IV/2, 225.

118. It is worth noting that Karl Barth writes, in the specific context of his statements on illness as a reality that is resistant to human effort, "God is indeed the basis of all reality. But He is not the only reality. As Creator and Redeemer He loves a reality which is different from Himself, which depends upon Him, yet which is not merely a reflection nor the sum of His powers and thoughts, but which has in face of Him an independent and distinctive nature and is the subject of its own history, participating in its own perfection and subjected to its own weakness." (CD III/4, 365).

119. On the underlying understanding of creation sketched out here, cf. Welker,

"And God said, Let the earth bring forth the living creature after its kind, cattle, and creeping thing, and beast of the earth after its kind: and it was so." (Gen 1:24) Even plants and animals develop and reproduce by themselves. One could say that God intended his creation to develop on its own and to explore its own possibilities. At the same time, this means that God has given freedom to his creatures. This is why the possibility exists for life processes—even at the organic level—to fail and to take on harmful forms: "the same biochemical processes which enable germ cells to produce new forms of life will also allow somatic cells to mutate and become malignant. That there is cancer in creation is not something that a more competent or compassionate Creator could easily have eliminated, but it is the necessary cost of a creation allowed to make itself."[120] The possibility of being taken ill is part of God's good creation. However, Jesus' healing of the sick makes it clear that the realization of this possibility is not the will of God.

To put it another way: Jesus' healing of the sick demonstrates that understanding God's will solely on the basis of creation theology is insufficient. When, in John 5, Jesus responds to the criticism that he is performing healing on the Sabbath, saying, "My Father is still working, and I also am working" (John 5:17), he makes it clear that the father's protective and permissive actions correspond to the son's saving actions. Only in their union—according to the statement "The Father and I are one!" (John 10:30)—do they represent the actions of God. The creator justifies himself through Jesus' healing of the sick, turning toward those who suffer from the arbitrariness of his creation. Thus the will of God—overcoming illness and pain—becomes visible to his creation.

AN OBJECTION FROM DISABILITY STUDIES

At this place it is helpful to recall the aforementioned critique by Sharon V. Betcher: a church driven by the narratives of healing to support the medical fight against sickness promotes a "'pick up your bed and walk' mentality . . . that circulates in Western cultures as the ethos of morality [. . .] and intact economic resource, i.e., labor power."

Given this critique, it is theologically relevant to note significant differences between biblical traditions. While in his earthly life Jesus did not deny care and healing to anyone who asked for it, the exalted Christ refuses Paul's petition to be liberated from a disease that Paul perceived as a "thorn in the flesh" (2 Cor 12:7–8). In our view, the synoptic traditions indeed support

---

Creation nad Reality.
   120. Polkinghorne, *Science and the Trinity*, 172.

efforts to help people and heal them via Christian social work and the medical system. Certainly, health must not be considered as the highest good and thus be revered as a deity, which would constitute idolatry. Where health is venerated in a religious manner, sick persons end up stigmatized. By contrast, Paul reminds us that the Christian congregation must not perceive the disabled body merely as a deficient body. Instead, its specific capacities contribute to the building up of the congregation.

The congregation in Corinth criticized Paul for the contrast between his appearance and what the "strong" members of the congregation had expected. "For they say, 'His letters are weighty and strong, but his bodily presence is weak, and his speech contemptible.'" (2 Cor 10:10) In his own letters Paul admits that he proclaimed the gospel "in spite of a physical infirmity." (Gal 4:13, see 1 Cor 2:3) Neither does he conceal that this physical weakness caused him to suffer and that he prayed to the Lord for it to be removed (see 2 Cor 12:7f.). Presumably, Paul was afflicted by "a physical deficiency that adversely affected his rhetorical performance."[121] Potentially this was the result of physical abuse he had endured during his missionary work. By the standards of the ancient world, his body manifested the lowly and disreputable condition of the apostle. For in Roman culture "a beaten body was a dishonored body."[122] Yet Paul was denied his wish that this weakness be removed. Instead, Paul was meant to embody Christ's word, "My grace is sufficient for you, for my power is made perfect in weakness [illness]." (2 Cor 12:9) The supposedly deficient body of the apostle thus comes to embody the word of the cross and thus participates in the transvaluation of all values that emerges from this word of the Lord.

Paul indeed interprets his physical weakness as a manifestation of Jesus' suffering and death. As he writes in 2 Cor 4:10–12, we are "always carrying in the body the death of Jesus, so that the life of Jesus may also be made visible in our bodies. For while we live, we are always being given up to death for Jesus' sake, so that the life of Jesus may be made visible in our mortal flesh. So death is at work in us, but life in you." The apostle's maltreated body reveals Jesus' life for the benefit of the life of the congregation.

Paul gains this insight only during the course of his missionary work. Between his plea for his suffering to be removed so his proclamation would no longer be hampered and the insight that Christ is revealed precisely in Paul's weakness, there is a process in which Paul gains a deeper insight, and something becomes explicit that had only been implicit before. Paul discovers that precisely his supposedly deficient body contributes to the

---

121. Martin, *The Corinthian Body*, 54.
122. Glancy, *Corporal Knowledge*, 41.

transformation of societal expectations and interactions. Even before Paul becomes aware of this, his body, his physical appearance, contributed to the build up of a community, which says of itself, "those members of the body that we think less honorable we clothe with greater honor" (1 Cor 12:23). Thus, even before Paul became aware of this, the apostle's appearance in Corinth had embodied, "a version of Christ's body in which status indicators are reversed, with greater honor given to those normally regarded as having lower status and less prestige accorded to those normally accorded badges of honor."[123]

Paul's theology makes it possible to discover life not only in health, but also in sickness. According to Paul, Jesus' life is revealed in Paul's weakness. This change of perspective helps emancipate people from common value judgments. The apostle's scars from beatings may overturn common perceptions about what God trusts a person so "scarred" to accomplish. Paul's appearance corrects the cultural constructs that disable people and that marginalize persons with disabilities. Being thus liberated from common perceptions of value, people discover a life that is no longer determined by the power of classic stereotypes. Thus, Paul can say that Christ's life in all its weakness is revealed for the benefit of the life of the congregation. The congregation profits from the unsettling of their usual worldview in which disability is associated with disgrace and is thus something to be ashamed of and concealed. The disabled body of Christ, which is embodied in the beaten body of Paul, "serves as an effective contrast to the idealized and commercialized images of the body,"[124] thus liberating people to live a life no longer circumscribed by the images of the body in the media.

The transformative power of supposedly disabled bodies can also be perceived from a secular perspective. This is illustrated by Denis Diderot's "Letter on the Blind for the Use of Those Who See." In this writing, "one of the exceedingly rare instances of a philosopher treating an impairment as something other than a deficit, the eighteenth century experimentalist philosopher Denis Diderot investigated blind people's ways of knowing. Taking a stance that resembles, if not prefigures, recent feminist criticisms of Descartes, Diderot, in his 'Letter on the Blind for the Use of Those Who See,' describes how blind people know about the world to show the shortcomings of Cartesian overreliance on metaphors that associate reason with light or sight and Cartesian reliance on visual rather than tactile ways of knowing."[125]

---

123. Martin, *The Corinthian Body*, 102.
124. Rappmann, "The Disabled Body of Christ as a Critical Metaphor," 25.
125. Cf. Silvers, "Feminist Perspectives on Disability."

Churches and ecclesial communities would do well to draw inspiration from both the synoptic traditions of Jesus healing the sick and from Paul's discovery of how the stricken body builds up the congregation. Faith communities can both support an ethos that aims at healing a disease—as long as this does not idolize health—and realize how persons with disability contribute to an enhancement of life by fundamentally overturning common stereotypes. Both of these orientations come together in the struggle against the social evil of the marginalization of persons with disease and disability.

BIBLIOGRAPHY

Anderson, Allan. *An Introduction to Pentecostalism: Global Charismatic Christianity.* Cambridge: Cambridge University Press, 2004. [2nd ed., 2014]

Ashby, Thomas. "Roman Malta." *JRS* 5 (1918) 23–80.

Atkinson, David. *The Church's Healing Ministry: Practical and Pastoral Reflections.* Norwich, UK: Canterbury, 2011.

Bachmann, Margot. "Die Nachwirkungen des hippokratischen Eides: Ein Beitrag zur Geschichte der ärztlichen Ethik." Ph.D. diss., Univerisity of Würzburg, 1952.

Barnes, Colin. "A Legacy of Oppression: A History of Disability in Western Culture." In *Disability Studies: Past, Present and Future*, edited by Len Barton and Mike Oliver, 3–24. Leeds: Disability Press, 1997.

Barth, Karl. *The Church Dogmatics*, III/4. Edinburgh: T. & T. Clark, 1961.

———. *The Church Dogmatics*, IV/2. Edinburgh: T. & T. Clark, 1958.

Baumgarten, Joseph M., and Michael T. Davis. "Cave IV, V, VI Fragments." In *The Dead Sea Scrolls II: Damascus Document, War Scroll, and Related Documents*, edited by James H. Charlesworth, 59–79. Tübingen: Mohr/Siebeck, 1995.

Bawell Weber, Susan. "Erfahrungen mit Spiritual Care in Deutschland und den USA." In *Spiritualität und Medizin: Gemeinsame Sorge für den kranken Menschen, Münchner Reihe Palliativ Care* 4, edited by Eckhard Frick and Traugott Roser, 202–9. Stuttgart: Kohlhammer, 2009.

Bendemann, Reinhard von. "Christus der Arzt—Krankheitskonzepte in den Therapiererzählungen des Markusevangeliums." In *Heilungen und Wunder: Theologische, historische und medizinische Zugänge*, edited by Josepf Pichler and Christoph Heil, 105–29. Darmstadt: WBG, 2007.

Betcher, Sharon. "Disability and the Terror of the Miracle Tradition." In *Miracles Revisited: New Testament Miracle Stories and Their Concepts of Reality*, edited by Stefan Alkier and Annette Weissenrieder, 161–81. Studies of the Bible and Its Reception 2. Berlin: de Gruyter, 2013.

———. *Spirit and the Politics of Disablement.* Philadelphia: Fortress, 2007.

Böhm, Martina. *Samarien und die Samaritai bei Lukas: Eine Studie zum religionshistorischen Hintergrund der lukanischen Samarientexte und zu deren topographischen Verhaftung.* WUNT 2/111. Tübingen: Mohr/Siebeck, 2001.

Bovon, Francois. *Das Evangelium nach Lukas 1,1—9,50.* EKK 3/1. Neukirchen: Neukirchener, 1989.

Brandt, Sigrid. "Sünde: Ein Definitionsversuch." In *Sünde: Ein unverständlich gewordenes Thema*, edited by Sigrid Brandt et al., 13–34. Neukirchen-Vluyn: Neukirchener, 1997.

Brennecke, Hanns Christof. "Heilen und Heilung in der Alten Kirche." In *Eschatologie und Schöpfung: Festschrift für Erich Gräßer zum siebzigsten Geburtstag*, edited by Martin Evang et al., 23–45. BZNW 89. Berlin: de Gruyter, 1997.

Brock, Nadia van. *Recherches sur le vocabulaire médical du grec ancien: Soins et guérison*. Études et Commentaires 41. Paris: Klincksieck, 1961.

Calvin, John. *Commentary on John*. Vol. 1. http://www.ccel.org/ccel/calvin/calcom 34.pdf.

Chaniotis, Angelos. "Illness and Cures in the Greek Propitiatory Inscriptions and Dedications of Lydia and Phrygia." In: *Ancient Medicine in its Socio-Cultural Context. Papers Read at the Congress Held at Leiden University*, 13–15 April 1992, edited by H.F.J. Hormannshoff et. al., 323–344. Amsterdam-Atlanta: Rodopi, 1995.

Chesnut, R. Andrew. *Born again in Brazil: The Pentecostal Boom and the Pathogens of Poverty*. New Brunswick, NJ: Rutgers University Press, 1997.

Church of England. House of Bishops. *A Time to Heal. A Contribution towards the Ministry of Healing*. London: Church House Publishing, 2004.

The Church's Ministry of Healing. Report of the Archbishops' Commission. Westminster: Church Information Board, 1958.

Cockerham, William C., Thomas Abel, and Gunther Lüschen. "Max Weber, Formal Rationalities, and Healthy Lifestyles." *Sociological Quarterly* 34 (1993) 413–28.

Deichgräber, Karl. *Der hippokratische Eid: Griechischer und deutscher Text des Eides mit einem Essay über das alte Dokument: Text griechisch und deutsch*. 4th ed. Stuttgart: Hippokrates Verlag, 1983 (1st ed., 1955).

Diller, Hans, ed. *Hippokrates, Schriften: Die Anfänge der abendländischen Medizin*. Reinbek b. Hamburg: Rowohlt, 1962.

Dörnemann, Michael. *Krankheit und Heilung in der Theologie der frühen Kirchenväter*. StAC 20. Tübingen: Mohr/Siebeck, 2003.

Duminil, Marie-Paule. *Le sang, les vaisseaux, le cœur dans la Collection hippocratique: Anatomie et physiologie*. Paris: Les Belles Lettres, 1983.

Edelstein, Emma, and Ludwig Edelstein. *Asclepius: Collection and Interpretation of the Testimonies*. Baltimore: John Hopkins University Press, 1945. Reprinted, 1998.

Edelstein, Ludwig. *Ancient Medicine: Selected Papers of Ludwig Edelstein*. Edited by Owsei Temkin and Lillian Temkin. Baltimore: John Hopkins University Press, 1967.

Ergänzungsband zum Evangelischen Gottesdienstbuch für die Evangelische Kirche der Union und für die Vereinigte Evangelisch-Lutherische Kirche Deutschlands. Edited by Kirchenleitung der VELKD and Rates von der Kirchenkanzlei der EKU. Berlin: Evangelische Haupt-Bibelgesellschaft und von Cansteinsche Bibelanstalt, 2002.

Eijk, Philip J. van der. "Aristotle and His School." In *Medicine and Philosophy in Classical Antiquity: Doctors and Philosophers on Nature, Soul, Health and Disease*. Edited by Ph. J. van der Eijk. Cambridge: Cambridge University Press, 2005.

———. *Aristoteles: De insomniis. De divination per somnum übersetzt und erläutert*. Aristoteles: Werke in deutscher Übersetzung 14,3. Berlin: Akademie Verlag, 1994.

———. "The Theology of the Hippocratic Treatise on the Sacred Disease." In *Medicine and Philosophy in Classical Antiquity: Doctors and Philosophers on Nature, Soul,

Health and Disease. Edited by Philip J. van der Eijk. Cambridge: Cambridge University Press, 2005.
Ernst, Katharina. *Krankheit und Heilung: Die medikale Kultur württembergischer Pietisten im 18. Jahrhundert*. Veröffentlichungen der Kommission für geschichtliche Landeskunde in Baden-Württemberg B 154. Stuttgart: Kohlhammer, 2003.
Ernsting, Heike. *Salbungsgottesdienste in der Volkskirche: Krankheit und Heilung als Thema der Liturgie*. Leipzig: EVA, 2012.
Etzelmüller, Gregor. "Christentum als Religion der Heilung: Zur Verhältnisbestimmung von moderner Theologie und Krankenbehandlung." In *Krankheitsdeutung in der postsäkularen Gesellschaft: Theologische Ansätze im interdisziplinären Gespräch*, edited by Günter Thomas and Isolde Karle, 448–64. Stuttgart: Kohlhammer, 2009.
———. "Der kranke Mensch als Thema christlicher Anthropologie. Die Herausforderung der Theologie durch die anthropologische Medizin Viktor von Weizsäckers." *ZEE* 53 (2009) 163–76.
———. "Leib, Seele, Umwelt Die interdisziplinäre Anthropologie Viktor von Weizsäckers und ihr Verhältnis zur paulinischen Anthropologie." In *Interdisziplinäre Anthropologie: Leib, Geist, Kultur*, edited by Thiemo Breyer, Gregor Etzelmüller, Thomas Fuchs and Grit Schwarzkopf, 287–313. Schriften des Marsilius-Kollegs 10. Heidelberg: Winter, 2013.
Fantuzzi, Marco. "Varianza e tenacia del polar thinking nel De Prisca Medicina pseudo-ippocartico." In *Formes de pensée dans la Collection Hippocratique Actes du Ive Colloque International Hippocratique* (Lausanne 21–26 Septembre 1981), 21–26. Geneva: Droz, 1983.
Glancy, Jennifer A. *Corporal Knowledge: Early Christian Bodies*. Oxford: Oxford University Press, 2010.
Grensemann, Hermann, ed. *Die hippokratische Schrift "Über die heilige Krankheit."* AM II 1. Berlin: de Gruyter, 1968.
Harnack, Adolf von. *Medicinisches aus der Ältesten Kirchengeschichte*. Leipzig: Hinrichs, 1892.
Heinimann, Felix. *Nomos und Physis: Herkunft und Bedeutung einer Antithese im griechischen Denken des 5. Jahrhunderts*. 1945. Reprinted, Darmstadt: WBG, 1978.
Herter, Hans. "Die kulturhistorische Theorie der hippokratischen Schrift 'Von der alten Medizin.'" *Maia* NS 15 (1963) 464–83.
Hippocrate. *L'Art de la médecine: Serment, ancienne médecine, art, airs, eaux, lieux, maladie sacrée, nature de l'homme, pronostic, aphorismes*. Edited by Jacques Jouanna and Caroline Magdelaine. Geneva: Fondation Hardt, 2003.
Holtz, Sabine. "Die Unsicherheit des Lebens: Zum Verständnis von Krankheit und Tod in den Predigten der lutherischen Orthodoxie." In *Im Zeichen der Krise: Religiosität im Europa des 17. Jahrhunderts*, edited by Hartmut Lehmann and Anna-Charlott Trepp, 135–57. Veröffentlichungen des Max-Plank-Instituts für Geschichte 152. Göttingen: Vandenhoeck & Ruprecht, 1999.
Hutchinson, Nichola. "Disabling Beliefs? Impaired Embodiment in the Religious Tradition of the West." *Body & Society* 12.4 (2006) 1–23.
Jones, W. H. S. *The Doctor's Oath: An Essay in the History of Medicine*. Cambridge: Cambridge University Press, 1924.
Jones, W. H. S. et. al., eds. *Hippocrates I–X* (1–4 1923–1931). Cambridge: Harvard University Press, 1979–2010.

Kahl, Brigitte. "Jairus und die verlorenen Töchter Israels. Sozioliterarische Überlegungen zum Problem der Grenzüberschreitung in Mk 5,21–43." In *Von der Wurzel getragen: Christlich-feministische Exegese in Auseinandersetzung mit Antijudaismus*, edited by Luise Schottroff and Marie-Theres Wacker, 61–78. Biblical Interpretation Series 17. Leiden: Brill, 1996.

Kasper, Helmut. *Griechische Soter-Vorstellungen und ihre Übernahme in das politische Leben Roms.* Munich: Mikrokopie, 1961.

Kee, Howard Clark. *Medicine, Miracle and Magic in New Testament Times.* SNTSMS 55. Cambridge: Cambridge University Press, 1986.

Kleinman, Arthur. *Patients and Healers in the Context of Culture: An Exploration of the Borderland between Anthropology, Medicine, and Psychiatry.* Comparative Studies of Health Systems and Medical Care 3. Berkeley: University of California Press, 1995.

Kleinman, Arthur, and Lilias H. Sung. "Why Do Indigenous Practitioners Successfully Heal?" *Social Science and Medicine* 13B (1979) 7–26.

Kliewer, Stephen. "Allowing Spirituality into the Healing Process." *Journal of Family Practice* 53 (2004) 616–24.

Koenig, Harold G., et al. *Handbook of Religion and Health.* Oxford: Oxford University Press, 2001.

Körtner, Ulrich H. J. "Für einen mehrdimensionalen Spiritualitätsbegriff: Eine interdisziplinäre Perspektive." In *Spiritualität und Medizin: Gemeinsame Sorge für den kranken Mensche*, edited by Eckhard Frick and Traugott Roser, 26–34. Münchner Reihe Palliativ Care 4. Stuttgart: Kohlhammer 2009.

Kollesch, Jutta, and Georg Hartwig. "Der hippokratische Eid: Zur Entstehung der antiken medizinischen Deontologie." *Philologus* 122 (1978) 253–326.

Kollmann, Bernd. *Jesus und die Christen als Wundertäter: Studien zu Magie, Medizin und Schamanismus in Antike und Christentum.* FRLANT 170. Göttingen: Vandenhoeck & Ruprecht, 1996.

Krämer, Sybille. *Medium, Bote, Übertragung: Kleine Metaphysik der Medialität.* Frankfurt: Suhrkamp, 2008.

Kütemeyer, Mechthilde. "Neurologie und Psychosomatik. Erinnerung an die Janz'sche Klinik." In *Die Wahrheit der Begegnung. Anthropologische Perspektiven der Neurologie: Festschrift für Dieter Janz*, edited by Rainer-M. E. Jacobi et al., 191–214. Beiträge zur medizinischen Anthropologie 3. Würzburg: Königshausen & Neumann, 2001.

Kudlien, Fridolf. *Der Beginn des medizinischen Denkens bei den Griechen von Homer bis Hippokrates.* Bibliothek der alten Welt. Stuttgart: Artemis, 1967.

"Les Ordonnances ecclésiastiques de 1561/ Die Kirchenordnung von 1561." In *Calvin-Studienausgabe.* Vol. 2: *Gestalt und Ordnung der Kirche*, edited by E. Busch et al., 238–279. Neukirchen-Vluyn: Neukirchener, 1997.

Malia, Linda M. *Healing Touch and Saving Word: Sacraments of Healing, Instruments of Grace.* Eugene, OR: Pickwick Publications, 2013.

Markschies, Christoph. "Gesund werden im Schlaf: Einige Rezepte aus der Antike, Akademische Causerie am 18. Oktober 2005." *Berichte und Abhandlungen* 12 (2006) 187–216.

Martin, Dale B. *The Corinthian Body.* New Heaven: Yale University Press, 1995.

———. *Inventing Superstition: From the Hippocratics to the Christians.* Cambridge: Harvard University Press, 2004.

Marty, Martin E. "Foreword." In *Caring and Curing: Health and Medicine in the Western Religious Traditions*, edited by Ronald L. Numbers and Darrel W. Amundsen, vii–ix. Baltimore: Johns Hopkins University Press 1998.

Mathews, Thomas F. *The Clash of Gods. A Reinterpretation of Early Christian Art*. Princeton: Princeton University Press, 1993.

Mieth, Dietmar. "Der behinderte Mensch aus theologisch-ethischer Sicht." In *Inklusive Kirche*, edited by Johannes Eurich and Andreas Lob-Hüdepohl, 113–30. Stuttgart: Kohlhammer, 2011.

Miller, William R., and Carl E. Thoresen. "Spirituality, Religion, and Health: An Emerging Research Field." *American Psychologist* 58 (2003) 24–35.

Morgenstern, Andrea. "Trauer zwischen Schuld und Scham." In *Krankheitsdeutungen in der postsäkularen Gesellschaft: Theologische Ansätze im interdisziplinären Gespräch*, edited by G. Thomas and I. Karle, 593–602. Stuttgart: Kohlhammer, 2009.

Moss, Candida R., and Jeremy Schipper. "Introduction." In *Disability Studies and Biblical Literature*, edited by Candida R. Moss and Jeremy Schipper, 1–11. New York: Palgrave Macmillan 2011.

Murken, Sebastian, and Claudia Müller. "Gott hat mich so ausgestattet, dass ich den Weg gehen kann: Religiöse Verarbeitungsstile nach der Diagnose Brustkrebs." *Lebendiges Zeugnis* 62 (2007) 115–28.

Nowak, Kurt. *Schleiermacher: Leben, Werk und Wirkung*. UTB für Wissenschaft. Göttingen: Vandenhoeck & Ruprecht, 2002.

Oeming, Manfred. "Behinderung als Strafe: Zum biblisch fundierten seelsorglichen Umgang mit dem Tun-Ergehen-Zusammenhang." In *Behinderung—Profile in-klusiver Theologie, Diakonie und Kirche*, edited by Johannes Eurich and Andreas Lob-Hüdepohl, 98–126. Behinderung—Theologie—Kirche 7. Stuttgart: Kohlhammer 2014.

———. "Krankheit." In *Wörterbuch alttestamentlicher Motive*, edited by Michael Fieger, 290–94. Darmstadt: WBG, 2013.

Padilla, Carlos E., and Walter V. Moczynski. "Navigating the Institutional Culture: Chaplains as Members of the Medical Team." In *Medical Ethics in Health Care Chaplaincy: Essays*, edited by Walter Moczynski et al., 33–49. Medical Ethics in Health Care Chaplaincy 1. Münster: LIT Verlag, 2009.

Polkinghorne, John. *Science and the Trinity: The Christian Encounter with Reality*. New Haven: Yale University Press, 2004.

Popkes, Enno Edzard. "Die Heilungen Jesu und die Anfänge der Jesusbewegung: Beobachtungen zu den synoptischen Erzählungen von den ersten Heilungen Jesu." In *Krankheitsdeutungen in der postsäkularen Gesellschaft: Theologische Ansätze im interdisziplinären Gespräch*, edited by Günter Thomas and Isolde Karle, 186–202. Stuttgart: Kohlhammer, 2009.

Powell, Lynda H., Leila Shahabi, and Carl E. Thoresen. "Religion and Spirituality: Linkages to Physical Health." *American Psychologist* 58 (2003) 36–52.

Rappmann, Susanne. "The Disabled Body of Christ as a Critical Metaphor-Towards a Theory." *Journal of Religion, Disability & Health* 7 (2004), 25–40.

Ritschl, Dietrich. *Zur Theorie und Ethik der Medizin: Philosophische und theologische Anmerkungen*. Neukirchen-Vluyn: Neukirchener, 2004.

Roser, Traugott. "Innovation Spiritual Care: Eine praktisch-theologische Perspektive." In *Spiritualität und Medizin: Gemeinsame Sorge für den kranken Menschen*, edited by Eckhard Frick and Traugott Roser, 45–55. Münchner Reihe Palliativ Care 4. Stuttgart: Kohlhammer, 2009.

Sax, William S. "Heilen Rituale?" In *Die neue Kraft der Rituale*, edited by Axel Michaels, 213–35. Heidelberg: Winter, 2007.

———. "Healing rituals. A critical performative approach." *Anthropology & Medicine* 11 (2004) 293–306.

Schaeffer, Denise. "Wisdom and Wonder in 'Metaphysics' A: 1–2." *Review of Metaphysics* 52 (1999) 641–56.

Silvers, Anita. "Feminist Perspectives on Disability." *The Stanford Encyclopedia of Philosophy*. Fall 2013. http://plato.stanford.edu/archives/fall2013/ entries/feminism-disability.

Schleiermacher, Friedrich. *The Christian Faith*. Edited by H. R. Mackintosh and J. S. Stewart. London: T. & T. Clark, 1989.

Schreiner, Susan E. *The Theatre of His Glory: Nature and the Natural Order in the Thought of John Calvin*. Durham, NC: Labyrinth, 1991.

Schubert, Charlotte. *Der Hippokratische Eid: Medizin und Ethik von der Antike bis heute*. Darmstadt: WBG, 2005.

Silvers, Anita, "Feminist Perspectives on Disability." The Stanford Encyclopedia of Philosophy (Winter 2016 Edition), edited by Edward N. Zalta (ed.), forthcoming URL = http://plato.stanford.edu/archives/win2016/entries/feminism-disability/.

Smit, Dirk J. "On Illness and Providence: Questions from the Reformed Tradition." In *Essays on Being Reformed: Collected Essays* 3, edited by Robert Vosloo, 141–64. Stellenbosch: SUN MeDIA, 2009.

Staden, Heinrich von. "Incurability and Hopelessness: The Hippocratic Corpus." In *La maladie et les maladies dans la collection hippocratique : Acts du VIe Colloque International Hippocratique*, edited by P. Potter, 75–112. Quebec: Sphinx, 1990.

Temkin, Owsei. *The Falling Sickness: A History of Epilepsy from the Greeks to the Beginnings of Modern Neurology*. Publications of the Institute of the History of Medicine 1/4. Baltimore: John Hopkins University Press, 1945.

Tieleman, Teun. *Galen and Chrysippus on the Soul: Argument and Refutation in the "De placitis," Books II–III*. Philosophia Antiqua 58. Leiden: Brill, 1996.

———. "Religion und Therapie in Galen." In *Religion und Krankheit*, edited by Gregor Etzelmüller and Annette Weissenrieder, 83–95. Darmstadt: WBG, 2010.

Thomas, Christine et. al. "Einfluss verschiedener Formen von Religiosität auf die Schwere und den Verlauf der Depression im Alter." In *Religion und Krankheit*, edited by Gregor Etzelmüller and Annette Weissenrieder, 283–91. Darmstadt: WBG, 2010.

Thomas, Günter. *Neue Schöpfung: Systematisch-theologische Untersuchungen zur Hoffnung auf das 'Leben in der zukünftigen Welt'*. Neukirchen-Vluyn: Neukirchener, 2009.

Waldschmidt, Anne. "Warum und wozu brauchen die Disability Studies die Disability History?" In *Disability History: Konstruktion von Behinderung in der Geschichte. Eine Einführung*, edited by E. Bösl et al., 13–27. Bielefeld: transkript 2010.

Weissenrieder, Annette. "'Er ist ein Gott!' Paulus, ein christlicher Asklepios?" In *An Leib und Seele gesund*, edited by Christof Gestrich, 79–101. Beihefte zur Berliner Theologischen Zeitschrift. Berlin: Wichern, 2007.

———. "'He Is a God!': Acts 28:1–9 in the Light of Iconographical and Textual Sources Related to Medicine." In *Picturing the New Testament: Studies in Ancient Visual*

Images, edited by Annette Weissenrieder et al., 134-56. WUNT 2/193. Tübingen: Mohr/Siebeck, 2005.

———. *Images of Illness in the Gospel of Luke. Insights of Ancient Medical Texts*. WUNT 164. Tübingen: Mohr/Siebeck 2003.

———. "The Plague of Uncleanness? The Ancient Illness Construct 'Issue of Blood' in Luke 8:43-48." In *Jesus and the Gospels*, edited by Wolfgang Stegemann et al., 207-22. Stuttgart: Kohlhammer.

———. "Stories Just under the Skin. Lepra in the Gospel of Luke,." In *Miracles Revisited: New Testament Miracle Stories and Their Concepts of Reality*, edited by Stefan Alkier and Annette Weissenrieder, 73-100. Studies of the Bible and Its Reception 2. Berlin: de Gruyter, 2013.

Weissenrieder, Annette, and Gregor Etzelmüller. "Christlicher Glaube und Medizin: Stationen einer Beziehung / Christian Beliefs and Medicine: Stations of Relationship." *DMW* 132 (2007) 2747-53.

Weissenrieder, Annette, and Karin. *Medizinische Verkörperungen in biblischen und paganen Texten der Antike: Ein Quellenbuch (forthcoming)*.

Weizsäcker, Viktor von. "Grundfragen medizinischer Anthropologie." In *Gesammelte Schriften 7*, edited by P. Achillles et al., 255-82. Frankfurt: Suhrkamp, 1987.

———. "Zur Frage der 'christlichen' Medizin" [1947]. In *Gesammelte Schriften 7*, edited by P. Achillles et al., 22132. Frankfurt: Suhrkamp, 1987.

———. "Stücke einer anthropologischen Medizin" [1926/1928]. In *Gesammelte Schriften 5*, edited by P. Achillles et al., 7-66. Frankfurt: Suhrkamp, 1987.

Welker, Michael. *Creation and Reality*. Translated by John F. Hoffmeyer. Minneapolis: Fortress, 1999.

Wienberg, Günther. "Von der sozialen Exklusion zur Inklusion von Menschen mit Behinderungen—eine sozialhistorische Skizze." *ZEE* 57 (2013) 169-82.

Wilhelm, Dorothee. "'Normal' werden—war's das? Kritik biblischer Heilungsgeschichten." *BiKi* 61 (2006) 103-5.

Wilson Nightingale, Andrea. "On Wandering and Wondering: 'Theoria' in Greek Philosophy and Culture." *Arion* 9 (2001): 23-58

Wohlers, Michael. "'Aussätzige reinigt!' (Mt 10,8). Aussatz in antiker Medizin, Judentum und frühem Christentum." In *Text und Geschichte: Facetten theologischen Arbeitens aus dem Freundes- und Schülerkreis. FS D. Lührmann*, edited by S. Maser and E. Schlarb, 294-304. MThS 50. Marburg: Elwert, 1999.

———. *Heilige Krankheit*. MThSt 57. Marburg: Elwert, 1999.

Zeppezauer, Dorothea. "Krankheitskonzepte in der Hagiographie." In *Krankheitsdeutungen in der postsäkularen Gesellschaft. Theologische Ansätze im interdisziplinären Gespräch*, edited by G. Thomas and I. Karle, 261-73. Kohlhammer: Stuttgart, 2009.

Zimmermann, Ruben. "Krankheit und Sünde im Neuen Testament am Beispiel von Mk 2, 1-12." In *Krankheitsdeutungen in der postsäkularen Gesellschaft. Theologische Ansätze im interdisziplinären Gespräch*, edited by Günter Thomas and Isolde Karle, 227-46. Kohlhammer: Stuttgart, 2009.

Zwingmann, C. et al. "Positive and Negative Religious Coping in German Breast Cancer Patients." *Journal of Behavioral Medicine* 29 (2006) 533-44.

14

Becoming a Doctor, Becoming a God
Religion and Medicine in Aelius Aristides' *Hieroi Logoi*[1]

—Georgia Petridou

PUBLIUS AELIUS ARISTIDES THEODORUS, one of the most renowned rhetoricians of the so-called second sophistic, was born in Northern Mysia in 117 CE. Out of Aristides' extant works, the *Hieroi Logoi*, five extant speeches and one fragmentary, which chronicle his long and volatile relationship with illness and healing, are the ones that have attracted the most interest. In particular, the last decade or so has seen some remarkable advances in our understanding of the *Hieroi Logoi* (henceforth *HL*) and its author.[2] The *HL*

---

1. I would like to thank wholeheartedly the 'Lived Ancient Religion' ERC Project at the Max-Weber Kolleg (Universität Erfurt) and it director Jörg Rüpke for funding my research project. I am indebted to Jan Bremmer and Jörg Rüpke as well as to the editors of the volume, Annette Weissenrieder and Gregor Etzelmüller, for their pertinent comments on an earlier draft of this article. I would also like to thank Paul Scade for improving the language of this study and Janet Downie (Princeton) for generously sharing with me the contents of her unpublished paper entitled 'The Therapeutic Dynamic in Aelius Aristides' *Sacred Tales*' delivered at the 2008 American Philological Association (APA) conference. Many thanks are also to be given to the team of the 'Medicine of the Mind-Philosophy of the Body' research project (Humboldt Universität zu Berlin) and especially to Philip van der Eijk, Manfred Horstmanhoff and Oliver Overwien, for discussing with me several aspects of the ancient medical discourse. Translations, unless otherwise stated, are mine. I have used Keil's edition, in which the six books (the first five are complete and the last one is fragmentary) of the *HL* appear as *Orationes* 47–52.

2 See, for instance, Horstmanshoff, "Did the god learn medicine?"; King, "Origins

are no longer thought of as the fevered fable of an incurable hypochondriac;[3] instead, they are considered as a rare first-person narrative, which, while extremely elaborate and self-conscious, offers a unique insight into the religious, medical and cultural life of the second century CE.[4]

Yet the predominant scholarly impression of Aristides is that of the paradigmatic patient who surrendered his physical and psychological health to Asclepius and spent a large part of his life in the temple of Asclepius at Pergamum blindly following divine orders on diet and regimen.[5] In that sense, Aristides fits Galen's description of the unwilling and uncooperative patient in his commentary on the Hippocratic *Epidemics*:

πρὸς τὴν τοιαύτην οὖν εὐπείθειαν αὐτὸς ὁ <Ἱπποκράτης> ἔλεγε καὶ τὰς προρρήσεις ὠφελεῖν ἡμᾶς καὶ ὅλως τὸ θαυμάζεσθαι τὸν ἰατρὸν ὑπὸ τοῦ κάμνοντος. οὕτω γέ τοι καὶ παρ' ἡμῖν ἐν <Περγάμῳ> τοὺς θεραπευομένους ὑπὸ τοῦ θεοῦ πειθομένους ὁρῶμεν αὐτῷ πεντεκαίδεκα πολλάκις ἡμέραις προστάξαντι μηδ' ὅλως πιεῖν, οἳ τῶν ἰατρῶν μηδενὶ προστάττοντι πείθονται. μεγάλην γὰρ ἔχει

---

of Medicine"; Pernot, "Rhetoric of Religion"; Harris and Holmes, eds., *Between Greece, Rome and the Gods*; Petsalis-Diomidis, *Truly Beyond Wonders*; Israelowich, *Society, Medicine, Religion*; Kouke, *Hieroi Logoi*; and Downie, *Limits of Art*. New discussions and editions of Aristides' work are also currently in preparation at the University of Strasbourg within the research framework of a project directed by Laurent Pernot.

3. Aristides as hypochndriac: Phillips, "A Hypochndriac and his God"; Behr, *Sacred Tales*, 162–64; Bowersock, *Sophists*, 72; and more recently, Harris, *Dreams and Experience*, 92. This anachronistic and largely ahistorical attribution of hypochondriasis to the *nosos* of Aristides has subsided in modern studies of the HL. Just as there is a plethora of chronic medical conditions modern doctors can neither identify nor treat, likewise there would have been many more analogous conditions which would have left the physicians of the ancient world perplexed and utterly unable to help. On Aristides' chronic pain and the burning issue of how we qualify and quantify pain, see King, "Chronic Pain." For a historical study of ancient *hypochondria*, as pain and discomfort "occurring in the region below the cartilage," which should be distinguished from the modern notion of hypochondria, see Leven, "Hypochonder" and van der Eijk, "Melancholia and 'Hypochondria.'"

4. On the self-consciousness of the narrative, see Petsalis-Diomidis, "Sacred writing, sacred reading"; Holmes, "Illegible Body"; and Downie, "Bathing and Oratory"

5. E.g.: Festugière, *Personal Religion*, 86–87, 98; Perkins, *Suffering Self*, ch. 7; Perkins, "The Self as Sufferer"; Cox Miller, *Dreams in Late Antiquity*, 192; Horstmanshoff, "Did the God Learn Medicine?"; King, "Origins of Medicine"; Israelowich, *Society, Medicine, Religion*, 37–132; and Κούκη, *Hieroi Logoi*, 13–57. There are, of course, exceptions to this rule. For example, a great deal of emphasis has been given to Aristides as a typical product of the *paideia* of the second century in Pernot, "Rhetoric of Religion" and "*Periautologia*"; Harris and Holmes, eds., *Between Greece, Rome and the Gods*; Petsalis-Diomidis, *Truly Beyond Wonders*; and Downie, *Limits of the Art*.

ῥοπὴν εἰς τὸ πάντα ποιῆσαι τὰ προστατόμενα τὸ πεπεῖσθαι τὸν κάμνοντα βεβαίως ἀκολουθήσειν ὠφέλειαν ἀξιόλογον αὐτῷ.⁶

> Concerning then this very concept of ready obedience Hippocrates himself used to say that public predictions and generally admiration towards the doctor on behalf of the patient benefit us. Thus, at any rate even among ourselves in Pergamum we see that those who are being treated by the god obey him, when on many occasions he orders them not to drink anything for fifteen days, while they obey none of the physicians who give this prescription. For it has great power on the patient's doing everything that has been prescribed, if he has been confidently persuaded that a substantial benefit for him will follow.

To be sure, this image of the submissive patient, who accepts and follows unquestioningly the medical prescriptions of the divine healer, the ultimate doctor as Aristides calls him in 1.4, is one that the orator himself advocates for rather ardently at the beginning of the *HL*, when he says: "therefore, in view of this, I decided to submit truly to the god, as to a doctor and do in silence whatever he wishes." In my mind, this is a deceptively simplistic tactic of self-representation and one that does not dovetail with a) Aristides' active involvement in his own treatment, b) his exegetical role in the interpretation of the dream-visions sent by the god, or c) the constant subordination of the medical views expressed by both the divine and the earthly healers to his own views.

This paper argues in favour of a more complex picture, which emerges from close reading of a number of extracts from the *HL* that cast Aristides in a very different light. In particular, the passages examined under section 3 (*Appropriating the powers of the mortal physicians: Aristides heals himself*) reveal a whole new aspect of Aristides' persona: that of the informed patient, who knows his medical literature and double-checks his physicians' instructions and accepts them only after much deliberation. Section 2 (*Appropriating Asclepius' healing powers: Aristides heals others*), on the other hand, discusses extracts from the *HL* in which Aristides proves to be as much of a challenge for his divine healer as he has been for his earthly physicians; while section 1 (*Aristides as the mirror image of Asclepius*) focuses on two dream-narratives which present Asclepius as the *catalyst* in Aristides' wondrous transformation from a suffering patient into a knowledgeable physician. In short, what I suggest here is that this new picture of

---

6. Gal. *In Hipp. Epid. VI comment.* 17b, 137 K. A more recent edition of the text can be found in Wenkebach, Ernst: *Galeni In Hippocratis Epidemiarum librum VI commentaria III–VI*, CMG V 10,2,2, 2. Aufl., Berlin 1956, 124–351.

Aristides' relationship to Asclepius is not one-directional nor does it involve total dependence; instead, both mortal patient and immortal physician are portrayed as bound together in a reciprocal exchange of gratitude (χάρις). Aristides offers a case of most complex and intricate illnesses for Asclepius to prove his interminable therapeutic abilities against, while Asclepius offers a unique tailor-made therapy for both Aristides' mind and body.[7]

The reader witnesses here a very peculiar version of what Susan Mattern described as "the patronage of therapeutics." I call this a divine patronage of therapeutics: just as high-ranked Roman citizens would take under their wings physicians of any social status (including low) and raise them to honourable positions, in the same way Asclepius adopts Aristides as a protégé and imparts to him a greater degree of medical knowledge and ability.[8] Thus, Aristides is elevated to the status of a potent physician.[9] Furthermore, Asclepius imparts to his devotee a certain degree of divinity, which raises Aristides above the level of the rest of his worshippers and provides him with the essential authority to ground his claims to healing powers analogous to those of the god. Or so Aristides would like us to believe.

An alternative interpretation of this intimate relationship between the divine healer and his eminent patient arises from examining it as an example of elite appropriation of Asclepius' healing powers, and, thus, as an excellent case-study for the "Lived Ancient Religion" (henceforth LAR) approach to the study of religions.[10] LAR lays extra emphasis on the individual appropriation of religious traditions and practices. Within such a research-framework, the *HL* are examined as a first-hand testimony of individual appropriation and evaluation of established ritual schemata and ritual performance.[11] The second section of this article focuses on how pre-

7. More on this topic in Pernot, "The Rhetoric of Religion."

8. Mattern, "The Patronage of Therapeutics," 1–18.

9. The status of the physician in the Roman world is a profoundly complex issue and one that has generated a great deal of scholarly debate. See Kudlien, *Die Stellung des Arztes*; Nutton, "Healers in the Medical Market Place" and "The Medical Meeting Place"; Pleket, "The Social Status of Physicians"; Lendon, *Empire of Honor*, 43–44; and Mattern, "The Patronage of Therapeutics."

10. To avoid methodological pitfalls of relying too much on elite descriptions of mass behaviour (Rüpke, "Lived Ancient Religion") in my monograph, I contrast Aristides' appropriation of the Asclepian cult with Alexander's populist approach in establishing the cult of *neos Asclepius-Glykon*, which is essentially an Asclepian religion with a distinct mysteric ambiance. It goes without saying that Alexander is discussed here as a composite figure and the focus is on the cultic realities behind Lucian's *Alexander the Pseudo-Prophet*. More on this topic in Petsalis-Diomidis, *Truly Beyond Wonders*, 14–41; and Gordon, "Individuality, Selfhood and Power."

11. In my forthcoming monograph *The Mysian Patient: Medicine and Mysticism in Aelius Aristides' Hieroi Logoi*, I consider the *HL* as both a *narrative of religious change*

cisely Aristides appropriates the ritual schema of supplication and incubation to portray himself as being in control of the specifics of sacred healing and as an erudite patient whose medical expertise suffices not only to heal himself but also others.

Furthermore, the LAR approach prioritizes the actual daily experience, practices, expressions, and interactions that can be related to "religion," and considers religious traditions to be the product of interaction between the individual religious participants and the providers of religious knowledge and services, the religious professionals. One of the main aims of LAR is to examine the role these professionals played in actively shaping the religious action, the ways they advanced, hindered, or simply diversified day-to-day religious experience in the imperial era. More importantly, LAR is interested in the ways the individual invents in order to contest and effectively bypass religious intermediaries and thus claim for himself the much-prized proximity with the divine. Aristides is, thus, of further interest to us, since in the narratives discussed below he portrays himself as not only having acquired the medical expertise of the medical practitioners, who frequented the Asclepieia of the second century, but also as being in possession of the healing powers of the divine healer himself.[12]

---

and as a *document of religious individuality*. In summary, I argue that Aristides in the *HL* appears to conceptualise illness in general and his two-year period of incubation (145–147 CE) at the Pergamene Asclepieion in particular (a period to which he refers to a "the kathedra"), as a dangerous and at times extremely painful initiatory process into a mystery cult of the type which have been extremely popular in the imperial era. Having said that, I would like to clarify that I do not necessarily take the cult of Asclepius at the Pergamene Asclepieion to be a mystery cult with formal initiation, a *hieros logos*, and inbuilt mechanisms of inclusion and exclusion; what I argue here is not that the cult of Asclepius at Pergamon was a mystery cult, but that—and this is far more important for the purposes of the *LAR* project—it was *lived* by Aristides *as such*. On *hieros logos* as an integral element of mystery cult see Festugière, *Personal Religion*, 88; and Petsalis-Diomidis, *Truly Beyond Wonders*, 125. On documents of religious individuality and on the concept of individuality in general, see the introduction in Rüpke and Woolf, eds., *Religious Dimensions of the Self*; and Rüpke, *The Individual in the Religions of the Ancient Mediterranean*.

12. On medical practitioners being present in the Asclepieion of Pergamum, see Israelowich, *Society, Medicine, Religion*, 90: "The world of the *Sacred Tales* has physicians offering medical care to the convalescents of the Asclepieion, providing them with authoritative advice with regard to the interpretation of dreams, performing medical procedures such as enemas and phlebotomies and even joining them in their journeys to undergo purges in certain divinely designated sites." cf. also ibid., 88–91. Aristides mentions some of his physicians: Asklepiacus (*HL* 2.35), Herakleon (*HL* 2.20), Porphyrion (*HL* 5.12), Satyros: (*HL* 3.8), Theodotos (*HL* 1.13, 1.55–57, 2.34, 4.21 and 5.57). Most of them, however, remain anonymous and get referred to in plural (οἱ ἰατροί), as in *HL* 2.39, 3.27 and elsewhere.

In essence, Aristides presents himself as both a physician of sorts (ἰατρός) and a sacred servant (θεράπων, διάκονος, θεραπευτής) of Asclepius, who enjoys a privileged relationship with the god.[13] It is certainly no coincidence that the term θεραπευτής can signify both the religious and the medical attendant, and that Aristides chooses especially this term as the crux of his self-definition in his dream encounter with the emperor Marcus (HL 1.23):[14]

> Ἕκτῃ ἐδόκουν ἅμα Ἀλεξάνδρῳ τῷ διδασκάλῳ προσιέναι τῷ αὐτοκράτορι, καθέζεσθαι δ' αὐτὸν ἐπί τινος βήματος. προσειπόντος δὲ αὐτὸν τοῦ Ἀλεξάνδρου προτέρου καὶ προσρηθέντος ὑπ' αὐτοῦ τε καὶ τῶν περὶ αὐτόν, ἅτε καὶ ἐκ πολλοῦ γνωρίμου καὶ συνήθους ὄντος, μετὰ τοῦτο προσῄειν ἐγώ. προσειπόντος δὲ κἀμοῦ καὶ στάντος ἐθαύμασεν ὁ αὐτοκράτωρ, ὡς οὐ καὶ αὐτὸς προσελθὼν φιλήσαιμι. κἀγὼ εἶπον ὅτι ὁ θεραπευτὴς εἴην ὁ τοῦ Ἀσκληπιοῦ· τοσοῦτον γάρ μοι ἤρκεσεν εἰπεῖν περὶ ἐμαυτοῦ. πρὸς οὖν τοῖς ἄλλοις, ἔφην, καὶ τοῦτο ὁ θεός μοι παρήγγειλε μὴ φιλεῖν οὑτωσί· καὶ ὅς, ἀρκεῖ, ἔφη. κἀγὼ ἐσίγησα. καὶ ὅς ἔφη, καὶ μὴν θεραπεύειν γε παντὸς κρείττων ὁ Ἀσκληπιός.

> On the sixth day, I dreamed that along with my teacher Alexander I approached the emperor, who sat upon a platform. When Alexander, since he was an old friend and acquaintance, first saluted him and was in turn saluted by him and his entourage,

---

13. θεραπευτής can denote both the "worshipper," the "servant of the god" (Plat. Phdr.252c; Leg.740c, IG11(4).1226 (Delos, 2nd BCE); and the "medical attendant" (Gorg. 517e; Resp. 369d and 341c). On διάκονος and διακονία, see below n. 36. Petridou, "Aristides as therapeutēs and the therapeutai of Asclepius at Pergamum" offers a comprehensive discussion of the cultic title of therapeutes in the works of Aelius Aristides and Galen.

14. Aristides was not alone in trusting his dreams as means of therapy. The author of the Hippocratic On Regimen considered dreams as an integral part of its subject matter, but he advised the patients to seek expert interpretation from skilled physicians not dream-interpreters (Vict. 87 Byl-Joly). On the integral role of dreams and dream-based healing in the Graeco-Roman Medicine in general see Oberhelman, "Dreams in Greco-Roman Medicine"; Harris, Dreams and Experience, 64–66; and the essays collected in Oberhelman, Dreams, Healing, and Medicine. In his Subfiguratio Empirica, ch. 10, 78 Deichgräber (not in Kuhn), Galen reports on a patient's successful healing in the Pergamene Asclepieion: the patient was given specific, albeit extraordinary, dietary advice in his dream encounters with Asclepius and was subsequently cured from epilepsy; while in De curandi ratione per venae sectionem (*De flebothomia) 11.314–315 K and MM 10.971–972 K the famous second century physician explains how he was himself directed to certain methods of treatment after divine dream injunctions. On dreams and their integral role in Aristides' illness and therapy as presented the HL, see Israelowich, Society, Medicine, Religion, 71–86; and Downie Limits of Art, 57–85 and "Dream Hermeneutics."

> I approached. And when I saluted and stood there, the emperor wondered why I too had not come forward and kissed him. And I said that I was a servant of Asclepius. For I was content to say that much about myself. "Therefore, in addition to other things," I said, "the god has instructed me not to kiss in this fashion." And he replied. "This suffices." And I remained silent. And he said, "Indeed, Asclepius is better than all to serve."

In that respect, Aristides models perhaps himself on Asclepiacus, a close-friend of his in Pergamum, who was said to have combined both the qualities of a health-care provider (ἰατρός) and those of a temple warden (νεωκόρος).[15] To be more specific, being a *therapōn* or a *therapeutēs*, that is a servant of the god, is not quite the same as being the god's priest, his ἱερεύς, but it is not long before Aristides dreams of acquiring that identity too. In particular, he dreams of being honoured by the priest of the god (HL 1.12–13) and in 1.15 he even dreams of wearing a priest's ceremonial outfit (ἐδόκουν ἐσθῆτα ἔχειν ἱερέως). Finally, in *HL* 1.41 the identification of the Mysian orator with the priest of Asclepius is complete and absolute. Aristides receives a letter from the Governor, which reads "Greetings to Aristides the priest! (Ἀριστείδῃ τῷ ἱερεῖ χαίρειν)." The priest of Asclepius was an extremely honourable office, held by a descendant of the Asclepiadae family for life.[16] More importantly, Aristides' religious *cursus honorum* does not stop there. Instead, Aristides' appropriation of Asclepian healing powers is a fairly gradual process that culminates with the orator's identification with the divine healer himself. The patient becomes the mirror-image of his divine physician. The two dream narratives narrated in *HL* 4.51–52 will flesh this out.

ARISTIDES AS THE MIRROR-IMAGE OF ASCLEPIUS

The first of the two seems central to Aristides' self-image as the god's chosen one and his perception of his relationship with the divine physician as reciprocal. It is worth noting that the dream-vision is delivered only after much deliberation, caution and a certain anxiety regarding its content and its suitability for the ears of a wider audience, a clever, perhaps rhetorical, device to draw the audience's attention to it.[17] Although the concept of close

---

15. Doctor: *HL* 3.25; temple warden: *HL* 1.47–49, 3.14 and 3.22.

16. Cf. *I.Perg*. no. 251; Arist. *Or*. 30.13–15, 25, 27 Keil.

17. This could also be explained as an exercise in false humility and prompted by Aristides' self-awareness about crossing certain boundaries in self-praise (*periautologia*) and appear extremely arrogant. An excellent discussion of the attractions and the dangers of *periautologia* in the *HL* and the work of Aristides as a whole can be found in

proximity with the divine is a central theme in the *HL*, as the ensuing section argues, this very same concept is taken here to the absolute extreme: our Mysian patient seems to be not simply close to the god but presents himself as enjoying a kind of mystic union with him:

> (50) τὰ δ' ἐντεῦθεν ἤδη, εἰ μὲν θέμις, εἰρήσθω καὶ γεγράφθω, εἰ δὲ μή, τοσοῦτον σοὶ μελήσειε, δέσποτα Ἀσκληπιέ, ἐπὶ νοῦν ἀγαγεῖν μοι διαγράψαι παντὸς δυσκόλου χωρίς. πρῶτον μὲν ὤφθη τὸ ἕδος τρεῖς κεφαλὰς ἔχον καὶ πυρὶ λαμπόμενον κύκλῳ, πλὴν τῶν κεφαλῶν· ἔπειθ' οἱ θεραπευταὶ προσειστήκειμεν, ὥσπερ ὅταν ὁ παιὰν ᾄδηται· σχεδὸν δὲ ἐν πρώτοις ἐγώ. κἀν τούτῳ νεύει ἔξοδον ὁ θεός, ἔχων ἤδη τὸ ἑαυτοῦ σχῆμα ἐν ᾧπερ ἕστηκεν. οἵ τε δὴ οὖν ἄλλοι πάντες ἐξῄεσαν κἀγὼ μετεστρεφόμην ὡς ἐξιών, καὶ ὁ θεός μοι τῇ χειρὶ προδείκνυσι μένειν. κἀγὼ περιχαρὴς τῇ τιμῇ γενόμενος καὶ ὅσον τῶν ἄλλων προὐκρίθην ἐξεβόησα, 'εἷς', λέγων δὴ τὸν θεόν. καὶ ὃς ἔφη· 'σὺ εἶ'. (51) τοῦτο τὸ ῥῆμα ἐμοί, δέσποτ' Ἀσκληπιέ, παντὸς ἀνθρωπίνου βίου κρεῖττον, τούτου πᾶσα ἐλάττων νόσος, τούτου πᾶσα ἐλάττων χάρις, τοῦτ' ἐμὲ καὶ δύνασθαι καὶ βούλεσθαι ζῆν ἐποίησε. καὶ ταῦτα μὲν ἡμῖν εἰρηκόσι μηδὲν ἔλαττον εἴη τῆς πρόσθεν τιμῆς παρὰ τοῦ θεοῦ. (52) Λόγον δέ ποτε ἤκουσα τοιόνδε φέροντα εἰς λόγους καὶ ὁμιλίαν θείαν. ἔφη χρῆναι κινηθῆναι τὸν νοῦν ἀπὸ τοῦ καθεστηκότος, κινηθέντα δὲ συγγενέσθαι θεῷ, συγγενόμενον δὲ ὑπερέχειν ἤδη τῆς ἀνθρωπίνης ἕξεως καὶ οὐδέτερόν γε εἶναι θαυμαστόν, οὔτε ὑπερέχειν θεῷ συγγενόμενον οὔθ' ὑπερσχόντα συνεῖναι θεῷ.

(50) As to what comes next, if it is appropriate, let it be said and written, and if not, may you be fully concerned, Lord Asclepius, to prompt me to describe it, without any quarrel. First the cult statue appeared having three heads and shining about with fire, except for the heads. Next we the worshippers stood in front of it, just like when the paean is sung. And I was almost among the first. At that point, the god, after having acquired the shape he has in his statues, signalled our departure. All the others were departing, and I was turning to depart too, and the God, with his hand, signalled me to stay. And I was delighted by the honour and the extent to which I was favoured from the others, and I shouted out, "(you are) the One", meaning the god. But he said, "It is you (who is the one)." (51) For me this statement, Lord Asclepius, meant more than human life itself, and every disease means little when compared to this, every reciprocal favour means very little in comparison to this, this made me able

---

Pernot *"Periautologia"* and Downie, *Limits of Art*, 141–47.

and willing to live. And now that we have said these things, may we have no less honour that before from the God. (52) Once I heard the following words, which pertained to my rhetoric and divine communion. He said that it was fitting that my mind be changed from its already established condition, and after having been changed, to associate with god, and by this association to be superior to the human condition, and that neither was to wonder at, neither by association with god, to be superior, nor by being superior, to associate with god.

Most scholars have focused on the so-called "henotheistic acclamation" of Asclepius as "the One," that is the only god, a ritual expression of distinction, which indicated Aristides' personal devotion to Asclepius.[18] The god manifesting himself in the form of his statue in the course of a dream or in waking reality is not unprecedented. In fact, it is a rather common phenomenon attested from the archaic to the Hellenistic and imperial period.[19] What is truly extraordinary is that Aristides encounters in his dream this uniquely teratomorphic effigies-epiphany of Asclepius, and that this statue is not only an outstanding shape-shifter (it changed to an image of the god's statue used as it appeared in Pergamum), but is also extremely body-conscious: it was the divine statue that signaled first the departure of the rest of the pilgrims and subsequently signalled to Aristides that he should be the only one to stay.[20] Asclepius' reply to Aristides: "It is you, who is the One!" is

---

18. On the liturgical acclamation εἷς θεός and henotheism, see Versnel, *Inconsistencies*, ch. 3; Markschies "Heis Theos?" and "Heis Theos—Ein Gott?" On *heis theos* and *megas theos* as ritual expressions of distinction and henotheism as a prominent religious feature of the imperial period, see Belayche, "ritual expressions of distinction"; Chaniotis, "*Megatheism*" and Gasparini, "Demonology vs. Henotheism." Although Downie, (*Limits of Art*, 149 n55) may be right in remarking that this exclamation is not a creedal statement (not at least the way we mean it today), one must be cautious not to regard Aristides' exclamation as devoid of religious significance. More significantly, the ritual acclamation *heis theos* is closely related to healing: Versnel (*Inconsistencies*, 50 n32), for instance, reminds us that εἷς is also reminiscent of ritual formulae of the type εἷς θεὸς ὁ βοηθῶν (βοηθός), which appear repeatedly in magical papyri that relate cases of successful divine interventions from deadly illness.

19. Cf. Van Straten "Daikrates' Dream"; Steiner, *Images in Mind*; Bremmer, "The Agency of Greek and Roman statues" and Petridou, *Divine Epiphany in Greek Literature and Culture*, ch. 1.

20. Behr (*Sacred Tales* ad loc.) thought that the statue with three heads "cannot be identified and should be assigned to the aberrancies of the dream world." Festugière (*Personal Religion*, 169 n22.), on the other hand, thought that the three headed creature could be read as an allusion to Kerberos, since the three headed dog that often accompanies statuary depictions of Sarapis. In this view, Aristides had "confused" Sarapis for Asclepius. In my view, this teratomorphic statuary manifestation of Asclepius supports the thesis (which I explore in detail in my forthcoming study) that Aristides' personal

in my mind indicative of the narrator's conscious effort to present himself as the counterpart and the mirror image of the god.[21] At that unique moment of extreme proximity with the divine, Aristeides transforms himself from a powerless worshiper to a potent god and a powerful divine physician. Aristides has somehow (via an oneiric mystic union with the god?) turned himself into a *new* Asclepius of sorts. Another analogous case of Aristides' presenting himself as the mirror image of Asclepius is the dream-vision narrated in 1.17, where the reader is told that Aristides dreams originally of a statue of Asclepius, which on closer inspection turns out to be a statue of himself! The god and his devotee are unified; the patient has become one with his divine physician.

It is certainly tempting to think that Aristides' transformation echoes the contemporary cultic realities of individual appropriation of Asclepian healing powers, such as those lurking in the cultic background of the oracular and healing cult of *neos Asclepius Glykon* ("The Sweet One"), which are accounted for in Lucian's *Alexander the pseudo-prophet*. Lucian's *Alexander* along with contemporary numismatic, epigraphic and sculptural evidence all attest to the rise of this powerful Asclepian cult, which first appeared in Abonouteichos (modern Inebolu) during the reign of Antoninus Pius (138–161 CE), and thrived well into the third century CE.[22] Galen himself seems to have been well acquainted with the cult of *neos Asclepius Glykon* (via Lucian's writings or personal knowledge?) and its popularity amongst the members of the Roman ruling class, who he vehemently chastises at 1.4 of his treatise *On examining the best physicians*.[23] In my mind, Galen may

---

concept of Asclepian functions and bodily physiognomy was much more complex and nuanced than our own, and even perhaps not far away from that of his Egyptian counterpart Sarapis. This latter interpretation can further be supported by the statuary triplex of Asclepius, Sarapis, and Isis, as seen by Pausanias (7.26.7) at the temple of the god in Aegina. More information on effigies epiphanies can be found in Petridou, *Divine Epiphany in Greek Literature and Culture*.

21. On Aristides as mirror image of Asclepius, see Cox Miller, *Dreams in Late Antiquity*, 203. Different aspects of Aristides' intimate relationship with Asclepius have been investigated by different scholars. See, for instance, the recent study of Israelowich, *Society, Medicine and Religion*, 113–21.

22. The cult of *neos Asclepius-Glykon* proved to be extremely popular with a geographical distribution that extends from the Greek mainland well into Pisidia and Mysia. Cf. G. Bordenache Battaglia "Glykon," in *LIMC* IV, 1, 279–83 and Petsalis-Diomidis, *Truly Beyond Wonders*, 12–66) with further bibliography. In the first chapter of her monograph, Petsalis-Diomidis offers an excellent analysis of the material evidence that attests to the popularity of this cult, both independently from and against the literary evidence provided by Lucian, and reaches the conclusion that "Asclepian pilgrimage could be the focus of intense contestation and religious polemic."

23. Galen's treatise *On examining the best physicians* survives only in Arabic and

also be thinking of the same Asclepian cult when, in his *On the Therapeutic Method,* he mocks Thessalos, the Methodist doctor, by saying that his rival fancies himself as the epiphany of a second Asclepius (Θεσσαλὸς, ὁ δεύτερος Ἀσκληπιὸς, εἰς ἀνθρώπους ἧκεν).[24]

In the same vein, we are told that Aristides' second oneiric encounter recounted in 4.52 pertained to Aristides' rhetorical speeches and fellowship with the divine (λόγους καὶ ὁμιλίαν θείαν). It revealed that there was one necessary and sufficient condition so as to attain union with the divine: a change of mind (χρῆναι κινηθῆναι τὸν νοῦν ἀπὸ τοῦ καθεστηκότος), a change of mind away from the ordinary, the *status quo*.[25] Having achieved this radical change in the way Aristides' mind worked, the orator would be free to συγγενέσθαι with the divine, that is to say, to achieve extreme proximity and intimacy with the divine, to converse with and become one with the god (κινηθέντα δὲ συγγενέσθαι θεῷ).[26] The term συγγίγνομαι means "to associate," "to keep company with," "to hold converse with," "to become acquainted

---

is translated by Iskandar, *Galeni De optimo medico cognoscendo* with Nutton, ("The Patient's Choice," 23–25). This cult's influence spread from the Black Sea to the centre of Pisidia and from there to the Roman court, if we are to judge by the fact (as reported by Lucian) that Rutilianus, a Roman senator, was keen to make the founder of the cult, Alexander, his son-in-law.

24. *De methodo medendi* 3,208 K: "But the most shameless Thessalos (ὁ δ᾽ ἀναισχυντότατος Θεσσαλὸς), who knows one thing alone—that you must fill the hollow wound—says his theories of medicine are established and firmly based. And yet all men know this, as I said before, and not only those of the present day, from the time when Thessalos, the second Asclepius, came among men, but also, I believe, those before Deukalion and Phoroneus, at least if those men were also Dogmatics. But in addition to knowing that the hollow wound or ulcer is something you must enflesh—they do still understand that—they realise that the one who knows the medications that are enfleshing such a wound is the doctor." On Pardalas and Galen, see Fischer "Galen, Pardalas, and Sundry Delights"; on Galen's relationship to Asclepius see *De opt. med. cogn.* i.1–4 with Nutton ("The Patient's Choice," 253–54). On Galen's religious belief in general see Kudlien, "Galen's religious Belief"; Frede, "Galen's Theology'" and, more recently, Pietrobelli, "Galien Agnostique."

25. The dream narrated in 4.52 is also narrated in more or less the same way, but in a completely different context and with very different ramifications, in yet another of Aristides' speeches entitled περὶ τοῦ παραφθέγματος (*Or.* 28.116 Keil).

26. Students and their master: Pl. *Phd.* 61d, *Men.* 91e; union and sexual intercourse: Xen. *Anab.* 1.2.12; Pl. *Rep.* 329c. Establishing strong bonds of συγγένεια (kinship) with the divine is the main endeavour in many initiation rituals. In the pseudo-Platonic *Axiochus* (371d), for instance, we find the notion of the initiand in Eleusinian *mystēria* being a γεννήτης θεῶν, a kinsman of the gods; while in Aristides' more intricate theology (as articulated in the oration he delivered in Smyrna in 142 CE in honour of Sarapis (*Or.* 45 Keil), a work heavily influenced by Platonic conceptions of the soul, as found in *Protagoras* and *Timaeus*) it is Sarapis who cleanses the *phychē* with wisdom, which is essentially the only thing that manifests the kinship of mortals with the gods: ἣ μόνη τὴν πρὸς θεοὺς συγγένειαν ἀνθρώποις δείκνυσι.

with," "to coexist." It can be used to describe a student's of disciple's relationship with their master, but it can also denote union and even sexual intercourse. In 4.27 HL Aristides delves further into this concept of *syggenestae* with the divine and its relation to illness: while enumerating the praise he received from the literati of his day, Aristides confides to the reader a piece of information he received in an exchange he had with the famous orator Pardalas: "and once that famous Pardalas, who, I would say, was the greatest expert of the Greeks of our time in the science of oratory, dared to say and affirm to me that he believed that I had become ill through some divine good fortune, so that by my association with the god, I might make this improvement (ἐτόλμησεν εἰπεῖν πρὸς ἐμὲ καὶ διισχυρίσασθαι, ἦ μὴν νομίζειν τύχῃ τινὶ θείᾳ συμβῆναί μοι τὴν νόσον, ὅπως τῷ θεῷ συγγενόμενος ἐπιδοίην ταύτην τὴν ἐπίδοσιν)."[27]

To return to our text, this close proximity with the divine would lead in turn to the fulfilment of all of Aristides' ambitions to excel and outdo not only his competitors, but his human *hexis*, his human "condition," "state," or "tenor" (συγγενόμενον δὲ ὑπερέχειν ἤδη τῆς ἀνθρωπίνης ἕξεως).[28] This notion of excelling or outshining is left deliberately vague and fluctuates between professional, intellectual and moral excellence as well as religious devotion. But the main focus of the narrative remains this much-prized proximity and conversation with the divine, which possesses an amazing transformative power for the individual, a power that is difficult to put into words. When in union with the divine, nothing remains the same. Can this power be so great as to transform a patient into a physician? It certainly seems so, if we are to judge from a wealth of passages in the HL where our renowned patient

---

27. The suggestion that his illness befell Aristides out of some favourable turn of luck or "some divine good fortune," and above all that this illness was thought to be a *conditio sine qua non* for attaining *syggeneia* with the divine, apparently came as a shock to Aristides. Or, at least, this is what the introductory verb *etolmēsen* seems to suggest. Whilst these words are put in the mouth of a third party, an objective observer of sorts, they do, nonetheless, reflect Aristides' own views on the utilitarian aspect of his illness as facilitating his direct contact with the divine.

28. The term *hexis* (from ἔχω, "to have," "to hold") is an interesting one. It means being in a certain state, a permanent condition as produced by *praxis* and can denote either a state of mind/soul (e.g., Pl. *Leg.* 650b) or a state of body (e.g., Xen. *Mem.* 1.2.4; Hp. *Alim.* 34). In Aristotle it denotes an acquired habit, as opposed to *energeia*, e.g.: *EN* 1098b33. However, it is more tempting to think that Aristides employs the Stoic term *hexis*, which is translated as "tenor" and refers to "the defining quality of a differentiated body." See, for instance, See, for instance, Simplicius, in *Cat.* 237.25–238.20 = LS 47S with Long and Sedley's commentary (1987, vol. 1, p. 289). Perhaps the meaning here is that Aristides is prompted to surpass the limitations of his human *hexis*, i.e. the human ways of thinking and acting, and thus approximate the divine *hexis*. I am grateful to Paul Scade for these references.

appears to be operating under the auspices of Asclepius as a divine healer himself. The following section discusses in detail three of those passages: first, Aristides' successful treatment of Zosimos, his foster father, secondly Aristides' successful medical intervention to save Philoumene, his nurse, and, finally, two cases out of the many examples of his self-healing. I also mention *en passant* several others passages of similar content.

APPROPRIATING ASCLEPIUS' HEALING POWERS: ARISTIDES HEALS OTHERS

In chapters 69–74 of the first book of the *HL*, Aristides and his trusty foster-father Zosimos are on a theoric voyage (θεωρία) to Pergamum, when a recurrent dream from the god interrupts their journey. Soon afterwards, Zosimos is sent to attend some business at one of his master's estates, and there he falls ill. His illness coincides with Aristides' illness. Despite his own medical troubles, when the god manifests himself, Aristides entreats him to Zosimos' welfare rather than his own. While there is nothing remarkable about a divine epiphany of a healing deity taking place at a moment of crisis, what are noteworthy in chapter 71 are the intensity and the vividness with which Aristides presents his proximity to Asclepius.[29] More significantly, Aristides presents himself as capable of bending Asclepius' will to his own in a scene of triple supplication (unparalleled in Greek literature) in which Aristides engages apparently not for his own sake, but for that of Zosimos:

> φανέντος δὲ τοῦ θεοῦ λαμβάνομαι τῆς κεφαλῆς ἐπαλλὰξ τοῖν χεροῖν, καὶ λαβόμενος ἐδεόμην σῶσαί μοι τὸν Ζώσιμον· ἀνένευσεν ὁ θεός. πάλιν οὖν τὴν αὐτὴν λαβὴν λαβόμενος ἐδεόμην ἐπινεῦσαι. αὖθις ἀνένευσε. τὸ τρίτον παραλαβὼν ἐπειρώμην πεῖσαι ἐπινεῦσαι· ὁ δὲ οὔτε ἀνένευσεν οὔτε ἐπένευσεν, ἀλλ' εἶχε δι' ἴσου τὴν κεφαλὴν καί μοι λέγει ῥήματα ἄττα, ἃ χρὴ λέγειν ἐν τοῖς τοιούτοις, ὡς ἀνύσιμα· ἐγὼ μνημονεύων οὐκ οἶμαι δεῖν ἐκφέρειν εἰκῇ. ἔφη δ' οὖν ὅτι ἐπαρκέσει τούτων λεχθέντων· ἓν δ' ἦν αὐτῶν 'φύλαξον'. τί οὖν ἀπέβη αὐτῷ μετὰ ταῦτα; (72) πρῶτον μὲν ἀνίσταται παρ' ἐλπίδας ἐξ ἐκείνης τῆς νόσου ὁ Ζώσιμος, καθαρθείς γε διὰ πτισάνης καὶ φακῆς, προειπόντος ἐμοὶ τοῦ θεοῦ ὑπὲρ αὐτοῦ, ἔπειτα ἐπεβίω μῆνας τέτταρας·

---

29. Even Behr (*Sacred Tales*, 34 n57), who denies the *HL* and Aristides' communication with Asclepius any real mystic aspect, is forced to admit that chapter 71 in Book 1 "points to something secret." On epiphany in crisis see Pfister, *RE*, s.v. "Epiphanie"; and more recently, Petridou, *Epiphany*, chs. 2 and 3. Platt, (*Facing the Gods*, 260–66) rightly considers the *HL* as "a narrative of epiphanic autopsy."

When the god appeared, I grasped his head with my two hands in turn, and having grasped him, I entreated him to save Zosimos for me. The god refused. Again having grasped him in the same way, I entreated him to assent. Again he refused. For the third time I grasped him and tried to persuade him to assent. He neither refused nor assented, but held his head steady, and told me certain phrases, which are proper to say in such circumstances since they are efficacious. And while I remember these, I do not think that I should reveal them purposelessly. But he said that when these were recited, it would suffice. One of them was: "Save(d)/ Preserve(d)"! What happened to him after this? (72) First of all Zosimos recovered beyond expectation from that disease, being purged with barley gruel and lentils, as the god foretold to me on his behalf, and next he lived four extra months.

The verb *ananeuō* ("to nod negatively") is employed twice in our narrative (ἀνένευσεν . . . αὖθις ἀνένευσε) to describe the twofold negative response of the divine healer, which arguably only makes the god's climactic consent to Aristides' appeal all the more dramatic, and takes the reader back to the heroic world of the Homeric poems, where an abundance of supplication scenes addressed both to mortals and immortals is to be found.[30] This scene carries all the traditional hallmarks of a supplication scene (ritualised request expressed in a way that creates moral obligation on behalf of the person entreated, physical contact between the entreated and the supplicant, etc.), but takes them to an entirely new level. The Mysian orator portrays himself as grasping not the god's knees, hand, beard, or any other bodily part of the person entreated that the supplicant could reach while positioned on a lower level (both literally and symbolically) by either crouching or kneeling. Aristeides, most surprisingly, grasps the god's head. Thus, Aristides the supplicant succeeds in presenting himself as attaining a unique proximity to the healing deity—which ultimately amounts to a kind of equality—whilst concurrently remaining in "a state of utter dependence." Thus, Aristides intensifies the urgency of the appeal, and significantly increases the chances of a favourable outcome.

30. The famous scene of *Iliad* 6 comes to mind, where the priestess Theano lays a fair robe on the knees of the statue of their poliadic goddess and vows luxurious sacrificial offerings in exchange for Diomedes' death. "Thus, she spoke, but Pallas Athena, denied her prayer," ἀνάνευε δὲ Παλλὰς Ἀθήνη (311). Cf. also *Il.* 22.205 and *Od.* 21.129. On supplication in general, see Gould, "*Hiketeia*"; Grotty, *The Poetics of Supplication* and Naiden *Ancient Supplication*. On supplication as a ritual act involving touching and carrying a certain power dynamic, see Kosak, "Healer's Touch." On incubation in Pergamon as supplication and incubants as suppliants, see Philostratus, *Vita Apollonii* 4.11.

What strikes at once is Aristides' pathos-laden description of his clutching the head of Asclepius, first with one hand and then with the other. This intense body language has the resounding pictorial and semantic dynamic of equality between two wrestlers, or even between two lovers rather than the inequality between the two agents involved in an act of supplication: the superior one (the one who grants the request) and the inferior one (the one who entreats). Aristides lays extra emphasis on this extraordinary form of supplication and on being on equal terms with the god by repeating the event in summary fashion in chapter 77 of the same book:

> ὁ δ' ἀπειθήσας ᾤχετο, ἐκ δὲ τούτου ἡ τελευτὴ ἐγένετο αὐτῷ. οὕτως ὅσον τε ἐπεβίω χάρις ἦν τοῦ θεοῦ, ὡς ἀληθῶς φυλάξαντος αὐτόν μοι, καὶ ἐτελεύτα παρὰ τὰ φανθέντα κινηθείς· καὶ τὰ κατ' ἀρχὰς ὑπὸ τοῦ θεοῦ δειχθέντα, ὅτε αὐτοῦ λαβόμενος τῆς κεφαλῆς ἱκέτευον, εἰς τοῦτο ἐτελεύτησε.

> But he disobeyed me and he left, and that became the cause of his death. Thus, whatever additional amount of living he got, it was a gift from the god, who truly kept him for my sake (or through my intervention) and he died because he moved about contrary to my revelations. That was how it ended what in the beginning was revealed to me by the god, when I grasped his head and supplicated him.

Chapters 71 and 72 make one thing obvious: Aristides is reluctant to comply with both the image of the helpless suppliant and, as a matter of fact, the image of the helpless patient. He may be ill and in need of a treatment, but, when he finally acquires the desired remedy from Asclepius, he is both literally and metaphorically on the same level with the god. Notice here the conspicuous position of the prepositional phrase: δι' ἴσου, which could mean that the god did not nod either negatively or positively and held his head stable, but it could also be taken to refer to Asclepius' positioning his head visually on the same level with Aristides' head, perhaps even looking his devotee straight in the eyes. It is at this moment of intense epiphanic activity, reciprocal visual exchange, and physical immediacy that the patient receives the remedy, and simultaneously appropriates the healing powers of his divine healer. Asclepius operates indirectly on Zosimos; the god heals Zosimos, but not on his own. Asclepius heals via the mediation of Aristides, who not only appropriates the god's healing powers—thus becoming a physician of sorts—but also appropriates the divine power and becomes a god of sorts.

To be sure, to engage in incubation for other peoples' illness was common enough.[31] However, what strikes the reader as odd is that all this intense and detailed description of how Aristides found out the way to cure Zosimos is followed by an anti-climax: Aristides withholds the precise wording of the divine diagnosis and prescription (presumably either of pharmaceutical nature, or, most likely, involving advice on regimen),[32] which usually follows the divine manifestation of the healing deity, and reveals nothing but the enigmatic verbal form φύλαξον. This verb could be read as an imperative of *phylattō* meaning "look after him!," "take care of him!," or "preserve him!"; or it could be read as an inaugmented epic aorist—we are after all in a supplication scene with distinctly heroic ambiance—meaning "I took care of him," "I preserved him."[33] The first is a direct order to Aristides to treat Zosimos the same way a physician would have, while the latter is a promise that the god himself has taken matters in his own hands.

Whatever it was that Aristides was told by the god, it turned out to be ἀνύσιμα "effectual" or "efficacious." Surprisingly enough, the divine prescription is revealed only partially, with much caution, and only after much deliberation: ἀγὼ μνημονεύων οὐκ οἴμαι δεῖν ἐκφέρειν εἰκῇ? Remembering the exact words is not a problem. Nonetheless, Aristides is reluctant to give us full access to the medical knowledge transmitted to him. There is an unmistaken air of esoteric knowledge conveyed from the deity to his human intermediary via a sort of supreme esoteric discourse, which is deemed communicable only to the ears of some and not of others.[34] Aristides makes his claims to medical knowledge acquired by means of divine revelation and even leaves a small opening in the curtains for us to peep through and get a glimpse of this divine truth and knowledge: the remedy contained the aforementioned purgation and it was effective. But soon the curtains are

---

31. Cf. the case of Arata from Lakedaimon, who suffered from dropsy (*IG* IV2, 1, nos. 121–22, B21). It was Arata's mother who slept in the temple of the god and dreamt of the god chopping off her daughter's head and successfully treating the disease. Cf. also the so-called Imouthes papyrus *POxy* 1381, which presents many interesting parallels with the *HL*. More on this topic in Hanson "'Dreams and Visions'"; Pearcy "Dream, Theme, and Narrative"; and Holmes "Illegible Body."

32. Cox-Miller, *Dreams in Late Antiquity*, 114; Behr, *Sacred Tales*, 36–40; Horstmanshoff, "Did the God Learn Medicine?," 282.

33. Holmes, "Illegible Body" offers an excellent discussion of the epic overtones of the *HL* as a whole and in particular the ways Aristides adopts for himself the Odyssean ethos and narrative model (a self-conscious narrator who constantly alludes to a multitude of alternative narratives offered by other characters in the story).

34. This is a recurrent motif that underlies the entirety of the *HL* and one I explore more in detail in my forthcoming study on Aristides' *Hieroi Logoi*.

drawn again and the reader is forced to take Aristides' authority on these medical matters for granted.

In chapter 74 of the same book, Zosimos is said to be in debt both to Asclepius for his divine providence and to Aristides himself for his intermediary service (τῷ τε θεῷ χάριν ἔχων τῆς προνοίας καὶ τῆς διακονίας ἐμοί). The term *diakonia*, as it balances precariously between the generic notion of service and that of the specific religious office, keeps Aristides protected against any possible accusations of impiety, whilst simultaneously emphasising the indispensability of his liaison with the divine healer.[35] Zosimos was saved by Asclepius *via* Aristides, who appears here to control and channel the god's healing powers at will. Through the god's divine providence and via Aristides' intermediary Zosimos has earned four extra months of life, while Aristides seems to have acquired some more or less permanent healing powers. It is this act of appropriating Asclepius' healing powers that apparently gives Aristides the right to order his patients around and dictate to them the recommended course of action and regimen. Notice, for example, the emphasis that our text lays on the very cause of Zosimos' eventual death: Zosimos died because he disobeyed Aristides,[36] disregarded his medical advice not to move: ὁ δ' ἀπειθήσας ᾤχετο, ἐκ δὲ τούτου ἡ τελευτὴ ἐγένετο αὐτῷ.[37]

The first book of the *HL* ends with yet another instance of what we called in the introductory section the "divine patronage of therapeutics." Only this time, our Mysian patient is transformed into a physician via what can be described as "an epistolary prescription." Aristides is said here to

35. For διακονία as "service," see Thuc. 1.133 (pl.), Pl. *Res*.371c, Aeschin. 3.13. It can also denote "religious service," "attendance on a religious duty," "ministration," as in Dem. 18.206; *Act.Ap.* 6.1, etc. In Polybius (15.25.21) the same term is used to denote "a body of servants" or "attendants." On *diakonia* and *diakonos* see Blasi, "Office Charisma," 249–50. The term *diakonos* is synonymous, at least in certain contexts, to the term *therapeutēs*, on which see Pleket, "The Social Status of Physicians," 159–61.

36. Extra emphasis is also laid by Galen in his commentary on the Epidemics (see above n. 5) on the subject of the patient's εὐπείθεια "ready obedience," or "compliance" with the doctor's orders. It is precisely this essential quality for a successful patient-physician cooperation that Zosimos is lacking. On the great significance of belief in the therapeutic capacity of a healer and the efficacy of a recommended course of therapy for a healing event to take place both in antiquity and in modern times, see the interdisciplinary study of van Schaik, "It may not cure you."

37. Sosimos' motives for such disobedience are clarified in chapter 75. Sosimos heard about the illness of one of Aristides' favourite servants and against Aristides' stern warnings acted as a medical practitioner on that patient, because as we are explicitly told, Zosimos was also "skilled in the art of medicine" (τὴν τέχνην ἀγαθός τὴν ἰατρικήν). We may be witnessing here a case of layman medicine of the kind that was not uncommon in the second century Roman Empire. More on the topic in Draycott "Lay Medical Theory, Method, and Practice."

have become the recipient of a "Himmelsbrief," a god-sent letter found right in front of the statue of Zeus-Asclepius, which in all likelihood contained the recommended treatment for his beloved nurse Philoumene. Aristides is subsequently dispatched from Pergamum (note the urgency the participle *ekpempsas* conveys) to raise Philoumene, from the bed of sickness. The term *symbolon* is also of interest here. It probably means that Aristides took this epistolary tablet to be a token, a sign from the god that prompted him to immediate action. Once again, our Mysian patient takes his cue from the divine physician and becomes himself a most effective healer.

> (78) τὴν τοίνυν τροφὸν τὴν ἀρχαίαν, ἧς οὐδέν μοι φίλτερον—Φιλουμένη ἦν ὄνομα αὐτῇ—μυριάκις μὲν ἔσωσε παρ' ἐλπίδας, κειμένην δέ ποτε ἀνέστησεν ἐκπέμψας ἐμὲ ἀπὸ Περγάμου, προειπὼν ὅτι καὶ τὴν τροφὸν ἐλαφροτέραν ποιήσοιμι. καὶ ἅμα λαμβάνω τινὰ ἐπιστολὴν πρὸ ποδῶν κειμένην τοῦ Διὸς Ἀσκληπιοῦ, σύμβολον ποιούμενος· εὗρον οὖν μόνον οὐ διαρρήδην ἕκαστα ἐγγεγραμμένα. ὥστε ἐξήειν ὑπερχαίρων καὶ καταλαμβάνω τὴν τροφὸν τοσοῦτον ἀντέχουσαν ὅσον αἰσθέσθαι προσιόντος. ὡς δ' ᾔσθετο, ἀνέκραγε τε καὶ ἀνειστήκει οὐκ εἰς μακράν.

> My old nurse, named Philoumene—none was dearer to me than her—whom he saved myriad times and beyond my expectations, was once lying ill in bed, and he restored her to health after having dispensed me from Pergamum by foretelling that I would relieve my nurse. And at that point, I found a letter lying before my feet in the Temple of Zeus Asclepius, and made it a sign. For not only did I discover every single thing written in it, but they everything was written explicitly too. So I departed overjoyed, and I found my nurse with only enough strength left in her to perceive my arrival. And as soon as she sensed my presence, she cried out and got up not too long afterwards.

Behr and others have interpreted this epistolary prescription as a feature of Aristides' dream, not a material object that Aristides actually picks up, but it does not have to be so.[38] These "Himmelsbriefe" are closely associated with both oracular and healing cults and feature prominently both in literary sources and inscriptions, especially those relating the foundation of a new healing cult.[39] These inscriptions are of great interest to the LAR research

---

38. Behr, *Sacred Tales*, 194; and *Collected Works*, 428 n103.

39. More examples in Sokolowski "Propagation" and Busine "The Discovery of Inscriptions." However, one must not forget that Himmerlsbriefe were also a standard feature of Hellenistic and Imperial aretalogies, and the *hieroi logoi* has long been recognised as a narrative with a distinct aretalogical flavour to it. On Himmelsbriefe as a typical element of Hellenistic aretalogies see Chaniotis, *Historie und der Historiker*, 68–69.

programme, because they legitimise the individual's claims to religious knowledge and power and thus allow for either perpetuation of pre-existing power-structures or the establishing of new socio-economic hierarchies via intense contestation of the old ones. By presenting himself as being in possession of one these divine epistolary inscriptions, Aristides bypasses the intermediary services of both temple physicians and dream-interpreters and makes claims to both divine omnipotence and medical expertise.[40]

The materiality of these god-sent epistolary remedies is their most prized feature: they connect the oneiric world of the dreamer with the hard facts of the illness and the need for therapy. Out of the many examples, the story Pausanias (10.38.13) reports about Asclepius appearing in a dream to the poetess Anyte and handing to her written tablets that contained the prescribed remedy for the treatment of a blind man named Phalysios is perhaps the one that forms the closest parallel to our case.[41] Anyte woke up from her dream vision only to find the same epistolary prescription she had dreamt of in her hands. The blind man opened the tablets and read them and this is how his vision was restored.

It is worth noticing that Pausanias found the story in the archive of inscribed miraculous healing narratives contained in the sanctuary of Epidaurus. Perhaps Aristides was inspired by analogous inscribed *ex-votos* in the temple of the god in Pergamum, but my main point is that we need not suppose that the letter which contained the remedy for his beloved nurse was part of his dream rather than a physical object Aristides brought with him to his meeting with Philoumene.

The narrative that contains Philoumene's treatment comes as further elaboration on the theme of Aristides operating as Asclepius' intercessor and acting as a physician himself. If one compares it to the ekphrastic description of Zosimos' salvation, Philoumene's case might seem less elaborate, but it is equally explicit and certainly telling of how our distinguished patient once again appropriated the divine healer's powers, became himself the doctor and saved his nurse.

Other cases of Aristides' appropriating the god's healing powers and acting as physician himself are reported in more or less summary fashion.

---

40. Often referred to as ὀνειροπόλοι or ὀνειροκρίται. These *oneirokritai* operated in the temples of other healing deities, where incubation was practised. Cf., for instance, *I.Delos* 2071, 2072, 2073, 2105, 2110, 2120, 2151, and 2619.

41. Asclepius' oneiric epiphany to Anyte is a typical example of what E. R. Dodds calls a "rapport epiphany": i.e. the deity appears to the perceiver, who after the revelation is left with a token, a visible mémoire of the divine visitation. See Dodds, *Greeks and the Irrational*, 102ff. For a more recent discussion of Asclepius' epiphany to Anyte, see Platt, *Facing the Gods*, 290–92; and Petridou, *Epiphany*, ch. 3.

In one of them Aristides dreams of being a priest at the temple of Asclepius and cures his limping friend by prescribing "rest" (1.15);[42] while a lengthy narrative from the third book of the *HL* takes the notion of "healing" to an entirely new level, and presents Aristides as saving the entire city of Smyrna and its citizens from an earthquake (3.38–43). The terminology used to describe the healing event is almost a word-for-word repetition of the description of the way Sosimos was healed by the gods' providence and power and Aristides' essential intermediary service: προνοίᾳ μὲν καὶ δυνάμει τῶν θεῶν, διακονίᾳ δ' ἡμῶν ἀναγκαίᾳ. Finally, in another excerpt (4.10) from the fourth book of the *HL*, upon his return to his ancestral estates Aristides is treated like the living embodiment of a healing deity the mere sight of whom is capable of restoring strength and vitality to his beloved old nurse.

APPROPRIATING THE POWERS OF THE MORTAL PHYSICIANS: ARISTIDES HEALS HIMSELF

Indeed, the entirety of the *HL* is interspersed with analogous instances, where Aristides presents himself as well-versed in medical matters and actively involved not only in the relief or recovery of others, but also in his own relief or recovery. As with the cases discussed above, some of these self-healing narratives are presented in a more synoptic way and others are more elaborate. For example, sandwiched between the two cases of Aristides' operating as a healer on both Zosimos and Philoumene lies a parenthetic narrative (1.74), which relates yet another instance of Aristides' appropriation of Asclepius' healing powers: this time, our distinguished patient-turned-physician dismisses the doctor's hesitation to give him an enema and persuades him to proceed with it regardless. In 3.20, on the other hand, Aristides refuses to follow the doctor's prescription to take some nourishment and instead decides to cure his high fever, convulsion and splitting headache by self-medicating intensive meditative contemplation of the statue of Zeus.

These brief references to Aristides' abilities for self-healing can be coupled with a number of more extensive passages where Aristides makes use of the same medical terminology as contemporary medical authors, and more interestingly, the same techniques of performative exhibition of his medical expertise. Chapters 49–50 of the fifth book of the *HL* provide an apt illustration of Aristides' self-healing abilities. They relate an oneiric

---

42. δεκάτῃ δ' ὑστέρᾳ ἐδόκουν ἐσθῆτα ἔχειν ἱερέως καὶ αὐτὸν παρόντα ὁρᾶν τὸν ἱερέα· ἐδόκουν δὲ καὶ τῶν ἐπιτηδείων τινὰ ὑποχωλεύοντα ἰδὼν ἐκ τῶν περὶ τὴν ἕδραν φάναι πρὸς αὐτὸν ὅτι ταῦτα ἡσυχίᾳ θεραπεύοι.

therapy that cured Aristides from being immobile in the autumn of 170 CE. Aristides dreams of a meeting with not one but two doctors, who recite a remedy attributed to Hippocrates. The prescription involves strenuous running followed by jumping in the cold sea:

ὅσον δὲ κἂν τούτῳ συνέβη καμεῖν ἡμέρας τινάς, θαυμαστῶς ὡς ὁ θεὸς καὶ ἅμα εἰωθότως ἰάσατο. βορέας μὲν γὰρ ὀπωρινὸς ἦν, εἶχον δὲ ἀδυνάτως κινεῖσθαι, ὥστε καὶ τὰς ἀναστάσεις ὤκνουν· ὁ δ' ἐπιτάττει. βέλτιον δ' ἴσως αὐτὸ τὸ ὄναρ διηγήσασθαι, καὶ γὰρ ἔναυλόν τέ ἐστι καὶ οὐκ ἀνάγκη παραλιπεῖν. ἠκέτην ἰατρὼ δύο καὶ διελεγέσθην ἐν τῷ προθύρῳ ἄλλα τέ μοι δοκεῖν καὶ περὶ ψυχροῦ λουτροῦ ἠρώτα μὲν ὁ ἕτερος, ὁ δ' ἀπεκρίνετο, τί λέγει, ἔφη, Ἱπποκράτης; τί δ' ἄλλο γε ἢ δραμόντα δέκα σταδίους ἐπὶ θάλατταν οὕτως ῥῖψαι; Ταῦτα μὲν δὴ ὡς ὄναρ πεφάνθαι ἐδόκουν. μετὰ δὲ τοῦτο ἐπελθεῖν ὡς ἀληθῶς αὐτοὺς τοὺς ἰατρούς, θαυμάσαι τε δὴ τοῦ ἐνυπνίου τὴν ἀκρίβειαν καὶ πρὸς αὐτοὺς εἰπεῖν, ἄρτι γε ὑμᾶς ἐδόκουν ὁρᾶν καὶ ἄρτι ἥκετε, καὶ δῆτα ὁπότερος μὲν ὑμῶν, ἔφην, ὁ ἐρωτῶν ἦν καὶ ὁπότερος ὁ ἀποκρινόμενος οὐκ ἔχω λέγειν· ἡ δ' ἀπόκρισις οὕτως εἶχεν, ὡς ἄρα Ἱπποκράτης κελεύοι δέκα σταδίους θεῖν τὸν μέλλοντα λοῦσθαι ψυχρῷ. ἅμα δὲ ἐμαυτῷ μετέβαλον τὸ ἐπὶ θάλατταν, ὡς δηλοῦν τὸ κατὰ φύσιν τῷ ποταμῷ, καὶ οὕτως εἶπον, δέκα σταδίους θεῖν τῷ ποταμῷ συμπαραθέοντα. ἐνεθυμήθην δ' αὐτὸ διὰ τὸ εἶναι ἐν μεσογείᾳ, ἐδόκει σαφὲς εἶναι καὶ χρῆναι οὕτω ποιεῖν.

In so far as even in this time I happened to fall ill for some days, the god cured me most wondrously and in his usual way. (49) For there was an autumnal north wind, and I was unable to move, so that I even hesitated to get up. But he ordered it. Perhaps it is better to narrate the dream itself, for it is still ringing in my ears and there is no need to omit it. "Two doctors came and at the doorway, among other things, discussed, I believe, a cold bath. One asked the question, and the other answered. "What does Hippocrates say?", he said. "What else, but to run ten stades to the sea and then jump in?" I dreamed that these things had appeared in my dream. (50) After this, the doctors themselves, in fact came in, and I marvelled at the precision of the dream, and said to them, "Just now I dreamed that I saw you and just now you have come. Indeed, which one of you," I said, "was the one who inquired and which one who answered, I cannot say. But the answer was as follows: "That Hippocrates ordered one who intended to take a cold bath, to run ten stades." At the same time I changed in my own interest the phrase "to the sea," as if I were making clear the descent to the river. And so I said, "to run ten stades, by running parallel to the river." I thought of this because of being inland. It seemed to be clear and to be necessary to do this.[43]

Schröder maintains that there is no mention of treating *opisthotonos* with cold baths in the Hippocratic corpus; hence, he thinks this Hippocratic remedy is a spurious one.[44] He does, however, mention the effects of cold baths as described in the second book of the *Regimen* (*Vict.* II.57 Joly-Byl).[45] However, in the third book of the *Diseases* (*Morb.* III.13.2 Potter) it is stated clearly that one possible treatment of *opisthotonos* includes showers with icy-cold water:

> Ἢν δὲ βούλῃ, καὶ ὧδε ποιέειν· ὕδωρ ὡς πλεῖστον ψυχρὸν καταχέας, ἔπειτα ἱμάτια λεπτὰ καὶ καθαρὰ καὶ θερμὰ ἐπιβάλλειν, πῦρ δὲ τότε μὴ προσφέρειν. Οὕτω χρὴ ποιέειν καὶ τοὺς τετάνους καὶ τοὺς ὀπισθοτόνους.

> If you like, you can also do the following: shower down with much cold water as possible, and then put on thin, clean and warm garments, but do not offer any heat at that point. Thus you must do also when treating cases of convulsive tetanus and *opisthotonos*.

Of course, it is difficult to conclude with any certainty that Aristides had read the exact same text with us, but given the wider philological and philosophical interest these texts held for the literati of the second century AD and Aristides' active engagement in the medical discourse of his time, such a suggestion should not be ruled out either.[46] Indeed, there are other passages in the *HL* which demonstrate clearly that Aristides was an avid reader of medical literature. I have in mind here Aristides' discussion of

---

43. Trans. Behr with emendations.

44. *opisthotonia* or *opisthotonos* is an extremely painful type of tetanic recurvation in which the body is drawn backwards and stiffens. The word and its cognates appear about 20 times in the Galenic corpus. Aristides seemed to have suffered at least once from this disease (3.21 *HL*), perhaps sometime in February of 148 CE.

45. Schröder, (*Heilige Berichte*, 136 n100): "Diese Antwort findet sich nicht in den Schriften des Hippokrates, verständlicherweise, da es sich um einen Traum des Aristides handelt. Doch werden wenigstens die Wirkungen der kalten Bäder bei Hipp. *de vict.* 2, 57, 2 erwähnt." Cf. also Festugière, *Personal Religion*, 94–95; and Behr, *Sacred Tales*, ad loc. None of the aforementioned scholars mentions the passage from the *de morbis*, which was brought to my attention by Oliver Overwien. On the diagnosis of *opisthotonos* in 3.12, see also Gourevitch, *Le Triangle Hippocratique*, 56–58.

46. On the popularity of these texts in the second sophistic see King, "Origins of Medicine."

Anthisthenes' treatise *On the use of wine* (3.33).⁴⁷ At any rate, by quoting a Hippocratic text, Aristides presents himself as well-versed in medical matters, an image that, as seen above, was a highly prized *desideratum* for the author of the *HL*.

The passage has been discussed in detail by Janet Downie in a paper titled "The Therapeutic Dynamic in Aelius Aristides' *Sacred Tales*." In her discussion, Downie lays emphasis on Aristides revisionist attitude towards the actual treatment and the mortal physicians who prescribe them: the patient spends more time narrating his own interpretation of the prescription and which parts of the original were replaced with others he considered as more appropriate; the sea is replaced by the river and the ten *stadia* prescribed running needs to be done parallel to the river bank for reasons only known to Aristides. More importantly, the discussion between the two ordinary physicians is recast in his complex and unique conceptual universe as a dream Asclepius sent long before the two doctors had their actual conversation. What is really significant for our purposes, however, is that by prioritising his own interpretation of the medical prescription itself over the one offered by the two physicians, Aristides draws attention to the central role he plays in his own therapy.⁴⁸ Rather than presenting himself as a submissive patient, Aristides portrays himself as a competent and erudite physician.⁴⁹ It seems that our Mysian patient was keen on appropriating not only the healing powers of the divine physician, but the medical expertise of his earthly physicians too.

The list of such examples could be easily extended, precisely because Aristides attempts to heal himself on several occasions, with that described in chapters 19–23 of the second book of the *HL* being perhaps the most striking. Contrary to the physician Herakleōn's ominous prediction that he would construct *opisthotonos*, and while still warm in his heart from having just experienced Asclepius' epiphany, Aristides' bathes in the ice-cold water of river Meletas, which in his own words felt like the gentle and well-tempered water of a bathing pool (ὥσπερ ἐν κολυμβήθρᾳ καὶ μάλα ἠπίου καὶ κεκραμένου ὕδατος). Bathing in the river Meletas not only did not destroy his physical health, but it seemed to have given his body a healthy pink tone and a sense of lightness.⁵⁰ Throughout the rest of the day and the night

---

47. The title of book is also mentioned by Diogenes Laertius (50.6.18): Περὶ οἴνου χρήσεως ἢ περὶ μέθης ἢ περὶ Κύκλωπος.

48. Cf. here Downie, *Limits of Art*, 89–102.

49. On this episode and Hippocrates as a medical authority in the *HL* and the work of Aristides as a whole, see Horstmanshoff, "Did the God Learn Medicine?"; and King, "Origins of Medicine."

50. On this episode see also Cox Miller, *Dreams in Late Antiquity*, 184–85; and

his body apparently retained this warmth and the kind of perfect balance of elemental qualities, a balance which could not have been achieved by human contrivance.[51] It is this state of perfectly balanced mixture of the four elemental qualities (wetness, dryness, hotness and coldness) in the human body that Galen calls "perfect mixture," εὐκρασία, in his treatise *On the Mixtures*.[52] It is anyone's guess as to whether Aristides had read his Galen or medical treatises of analogous content, but, I think, few would argue against the technical language of his account and the fact that this description is the product of a learned and well-informed patient. This description comes from a patient who hoped to emulate, if not surpass in erudition, the physicians of his time, and thus appropriate a fair share of their powers.

Given all the aforementioned evidence for Aristides' keen interest in medicine and his active involvement in the healing process either via appropriation of the god's healing powers, constant reinterpretation of his advice on regiment or via contestation of the views of his attending physicians, it seems that this new picture of Aristides resembles less and less the typical suppliant of the numerous healing shrines Galen criticizes in his commentary to the Hippocratic *Epidemics*. In fact, this new picture of Aristides resembles more the portrayal of a very different kind of informed patient—a typical product of the second century *paideia*—who trusts in the

---

Brown, *The Making of Late Antiquity* (1974, 54), where Aristides is ironically called "the pink professor." On *kouphotēs* ("lightness") as a medical term commonly attested in contemporary medical authors like Galen, see van Brock, "Recherches sur le vocabulaire médical," 211–12, no. 41.

51. *HL* 2.22–23: καὶ οὔτε τι ξηροτέρου οὔτε ὑγροτέρου τοῦ σώματος ᾐσθόμην, οὐ τῆς θέρμης ἀνῆκεν οὐδέν, οὐ προσεγένετο, οὐδ᾽ αὖ τοιοῦτον ἡ θέρμη ἦν, οἷον ἄν τῳ καὶ ἀπ᾽ ἀνθρωπίνης μηχανῆς ὑπάρξειεν, ἀλλά τις ἦν ἀλέα διηνεκής, δύναμιν φέρουσα ἴσην διὰ παντὸς τοῦ σώματός τε καὶ τοῦ χρωτός. 23 παραπλησίως δὲ καὶ τὰ τῆς γνώμης εἶχεν. οὔτε γὰρ οἷον ἡδονὴ περιφανὴς ἦν οὔτε κατ᾽ ἀνθρωπίνην σωφροσύνην ἔφησθα ἂν εἶναι αὐτό, ἀλλ᾽ ἦν τις ἄρρητος εὐθυμία, πάντα δεύτερα τοῦ παρόντος καιροῦ τιθεμένη, ὥστε οὐδ᾽ ὁρῶν τὰ ἄλλα ἐδόκουν ὁρᾶν· οὕτω πᾶς ἦν πρὸς τῷ θεῷ. "During all the rest of the day and night till bed time, I preserved the condition which I had after the bath, nor did I feel any part of my body to be drier or moister. None of the warmth left me, none was added, nor again was the warmth such as one would have from a human contrivance, but it was a certain continuous body heat, producing the same effect throughout the whole of my body and during the whole time. (23) My mental state was also nearly the same. For there was neither, as it were, conspicuous pleasure, nor would you say that it was like a human joy. But there were a certain inexplicable contentment, which regarded everything as less than the present moment, so that when I saw other things, I seemed not to see them. Thus I was wholly with the God." Trans. Behr with emendations.

52. Cf. for instance, *De Temper.* 37.17–32.4 Helmreich = K. I.558–559 with P. J. van der Eijk, "Galen on the Nature of Human Being." A comparison between the aforementioned passage from Galen's treatise *On the Mixtures*, or *On the Proportions* and the passage from the *HL* quoted above is an issue I would like to revisit on a future occasion.

healing deity only partly; relies exclusively only on his own knowledge of medicine and dialectics and who scrutinizes dietary regimes and regimen as much as he does his attending physicians, both on the basis of medical practice and theory.[53]

SYNOPSIS

This study has offered a close reading of a selection of passages from the *HL*, which cast Aristides, the famous second-century patient, in a new light. Far from being a submissive patient who idly resided in the Pergamene Asclepieion and relied exclusively on the therapeutic powers of divine healers, Aristides is shown here as an informed patient and one who is not only in possession of the basics of the medical discourse but who also functions as a physician of sorts and takes both his own life and the lives of others into his hands. Instead of the traditional scholarly view of Aristides as a passive patient, this paper has argued for a fresh view of our Mysian orator as the active agent in his own healing process. Furthermore, the passages discussed above demonstrate Aristides' attempt to bypass the religious intermediaries of the healing temple, appropriate their religious offices, and claim for himself extra honour (the symbolic capital of the second century elite) as well as direct (unmediated) contact with the divine. More significantly, by appropriating the religious roles of the temple's priestly personnel (priests and dream-interpreters) and the traditional ritual schemata of supplication and incubation, Aristides gets one step closer to his ultimate goal of appropriating Asclepius' healing powers and becoming himself the divine physician. This was by no means unprecedented but, as I have argued, it was never done so artfully and so subtly: by appropriating medical knowledge and expertise, Aristides effectively lays claim to a type of divinity; by becoming a doctor, Aristides becomes a god.

53. On the audience of the treatise, see Nutton, "Patient's Choise," 243–44. The passages discussed above are, in fact, only fragments of a wider emerging picture, which portrays a very different kind of patient mostly to be found amongst the members of the socio-political elite of the second century CE: the patient who values his body and has the time and the knowledge to attend to his physical and physic needs (both proactively and reactively). This patient does not relinquish control over his body and its functions, at least not easily at least, and certainly not before he tests the efficacy of the practitioner of the *technē iatrikē* and his methods. This patient/medical connoisseur and his like are perhaps the intended readers of such contemporary medical treatises on healthcare and healthcare specialists as Plutarch's *de sanitate tuenda praecepta* (ὑγιεινὰ παραγγέλματα), Galen's *de sanitate tuenda*, or his *On Examining the Best Physicians*. More on Galen's treatise *On Hygiene* in Wilkins, "Treatment of the Man"; on Plutarch's *Praecepta*, see Van Hoof "Plutarch's 'Diet-Ethics.'"

BIBLIOGRAPHY

Behr, Charles. A. *Aristides and the Sacred Tales*. Amsterdam: Hakkert, 1968.
———. *P. Aelius Aristides: The Complete Works*. 2 vols. Leiden: Brill, 1981–1986.
Belayche, Nicole. "*Deus deum* . . . *summorum maximus* (Apuleius): Ritual Expressions of Distinction in the Divine World in the Imperial Period." In *One God: Pagan Monotheism in the Roman Empire*, edited by Stephen Mitchell and Peter van Nuffelen, 141–64. Cambridge: Cambridge University Press, 2010.
Blasi, Anthony J. "Office Charisma in Early Christian Ephesus." *Sociology of Religion* 56 (1995) 245–55.
Bremmer, Jan N. "The Agency of Greek and Roman Statues from Homer to Constantine." *Opuscula* 6 (2013) 7–21.
———. *Initiation into the Mysteries of the Ancient World*. Münchner Vorlesungen zu antiken Welten 1. Berlin: de Gruyter, 2014.
Brock, Nadia van. *Recherches sur le vocabulaire médical du grec ancien*. Études et Commentaires 41. Paris: Klincksieck, 1961.
Brown, Peter. *The Making of Late Antiquity*. Cambridge: Harvard University Press, 1978.
Bowersock, Glen. W. *Greek Sophists in the Roman Empire*. Oxford: Clarendon, 1969.
Busine, Aude. "The Discovery of Inscriptions and the Legitimation of New Cults." In *Historical and Religious Memory in the Ancient World*, edited by Beate Dignas and R. R. R. Smith, 241–53. Oxford: Oxford University Press, 2012.
Cagnat, René. et al., eds. *Inscriptiones Graecae ad Res Romans Pertinentes*. Paris: Leroux, 1911.
Chaniotis, Angelos. "Megatheism: The Search for the Almighty God and the Competition of Cults." In *One God: Pagan Monotheism in the Roman Empire*, Stephen Mitchell and Peter van Nuffelen, 112–39. Cambridge: Cambridge University Press, 2010.
Deichgräber, Karl. *Die griechische Empirikerschule: Sammlung der Fragmente und Darstellung der Lehre*. Berlin: Weidmannsche, 1965.
Downie, Janet. *At the Limits of Art: A Literary Study of Aelius Aristides' Hieroi Logoi*. Oxford: Oxford University Press, 2013.
———. "Dream Hermeneutics in Aelius Aristides' Hieroi Logoi." In *Dreams, Healing, and Medicine in Greece: From Antiquity to the Present*, edited by Steven M. Oberhelman, 109–28. Burlington, VT: Ashgate, 2013.
———. "A Pindaric Charioteer: Aelius Aristides and His Divine Literary Editor (*Oration* 50.45)." *Classical Quarterly* 59 (2009) 263–69.
———. "Proper Pleasures: Bathing and Oratory in Aelius Aristides' Hieros Logo I and Oration 33." In *Aelius Aristides between Greece, Rome and the Gods*, edited by W. V. Harris and Brooke Holmes, 117–30. Columbia Studies in the Classical Tradition 33. Leiden: Brill, 2008.
Draycott, Jane. "Literary and Documentary Evidence for Lay Medical Theory, Method, and Practice in the Roman Republic and Empire." In *Homo Patiens: Approaches to the Patient in the Ancient World*, edited by Georgia Petridou and Chiara Thumiger, 432–50. SAM 45. Brill: Leiden, 2016.
Eijk, Philip J. van der. "Galen on the Nature of Human Beings." In *Galen and Philosophy*, edited by P. Adamson and J. Wilberding. London: Bulletin of the Institute of Classical Studies Supplements, forthcoming.

———. "Melancholia and 'Hypochondria'—Steps in the History of a Problematic Combination." In *Miroirs de la mélancolie = Mirrors of Melancholy*, edited by Hélène Cazes and Anne-France Morand, 13–28. Les Collections de la République des Lettres: Symposiums. Paris: Hermann, 2015.

Festugière, André-Jean. *Personal Religion among the Greeks*. Sather Classical Lectures 26. Berkeley: University of California Press, 1954.

Fischer, Klaus-Dietrich. "Galen, Pardalas, and Sundry Delights for the Student of Ancient Greek Medicine." *Galenos* 3 (2009) 161–76.

Frede, Michael. "Galen's Theology." In *Galien et la Philosophie*, edited by Jonathan Barnes and J. Jouanna, 73–130. Entretiens sur l'Antiquité Classique 39. Geneva: Fondation Hardt, 2003.

Fögen, Thorsten. "The Role of Verbal and Non-verbal Communication in Ancient Medical Discourse." In *Latin et langues romanes—Études de linguistique offertes à József Herman à l'occasion de son 80ème anniversaire*, edited by Sándor Kiss, Luca Mondin, and Giampaolo Salvi, 287–300. Tübingen: Niemeyer, 2005.

Gasparini, Valentino. "Isis and Osiris: Demonology vs. Henotheism?" *Numen* 58 (2011) 697–728.

Gordon, Richard L. "Individuality, Selfhood and Power in the Second Century: The Mystagogue as a Mediator of Religious Options." In *Religious Dimensions of the Self in the Second Century CE*, edited by Jörg Rüpke and Greg Woolf, 146–72. Studien und Texte zu Antike und Christentum 76. Tübingen: Mohr/Siebeck, 2013.

Gould, John. "Hiketeia." *Journal of Hellenic Studies* 93 (1973) 74–103.

Gourevitch, Danielle. *Le Triangle Hippocratique dans le Monde Gréco-Romain: Le Malade, sa Maladie et son Médecin*. Bibliothèque des écoles françaises d'Athènes et de Rome 251. Rome: Ecole française de Rome, 1984.

Graf, Fritz. "Heilgtum und Ritual: Das Beispiel der griechisch-römischen Asklepieia." In *Le Sanctuaire Grec*, edited by S. Albert, 159–203. Geneva: Fondation Hardt, 1992.

Grotty, Kevin. *The Poetics of Supplication: Homer's Iliad and Odyssey*. Myth and Poetics Ithaca, NY: Cornell University Press, 1994.

Hanson, John S. "Dreams and Visions in the Graeco-Roman World and Early Christianity." In *Aufstieg und Niedergang der römische Welt* II.23.1 (1980) 1395–427.

Harris, William V. *Dreams and Experience in Classical Antiquity*. Cambridge: Harvard University Press, 2009.

Holmes, Brooke. "Aelius Aristides' Illegible Body." In *Aelius Aristides between Greece, Rome and the Gods*, edited by W. V. Harris and Brooke Holmes, 81–113. Columbia Studies in the Classical Tradition 33. Leiden: Brill, 2008.

Hoof, Lieve van. "Plutarch's 'Diet-Ethics' *Precepts of Healthcare*: Between Diet and Ethics." In *Virtues for the People: Aspects of Plutarchan Ethics*, edited by G. Roskam and L. van der Stockt, 109–29. Leuven: Leuven University Press, 2011.

Horstmanshoff, Manfred H. F. J. "The Ancient Physician: Craftsman or Scientist?" *Journal of the History of Medicine and Allied Sciences* 45 (1990) 176–97.

———. "Did the God Learn Medicine? Asclepius and Temple Medicine in Aelius Aristides' *Sacred Tales*." In *Magic and Rationality in Ancient Near Eastern and Graeco-Roman Medicine*, edited by H. F. J. Horstmanshoff and M. Stol, 325–41. Studies in Ancient Medicine 27. Leiden: Brill, 2004.

Iskandar, Albert Z. "Galen and Rhazes on Examining Physicians." *Bulletin of the History of Medicine* 36 (1962) 362–65.

———. *Galeni De optimo medico cognoscendo libelli versio Arabica.* Corpus Medicorum Graecorum Supplementum Orientale IV. Berlin: Akademie, 1988.
Johnson, Luke Timothy. *Among the Gentiles: Greco-Roman Religion and Christianity.* Anchor Bible Reference Library. New Haven: Yale University Press, 2009.
King, Helen. "Chronic Pain and the Creation of Narrative." In *Constructions of the Classical Body*, edited by James I. Porter, 269–86. Ann Arbor: University of Michigan Press, 1999.
———. "The Origins of Medicine in the Second Century AD." In *Rethinking Revolutions through Ancient Greece*, edited by Simon Goldhill and Robin Osborne, 246–63. Cambridge: Cambridge University Press, 2006.
Kouke, Elisavet. Ἱεροὶ Λόγοι: Σώμα καὶ γλῶσσα στα ὄνειρα ενός ῥήτορα. Athens: Smile, 2012.
Kosak, Jennifer. "Interpretations of the Healer's Touch in the Hippocratic Corpus." In *Homo Patiens: Approaches to the Patient in the Ancient World*, edited by Georgia Petridou and Chiara Thumiger. SAM 45. Leiden, Brill, 2016.
Kudlien, Fridolf. "Galen's Religious Belief." In *Galen: Problems and Prospects*, edited by Vivian Nutton, 117–30. London: Wellcome Institute for the History of Medicine, 1981.
———. *Die Stellung des Arztes in der römischen Gesellschaft: Freigeborene Römer, Eingebürgerte, Peregrine, Sklaven, Freigelassene als Ärzte.* Forschungen zur antiken Sklaverei 18. Stuttgart: Steiner, 1986.
Lendon, Jon. E. *Empire of Honour: The Art of Government in the Roman World.* Oxford: Clarendon, 1997.
Leven, Karl-Heinz. "'At Times These Ancient Facts Seem to Lie before Me Like a Patient on a Hospital Bed'—Retrospective Diagnosis and Ancient Medical History." In *Magic and Rationality in Ancient Near Eastern and Graeco-Roman Medicine*, edited by H. F. J. Horstmanshoff and M. Stol, 269–84. Leiden: Brill, 2004.
———. "Hypochonder." In *Antike Medizin: Ein Lexikon*, edited by Karl-Heinz Leven, 448. Munich: Beck, 2005.
Markschies, Christoph. "*Heis Theos*—Ein Gott? Der Monotheismus und das antike Christentum." In *Polytheismus und Monotheismus in den Religionen des Vorderen Orients*, edited by M. Krebernik und J. van Oorschot, 209–34. AOAT 298. Münster: Ugarit-Verlag, 2002.
———. "*Heis Theos*? Religionsgeschichte und Christentum bei Erik Peterson." In *Vom Ende der Zeit: Geschichtstheologie und Eschatologie bei Erik Peterson. Symposium Mainz*, edited by Barbara Nichtweiss, 38–74. Religion-Geschichte-Gesellschaft 16. Münster: LIT Verlag, 2001.
Mattern, Susan P. *Galen and the Rhetoric of Healing.* Baltimore: Johns Hopkins University Press, 2008.
———. "Physicians and the Roman Imperial Aristocracy: The Patronage of Therapeutics." *Bulletin of the History of Medicine* 73 (1999) 1–18.
Miller, Patricia Cox. *Dreams in Late Antiquity: Studies in the Imagination of a Culture.* Princeton: Princeton University Press 1994.
Naiden, F. S. *Ancient Supplication.* Oxford: Oxford University Press, 2006.
———. "*Hiketai* and *Theoroi* at Epidaurus." In *Pilgrimage in Graeco-Roman and Early Christian Antiquity: Seeing the Gods*, edited by Jaś Elsner and Ian Rutherford, 73–96. Oxford: Oxford University Press, 2005.

Nutton, V. "Healers in the Medical Market Place: Towards a Social History of Graeco-Roman Medicine." In *Medicine in Society: Historical Essays*, edited by Andrew Wear, 15–58. Cambridge: Cambridge University Press, 1992.

———. "The Medical Meeting Place." In *Ancient Medicine in Its Socio-Cultural Context*, edited by Philip J. van der Eijk et al., 1:3–25. Amsterdam: Rodopi, 1995.

———. "The Patient's Choice: A New Treatise by Galen." *Classical Quarterly* 40 (1990) 236–57.

Obermann, Steven M. *Dreams, Healing, and Medicine in Greece: From Antiquity to the Present*. Burlington, VT: Ashgate, 2013.

———. "Dreams in Greco-Roman Medicine." In *Aufstieg und Niedergang der römischen Welt* II.37.1 (1993) 121–56.

Parker, Robert. "Theophoric Names and the History of Greek Religion." In *Greek Personal Names and Their Value as Evidence*, edited by Simon Hornblower and Elaine Matthews, 53–80. Proceedings of the British Academy 104. Oxford: Oxford University Press, 2000.

Pearcy, Lee. T. "Dream, Theme, and Narrative: Reading the Sacred Tales of Aelius Aristides." *Transactions of the American Philological Association* 118 (1988) 377–91.

Perkins, Judith. "The Self as Sufferer." *Harvard Theological Review* (1992) 245–272.

———. *The Suffering Self: Pain and Narrative Representation in the Early Christian Era*. London: Routledge, 1995.

Pernot, Laurent. "Periautologia: Problèmes et méthodes de l'éloge de soi-même dans la tradition éthique et rhétorique gréco-romaine." *RÉG* 111 (1998) 101–24.

———. "The Rhetoric of Religion." *Rhetorica* 24 (2006) 235–54.

Petridou, Georgia. "Contesting religious and medical expertise: The therapeutai of Pergamum as religious and medical entrepreneurs." In *Beyond Priesthood. Religious Entrepreneurs and Innovators in the Roman Empire*, edited by Richard Gordon, Georgia Petridou and Jörg Rüpke, 145–166. Berlin: DeGruyter, 2017.

Petridou, Georgia. *Divine Epiphany in Greek Literature and Culture*. Oxford: Oxford University Press, 2015.

Petridou, Georgia, and Chiara Thumiger, eds. *Homo Patiens: Approaches to the Patient in the Ancient World*. SAM 45. Leiden: Brill, 2016.

Petsalis-Diomides, Alexia. "Sacred Writing, Sacred Reading: The Function of Aelius Aristides' Self-Presentation as Author in the Sacred Tales." In *The Limits of Ancient Biography*, edited by Brian McGing and Judith Mossman, 351–94. Swansea: Classical Press of Wales, 2006.

———. *Truly Beyond Wonders. Aelius Aristides and the Cult of Asklepios*. Oxford: Oxford University Press.

Phillips, E. D. "A Hypochondriac and His God." *Greece & Rome* 61 (1952) 23–36.

Pietrobelli, Antoine. "Galien Agnostique: Un Texte Caviardé Par La Tradition." *Revue des études grecques* 126 (2013) 103–35.

Platt, Verity. *Facing the Gods: Epiphany and Representation in Graeco-Roman Art, Literature and Religion*. Greek Culture in the Roman World. Cambridge: Cambridge University Press, 2011.

Pleket, H. W. "The Social Status of Physicians in the Graeco-Roman World." In *Ancient Medicine in Its Socio-Cultural Context*, edited by Ph. J. van der Eijk et al., 1:27–34. Wellcome Insttitute Series in the History of Medicine. Amsterdam: Rodopi, 1995.

Rüpke, Jörg. *The Individual in the Religions of the Ancient Mediterranean*. Oxford: Oxford University Press, 2013.

———. "Lived Ancient Religion: Questioning 'Cults' and 'Polis Religion.'" *Mythos* 5 (2012) 191–204.

Schaik, Katherine van. "It May not Cure You, It May not Save Your Life, but It Will Help You." In *Homo Patiens: Approaches to the Patient in the Ancient World*, edited by Georgia Petridou and Chiara Thumiger, 471–95. SAM 45. Leiden: Brill, 2016.

Schmitz, Thomas A. *Bildung und Macht: Zur sozialen und politischen Funktion der zweiten Sophistik in der griechischen Welt der Kaiserzeit*. Zetemata 97. Munich: Beck, 1997.

Schröder, Heinrich Otto. *Heilige Berichte: Einleitung, deutsche Übersetzung und Kommentar*. Wissenschaftliche Kommentare zu griechischen und lateinischen Schriftstellern. Heidelberg: Winter, 1986.

Sokolowski, Franciszek. "Propagation of the Cult of Sarapis and Isis in Greece." *Greek, Roman and Byzantine Studies* 15 (1974) 441–48.

Staden, Heinrich von. "Galen and the Second Sophistic." *Bulletin of the Institute of Classical Studies* 41 (1997) 33–35.

Steiner, Deborah Tarn. *Images in Mind: Statues in Archaic and Classical Greek Literature and Thought*. Princeton: Princeton University Press, 2001.

Straten, Folker T. van. "Daikrates' Dream: A Votive Relief from Kos and Some Other Kat'Onar Dedications." *Bulletin Antieke Beschaving* 51 (1976) 1–38.

Versnel, Henk S. *Inconsistencies in Greek and Roman Religion*. Vol. 1, *Ter Unus: Isis, Dionysos, Hermes: Three Studies in Henotheism*. Studies in Greek and Roman Religion 6. Leiden: Brill, 1990.

Wilkins, John M. "Treatment of the Man: Galen's Preventive Medicine in the *De Sanitate Tuenda*." In *Homo Patiens: Approaches to the Patient in the Ancient World*, edited by Georgia Petridou and Chiara Thumiger, 413–31. SAM 45. Leiden: Brill, 2016.

15

Interior Views of a Patient
Illness and Rhetoric in "Autobiographical" Texts (L. Annaeus Seneca, Marcus Cornelius Fronto and the Apostle Paul)

—Annette Weissenrieder

Ὑγίαινε—LITERALLY: "BE HEALTHY!" IS a fixed formal element that became firmly established as a kind of *formula valetudinis* at the start and/or end of ancient letters. Heikki Koskenniemi investigated this conventional phraseology in Greek papyrus letters and noted that the words of greeting "clearly referred to the correspondents' well-being and health" in their expression of care and sympathy.[1] As a two-part formula, (εἰ ἔρρωσαι or ὑγιαίνεις, εὖ ἂ ἔχοι, καὶ αὐτὸς δ' ὑγίαινον), it is usually located after the prologue. It corresponds to the Latin *si valens, bene est, ego valeo*.[2] It is used both in personal letters and in business letters, where it is preceded by a mention of the ruler's well-being. Cicero uses an expanded formula, especially in the tearful letters written to his wife, daughter and his friend Atticus, when he writes: *Cura ut valeas et ita tibi persuadeas, mihi te carius nihil esse nec umquam fuisse*.[3] In

---

1. Koskenniemi, *Studien zur Idee und Phraseologie des griechischen Briefes*, 128. See for the following Weissenrieder, "Innenansichten eines Kranken."

2. Epicurus Fragment 176; on the royal letters, see Wellers RC 56, 58, 59, 61, 71 and 72; on the Latin version, see, for instance, Plautus *Persa* 502 (*si valetis, gaudeo. Ego valeo recte et rem gero et facio lucrum*) and Seneca *Epist.* 15.

3. "Take care of your health, and rest in the knowledge that nothing in the world is

addition to the direct addressee, writers also asked about the well-being of children and close relatives: καὶ ἡ θυγάτηρ σου καὶ τὰ παιδία [αὐτῆς].[4] Most of the letters, in addition to the formula at the start of the letter, also include a closing clause that exhorts the recipient to take care of his health: σεαυτοῦ (or τοῦ σώματος) ἐπιμέλου, ἵν᾿ ὑγιαίνῃς or the variation καλῶς ποιήσεις, εὐχαριστήσεις μοι or χαιριεῖ, χαρίζοιο—corresponding to the Latin *cura ut valeas*. Still, the addressee's health was not only discussed in these formulaic terms. In particular, the letters of the Imperial era provide detailed descriptions of illnesses.[5] Of course a certain amount of caution is required when reading the letters as forms of autobiographical writing, since the category of autobiography was unknown in ancient literary theory.[6] Modern terms

more important to me, or ever was, than you." Cicero XIV.3, Letter 9.

4. For instance in P. Flind. Petr. II 2.4; similarly, P. Tebt. III 948.4f. and P. Mich. Zen 55; P. Cairo Zen. III 59365.

5. It is difficult to concisely describe the importance of physical handicaps or disabilities in the ancient world, which is why I prefer to speak rather of illness instead of disability in the following. Scholars refer again and again to ancient medicine's lack of interest in disabilities. For instance, Bien [*Entstehung von Mißbildungen im physiologischen und medizinischen Schrifttum der Antike*, 16] states that there was no work in all of antiquity that exclusively dealt with deformities (some interpretations believe *De morbo sacro* in the Corpus Hippocraticum and Galen's *Puero Epileptico Cons.* to be exceptions). The definition of a handicap, however, is not merely based on the elaborations of medicine, but assumes a societal debate that did not exist in antiquity. Particularly in recent research, which focuses on "intersectionality," authors like Heike Raab have pointed out that handicaps not only affect medicine, but that a "multidimensional concept of disability" must be used as a basis, taking economic, legal and subjectivizing procedures into account as well as gender and sexuality. Showing this multidimensionality of disability does not seem to be possible for the present source material. See: http://www.zedis.uni-hamburg.de/wp-content/uploads/2007/01/intersectionality_raab.pdf

Another aspect may be that medicine's focus was aimed at preserving "normal" functionality. For instance, Garland [*The Eye of the Beholder. Deformity and Disablity in the Graeco-Roman World*, 123] writes: "The lack of interest, or at least lack of debate, was partly no doubt due to the fact that such conditions were incorrigible and partly to the fact that the majority of persons exhibiting these abnormalities would not have survived infancy." If one wanted to refer to physical deformities, the terms most commonly used were τέρας (miraculous sign) and the verbs πηρόω (to disfigure) and κωλύω (to hinder). It is also noteworthy that ancient medicine was more familiar with the state of being ill than with the illness itself. The terms νόσος, νόσημα and νοσεῖν, for example, are noticeably absent in Galen's writings. Instead, he refers to the affected body part. This may be due to a concept of nature that believes in nature's workmanship and sees illness merely as an unnatural condition (Galen *Die Inaeq. Intemper.* 5; VII 743 Kühn; *MM* X 41. 50f. 59.71 Kühn), but does not question nature's workmanship as such.

6. See also the arguments of Misch, *Geschichte der Autobiographie* Vol. 1.1, who, however, only mentions the concept in the title (see pages 3–21); also Bompaire, "Quatre styles d'autobiographie au IIe siècle après J.-C."; Aelius Aristide, Lucien, Marc-Aurèle, Galien," 199–209; the contribution by Petridou in this volume; Reardon,

like "self-awareness" and the "individual" are not necessarily compatible with the ancient understanding of the self. Instead, we can read the letters as a biography written by a first-person narrator.[7]

In the following I would like to sketch out three striking examples of ancient correspondence in which the authors' depictions of illness play an important role in understanding the respective letters. It can be seen that the depiction of illness varies according to the choice of literary genre: the letters range from reports to an individual person—the friendship letter—to the stylization and functionalization in the genre of the teaching letter to the genre of the tearful letter. What they all have in common is that the senders describe the illnesses from the perspective of the person who is affected; however, despite their clearly high level of education, they largely avoid using any specialized terminology. Instead, they simply describe and rhetorically reflect on the condition, which in some cases is life-threatening, using generally comprehensible terms.

L. ANNAEUS SENECA: SELF-REPRESENTATION IN ILLNESS AS EXISTENTIAL COMMUNICATION[8]

The following excerpt from the 54th letter of L. Annaeus Seneca to Lucilius clearly belongs to the genre of the teaching letter,[9] and pertains to the

---

"L'autobiographie à l'époche de la Seconde Sophistique: quelques conclusions," 279–84; Momigliano, *The Development of Greek Biography*, especially 23–42; Whitmarsh, *The Second Sophistic. Greece & Rome*, especially Ch. V. An overview of the imperial-era biography debate is found in Lewis, "Imperial Autobiography. Augustus to Hadrian," 629–706. See also the introduction by Niggl in *Die Autobiographie. Zu Form und Geschichte einer literarischen Gattung*.

Particularly worth mentioning are the *Confessiones* of Augustine and the *Carmen de vita sua* by Gregory of Nazianzus. Both use medical metaphors; however, illness plays a central role in the *Carmen*. Ultimately, it is illness that allows Gregory to withdraw from the office of bishop, which he hates; he writes that illness has saved him from the responsibility of acting as a "physician for suffering," while he himself is "overfull of illnesses" (see *Carmen* 883–885; 1336ff.; 1442; 1745; 1819–1821 passim). Unfortunately, there is no room in the context of this essay to go into further detail on this; however, see the further commentary by Jungck, *Gregor von Nazianz. De Vita Sua*.

7. See more extensively Goodwin, *Autobiography*, particularly extensive in the "Introduction."

8. This sub-heading is based on Cancik, *Untersuchungen zu Senecas Epistulae morales*, 89.

9. See: Cancik, *Untersuchungen zu Senecas Epistulae morales*, 75–89, Mazzoli, "Le 'epistulae Morales ad Lucilium' di Seneca. Valore letterario e filosofico," 1823–77; and Cugusi, *Evoluzione de Forme dell'Epistolografia Latina*, 196–206.

context of the sixth book of the collection, which is dedicated to the "good thought"[10]—a formula that is also used within the 54th letter.

> My ill-health had allowed me a long furlough, when suddenly it resumed the attack. "What kind of ill-health?" you say. And you surely have a right to ask; for it is true that no kind is unknown to me. But I have been consigned, so to speak, to one special ailment. I do not know why I should call it by its Greek name; for it is well enough described as 'shortness of breath.' Its attack is of very brief duration, like that of a squall at sea; it usually ends within an hour; . . . I have passed through all the ills and dangers of the flesh; but nothing seems to me more troublesome than this. And naturally so; for anything else may be called illness; but this is a sort of continued "last gasp." Hence physicians call it "practising how to die."

Seneca continues:

> Yet in the midst of my difficult breathing I never ceased to rest secure in cheerful and brave thoughts . . . I have never ceased to encourage myself with cheering counsels of this kind . . . then little by little this shortness of breath, already reduced to a sort of panting, came on at greater intervals, and then slowed down and finally stopped. Even by this time, although the gasping has ceased, the breath does not come and go normally; I still feel a sort of hesitation and delay in breathing.[11]

Even early medical writings document shortness of breath, or "asthma" (Papyri Ebers, approx. 1550 BCE), and this is also described in the

---

10. This is performed in the "final letter" 62: *mentiuntur qui sibi obstare ad studia liberalia turbam negotiorum videri volunt: simulant occupationes et augent et ipsi se occupant. Vaco, Lucili, vaco et ubicumque sum, ibi meus sum. Rebus enim me non trado, sed commodo, nec consector perdendi temporis causas; et quocumque constiti loco, ibi cogitationes meas tracto et aliquid in animo salutare converso.*

11. Seneca, *Moral Letters to Lucilius*, trans. Richard Mott Gummere, Loeb Classical Library, 1917, Vol. 1. *Londum mihi commeatum dederat mala valetudo; repente me inasit. 'Quo genere?' inquis. Prorsus merito interrogas: adeo nullum mihi ignotum est. Unit amen morbo quasi adsignatus sum, quem quare Graeco nomine appellem nescio; satis enim apte dici suspirium potest. Brevis autem valde et procellae similis est impetus; intra horam fere desinit; . . . Omnia corporis aut incommoda aut pericula per me transierunt: nullum mihi videtur molestius. Quidni? aliud enim quidquid est aegrotare est, hoc animam egerere. Itaque medici hanc 'meditationem mortis' vocant; . . . Ego vero et in ipsa suffocatione non desii cogitationibus laetis ac fortibus adquiescere . . . His et euismodi exhortationibus . . . adloqui me non desii; deinde paulatim suspirium illud, quod esse iam anhelitus coeperat, intervalla maiora fecit et retardatum est. At remansit, nec adhuc, quamvis desierit, ex natura fluit spiritus; sentio haesitationem quandam eius et moram.*

Corpus Hippocraticum and other medical corpuses. It was probably Aretaeus of Cappadocia who first classified asthma as an illness.[12] With the word *suffocatio*, Seneca refers to the state of suffocation that is often used as a *terminus technicus* in the literature but does not appear in medical texts.[13] However, Seneca's use of the genera verbi is noteworthy: passive verbs and dative or accusative personal pronouns (*per me transierunt, nullum mihi . . . molestius*) indicate that the author is subjected to the illness, and that his influence over its course is fairly limited. Such indications are further supported when we consider that he also names an anonymous crowd of doctors (*medici*) who care for him, rather than *his doctors*, as will be the case in Fronto. Naturally, that makes the switch to the first person (*ego*) within this section even more noteworthy. With this, Seneca completes the shift from his physical description to his mental strategy, that of "good thoughts." Consequently, Seneca also moves from a description of his physical condition to the kind of stylistically confident teaching letter that characterizes the Stoic. Among other things, this is indicated by the term *meditatio mortis*:[14] even if the author is marked by the illness and severely tested by it, he is still superior to it. Accordingly, he does not make any third-person statements in the methodological/philosophical sections, but rather self-assessments. Of course, these self-assessments are also—and particularly—a literary manifestation, a philosophical lesson about philosophizing as an "existential communication,"[15] and therefore they point to the wise man. Thus illness is not the patient's fault; instead, it acts as a sort of test of strength, a kind of self-education, and health is therefore the προηγμένον: the preferred state, but not good in and of itself. Living and suffering with one another is a form of philosophizing with one another.

This idea of the health and illness metaphor can be further expanded when we analyze Seneca's arguments in the *Epistulae morales* 114, where he combines anthropological, ethical and critical stylistic aspects. Here the text states, "The [human] properties of intellect and soul[16] have the same charac-

12. See more extensively Costa, *Seneca. 17 Letters with translation and commentary*, 170.

13. Only in Pliny are there two passages where the term refers to the ancient form of hysteria; see Plin. *NH* 20.30; 26.158.

14. The formulas *meditatio mortis* and *meditare mortem* are used frequently in Seneca. See, for instance, 4.5; 12.9; 26.7–9; 30.4 and 12; 36.8; 49.9–12: 61.4; 69.6; 70.2; 120.14; see also *Nat.Quest.* VI 32.8–9; *Brev.Vit.*VII 3. See also Cancik, *Untersuchungen zu Senecas Epistulae morales*, 109–12; Leeman, "Das Todeserlebnis im Denken Senecas," 322–33 (on page 333 with reference to the letter discussed here).

15. Cancik, *Untersuchungen zu Senecas Epistulae morales*, 91.

16. Seneca often uses *animus* in direct contrast to *corpus*. See the *Oxford Latin Dictionary* (hereafter abbreviated as *OLD*), which states, "the mind as opposed to the

ter: if the soul is healthy, if it is passionless, serious and considerate, then the intellect is also sober and clear. If the soul is burdened with faults, the intellect is also affected."[17] Seneca's idea of health is described through a series of adjectives: *compositus*—passionless,[18] *gravis*—serious and considerate,[19] *temperans*—temperate and cool-headed, all of which are part of the *animus*.[20] They share a connection with the ideal of apathy, whose ideal image is a life that cannot be affected by external influences and requires self-recognition and self-control. *Ingenium*, then, is a "natural talent" like "mental power, natural ability, talent, intellect."[21] Stoics consider these to be part of the preferred adiaphora. Seneca defines illness similarly to health: "Do you not see that if a man's soul has become sluggish, his limbs drag and his feet move indolently? If it is womanish, that one can detect the effeminacy by his very gait? That a keen and confident soul quickens the step? That madness in the soul, or anger (which resembles madness), hastens our bodily movements from walking to rushing? And how much more do you think that this affects one's ability, which is entirely interwoven with the soul,—being moulded thereby, obeying its commands, and deriving therefrom its laws!"[22] Certainly it is no coincidence that the body (*corpus*) is mentioned when the dimension of illness is being plumbed. The image and counterimage are arranged in climactic terms: a weak soul (*elanguit*) results in a feminine gait (*emminatus*),[23] and a fiery soul (*acer, ferox*) not only hastens the steps, but ends in furor (*nec ire sed ferri*) and a loss of control (*turbatum esse corporis motum*). A sick person (in other words one who is not focused on the

---

body, the mind is soul as constituting with the body the whole person." See also Pittet, *Vocabulaire Philosophique de Sénèque*, on *animus*.

17. Seneca *Epistula* 114.3: *Non potest alius esse ingenio, alios animo color. Si ille sanus est, si compositus, gravis, temperans, ingenium quoque siccum ac sobrium est: illo vitatio hoc quoque adflatur.*

18. See *OLD*: "mentally sound, sane, sensible, sober, reasonable."

19. See *OLD*: "[of persons, their ideas, etc.] not given to levity or frivolity, grave, serious, earnest, thoughtful, etc."

20. For a detailed analysis of the letter, see Costa, *Seneca*, 225–30.

21. *OLD* on the term *ingenium* 4a.

22. Seneca *Epist*. 114.3, trans. Richard Mott Gummere (Latin text edition cited by Costa, *Seneca*, 138): *non vides, si animus elanguit, trahi membra et pigre moveri pedes? Si ille effeminatus est, in ipso incessu apparere mollitiam? Si ille acer est et ferox, concitari gradum? Si furit aut, quod furori simile est, irascitur, turbatum esse corporis motum nec ire sed ferri? Quanto hoc magis accidere ingenio putas, quod totum animo permixtum est, ab illo fingitur, illi paret, inde legem petit?*

23. *OLD* on effeminatus: "imitating a woman in appearance or behaviour, effeminate."

good thought) is thus the counter-image of an ideal wise man.[24] The text is interpreted in the hermeneutic context as a "body-soul" construct, both of which are based on harmony, and in both cases it is true that the smallest bodily characteristics provide information about the person, his intellectual capacity and his health. And what is true for the body and for health is also true for style and rhythm, which can just as easily be influenced by the "good thought."

Seneca thus uses the opportunity afforded by the genre of the teaching letter, where the letter's situation also includes a personal description of his well-being, to describe the physical ailments that threaten to overtake his body. However, he describes this as a mere example of his philosophical insights: self-representation leads to an "existential message." He himself, of course, is the best witness to the form of the good thought. Even if he is gripped by illness, the message is that he is not sick, because the methodological dimension of the "good thought" does not affect his existential message, which has a literary effect. How greatly this distances Seneca from the genre of the personal letter can be seen by comparing his writings with the letters of the rhetorician Fronto, whose descriptions of illness are certainly unusual for the ancient era.

MARCUS CORNELIUS FRONTO: SELF-REPRESENTATION IN ILLNESS AS AN EXPRESSION OF PERSONAL RELATIONSHIP

Formally speaking, Seneca's collection of letters corresponds to those of the rhetorician Marcus Cornelius Fronto (90/95 until after 167 CE)[25] in the sense that both are teachers addressing their pupils. It is not clear from the texts whether Fronto also intended to publish his letters.[26] However, even a

---

24. Of course it must also be noted that the variations in gait and bodily feeling ultimately correspond to a rash style. See also: "For just as a less ostentatious gait becomes a philosopher, does a restrained style of speech, far removed from boldness." (Sen. *Epist.* 40.14., trans. Richard Mott Gummere, here and in the following). On the question of artistic style, see more explicitly Möller, *Talis oratio—qualis vita*, 176–82.

25. Date according to Michael P.J. van den Hout, *A Commentary on the Letters of M. Cornelius Fronto*; on the date, cf. also Edward Champlin, *Fronto and Antonine Rome*; for the text, I use *Marcus Cornelius Fronto. Epistulae* (ed. Michael P. J. van den Hout). With another numbering system, see also *The Correspondence of Marcus Cornelius Fronto* (trans. C. R. Haines; LCL; 2 vols.). Also helpful: Stowers, *Letter Writing in Greco-Roman Antiquity*, 81–82. K. Luchner, Philiatroi. *Studien zum Thema Krankheit in der griechischen Literatur der Kaiserzeit* (Göttingen: Vandenhoeck, 2004).

26. According to Cugusi, *Evoluzione de Forme dell' epistolografia Latina*, 246–247, Fronto wanted to publish the Copial books. A.S.L. Farquharson assumes in his

cursory glance at the numerous examples where various illnesses play a role guides us toward different interpretations of the two rhetoricians.

The dialogue between Fronto and Marcus Aurelius has often been referred to by scholars as "hypochondriac."[27] However, in my opinion, when the dialogue is integrated into Marcus Aurelius' hermeneutics, this interpretation does not hold. Thus the following will view the correspondence within the context of Marcus Aurelius' *Meditationes*.

The best-known example of illness in Fronto's body of letters is probably the following citation. The context for this depiction of illness is an apology for being unable to meet Marcus Aurelius earlier, thus following the *topos* of absence (ἀπουσία), which according to Thraede is a standard topic for letters;[28] however, in the correspondence between Fronto and Marcus Aurelius it stands out from the other letters in an unusual way: "The diarrhea and vomiting took so much out of me that I lost my voice, had trouble swallowing, then difficulty breathing; finally my blood vessels failed (Cael. Aurel. Acut. 3,2,8), and without adequate circulation I was doing very poorly indeed (see also Plaut. Mil. 1331). Finally, my relatives began to lament over me (see Luke 8:52; Liv. 4,40,3), and I was unconscious for some time; the doctors did not have any time or opportunity to revive me at least with a cold bath or food; only in the evening was I able to keep down a couple of pieces of bread dunked in wine. But that brought me right back to life. Still, I was unable to speak for three whole days afterward. But now I am again in good health, thanks to the help of the gods..."[29] Compared to Seneca's letters, the level of detail and the chosen tone are remarkable. His mention of the illness seems to play an emphatic function, which certainly expresses an undiminished bond. A comparable tendency can also be seen

---

introduction that Marcus Aurelius also wanted to publish his letters to Fronto [*The Meditations of the Emperor Marcus Aurelius Antoninus. Edited with translations and commentary. Vol I*, XI].

27. Whitehorne ("Was Marcus Aurelius a Hypochondriac?," 413–21) puts forth the thesis that the letters reflect Fronto's hypochondria rather than that of Marcus Aurelius (415). Whitehorne argues that about 30% of Fronto's letters are devoted to his reports on illness. Of the 45 known letters of Marcus Aurelius, he says, 27 are about Fronto's complaints, while a smaller percentage have to do with Marcus Aurelius' own health.

28. Klaus Thraede mentions the motif of absence due to illness in reference to Basil the Great (*Grundzüge griechisch-römischer Brieftopik*, 117, esp. n178).

29. Fronto *Ad M.Caes.* 5,55: *Cholera usque eo adflictus sum, ut vocem amitterem, singultirem, suspirio tum angerer, postremo venae deficerent, sine ullo pulsu venarum animo male fieret. Denique conclamatus sum a nostris; neque sensi aliquandiu; ne balneo quidem aut frigida aut cibo recreandi me ac fovendi medicis tempus aut occasio data; nisi post vesperam micularum cum vino destillatum gluttivi. Ita focilatus totus sum. Postea per continuum triduum vocem non reciperavi. Sed nunc deis iuvantibus commodissime valeo...*

in Demetrius' treatise *De stilo*, which uses the expression ἐπιστολαὶ φιλικαί, letters of friendship.[30] Admittedly, it is not merely the illness and the extensive description of the illness that constitute the genre of the friendship letter. Rather, this genre is clearly present when the author and the addressee are ill at the same time—a phenomenon that we notice in the context of the cited passage and that will be further shown by the following citations, which precede the abovementioned passage and give us more insight into the correspondence between Fronto and Marcus Aurelius:

Fronto: "I would like to know how you, Lord, passed the night. I was gripped by a pain in my neck."[31] Marcus Aurelius: "I seem to have gotten through the night without a fever; I ate something without vomiting, and now I feel much better. We will see what the [next] night brings. But my dear teacher: since you were recently worried about this affliction, you can surely understand how I felt upon hearing that you had neck pains."[32] Fronto: "My neck, Lord, hurts terribly, but the pain in my foot has vanished."[33] Marcus Aurelius: "If your neck pains should finally disappear on the third day as well, that will also help my gradually returning health, my dear teacher. Today I took a bath and went for a short walk, and I ate a bit more, though not without some stomach complaints."[34]

The letters reflect an encounter between two friends that uses the written form as a conversation and establishes a friendly connection over distance. The descriptions of illness illustrate an expression of empathy (*quomodo manseris ... scire copio; cervicium dolore te arreptum, quo animum didicerim; cervicum dolores si tertia quoque die remiserint, erit quod meam redeuntem valetudinem maiorem*) with the other person that affects the physical as well as the emotional state; as Marcus Aurelius writes, "As long as you are lying there, I too have the inward feeling that I am lying down."[35] It is certainly worth noting that the illness overcomes physical separation, for this unity within illness creates memory and remembrance. Thus we

30. See Thraede, *Grundzüge griechisch-römischer Brieftopik*, 21 and 24–25.

31. Fronto *Ad M.Caes.* 5,27: *Quomodo manseris, domine, scire cupio. Ego cervicum dolore arreptus sum.*

32. Fronto *Ad. M.Caes.* 5,28: *Noctem sine febri videor transmisisse; cibum non invitus cepi, nunc ago levissime. Nox quid ferat, cognoscemus. Sed, mi magister, cervicum dolore te arreptum, quo animum didicerim, profecto ex tua proxima sollicitudine metiris.*

33. Fronto *Ad M.Caes.* 5,29: *Cervicum, domine, dolore gravi sum correptus, de pede dolor decessit.*

34. Fronto *Ad M.Caes.* 5,30: *Cervicum dolores si tertia quoque die remiserint, erit quod meam redeuntem valetudinem maiorem in modum adiuvet, mi magister. lavi et hodie et ambulavi paulum, cibi paulo plus sumpsi nondum tamen libente stomacho.*

35. Fronto *Ad M.Caes.* 3,20.

have here the letter-specific *topos* of the "physically distant—yet nonetheless present."[36] This empathy in times of illness is also noteworthy in another sense: Thraede demonstrated at length that the form of the friendship letter more commonly takes place between a superior and a subordinate.[37] In addition, Marcus Aurelius clearly placed himself in the subordinate position of the concerned pupil, which did not at all correspond to the actual power balance; this further reinforces the topic of the friendship letter.[38]

One might now assume that, given this background of experiencing illness and communicating at length about it, care for the body would be of central importance. However, one of Fronto's comments is particularly worth noting: "[In my life] I have allowed concern for my soul to take precedence over concern for my body."[39] This traditional Stoic doctrine of temperate care for one's own body is also clearly expressed in Marcus Aurelius' *Meditationes*, where he adopts Epicurus' attitude:[40] "Epicurus says: During my illness I did not talk about the sufferings of my little body, nor did I speak about such topics with my visitors; instead, I focused entirely on the core messages of the natural philosophers."[41] It is certainly fundamental that Marcus Aurelius bases his text on a triadic form of anthropology: σῶμα, ψυχή and νοῦς. Even in 2,2,1–3, in his definition of the "self," he defines the three levels: "What I am, are little bits of fleshes [sic! plural[42]] and little breaths of air and the guiding principle ... and you should scorn the little meat as though you were already dying: impure blood, little bones and an

---

36. See Thraede, *Grundzüge griechisch-römischer Brieftopik*, 27.

37. Thraede, *Grundzüge griechisch-römischer Brieftopik*, 26–27.

38. Numerous examples, especially from late antiquity, prove that the motif of accepting an illness out of empathy is fairly common. At the same time, the power structure is rarely reversed. See, for example, Libanios *Epist*. 13: Τῇ διὰ τὴν σὴν ἀρρωστίαν λύπῃ καὶ αὐτοὶ πεπτώκαμεν εἰς ἀρρωστίαν. τί γὰρ ἡμῖν ἡδὺ σοῦ γε ἀνιωμένου; Σελεύκῳ Δὲ ἄρα ἔπεπε καὶ τοῦτο ἀγγεῖλαι τὸ ὡς ἐκπέφευγας τοῦ κακοῦ τὴν ἀκμήν. ᾗ δὴ καὶ πείθομαι τὸν Ἐντρέχιον εὐτυχῆ νομίζειν. ὄψεται γὰρ Βιθυνίαν, ὅτε βέλτιον. Βέλτιν δέ, ὅτε καὶ σοὶ τὸ σῶμα ἐν ὑγιείᾳ. χάριν δὲ εἰδότες σοι τοῦ φιλεῖν τὸν ἄνδρα χάριν ἑτέραν αἰτοῦμεν προσθεῖναι τὸ τόνδε καλεῖν. "Out of pain over your illness, I have now fallen victim to an illness myself. For what could be pleasant to me when you are doing badly? Seleucus also should have told me that you had already escaped the peak of the ailment. Therefore I am convinced that Entrechios can be considered lucky. For he will see Bithynia when it is better. By better, I mean when you are once again [completely] physically healthy. And I must now thank you for considering the man worthy of your friendship, but I ask for one more occasion for gratitude: invite him to visit you!"

39. Fronto *De nepote amisso* 9.1: *Animo potius quam corpori curando operam dedi*.

40. The following is based on Jäkel, *Marcus Aurelius's Concept of Life*, especially 5–21.

41. Marcus Aurelius *Med*. 9,41,1.

42. The plural form is also found in the Hippocratic text *De carnibus*.

interweaving of sinews, veins and arteries twined together." Naturally it is first worth noting that Marcus Aurelius speaks not only of the body using a diminutive, σάρκιον, but also applies this to the breath of air, πνευμάτιον, and the little soul, ψυχάριον. Body/flesh, breath and soul are seen in a strict Stoic sense as material components of the body, which are almost exclusively viewed with a diminutive tendency. Thus the world of the little body seems to be constantly shrinking. Rutherford mentions a "view from above" in this context.[43] Marcus Aurelius contrasts this with reason and with the internal (divine) force as ἡγεμονικόν, a type of "divine protected space" against the material world of the body. In contrast to Seneca, the internal space remains completely undamaged even during illness (see, e.g., *Med.* 3,16,3). If one relates these insights to the correspondence between Marcus Aurelius and Fronto, it becomes clear that the "temperate" care for one's own body is shared with none less than a close companion. This deep bond, like the reference to reason, seems to be a protective shield against the material world of the body. At the same time, however, the treatment of the body and of illness remains contradictory. On the one hand, it persists in direct, detailed descriptions of physical fragility, while on the other hand it is called into question by adapting traditional Stoic and Platonic philosophy and its relationship with reason, which makes the physical dimension the starting point for philosophical considerations. Consequently, illness is a sign of the ephemeral nature of human life.

Thus the correspondence between Fronto and Marcus Aurelius is also part of a special epistolary genre, that of the friendship letter, which in turn influences the depiction of illness. The letter is an expression of the spatial distance between friends; it facilitates the friendly bond and also acts as a protective shield against the power of illness and suffering.

THE APOSTLE PAUL: THE POWER OF GOD APPEARS IN THE MOMENT OF PHYSICAL WEAKNESS

In addition to Seneca, Fronto and Marcus Aurelius, the Apostle Paul is surely one of those authors whose letters can be read "autobiographically" with regard to the suffering self, especially the statements about his physical weakness in the second letter to the Corinthians.

The founding of the Corinthian community is described in the Acts of Paul, where he meets Priscilla and Aquila, who had left Rome in the context of Emperor Claudius' Jewish expulsions in 49 CE.[44] As the founder of the

43. Rutherford, *The Meditations of Marcus Aurelius*, 155ff.
44. For further discussion, see Klauck, *Ancient Letters and the New Testament.* On

community in Corinth, Paul attempts to fulfill his role as a leader even after his departure, in other words from his new location in Ephesus and Macedonia.[45] This spatial distance leads to an extensive correspondence, which is only available to us in fragmentary form. This correspondence with the Corinthians in particular depicts a Paul who must constantly reassure himself of his own presence, whether in writing or verbally, but especially with regard to his own physical weakness.[46]

There are two reasons why Paul may have reflected apologetically on his own presence: (1) fundamentally, a missionary was expected to demonstrate λογός and γνῶσις, as described in detail in 1 Cor 1–2. The λογός, the beauty and representation of speech, are a central aspect of his reflections. Of course, this aspect indicates the social status of the educated class, who were trained in the theory and practice of rhetoric[47] and for whom this was a way to distinguish themselves from the other classes[48] as well as a way to convey a political leadership claim.[49] Fundamentally, the public image of the educated person took place within the atmosphere of a competition; it was always directly or indirectly compared with that of other aspirants. In order to succeed, a certain amount of uniqueness was required here. A lack of same was met with hooting, groans, hissing, yelling or silence, or even throwing stones, as Philostratus describes graphically from his own experience.[50] Paul does not seem to have met this requirement for uniqueness, at least not in the sense of his physical weakness. (2) Paul paid a second personal visit to the community, which had been unsettled by missionaries whom he considered to have seriously called his authority into question. However, it

---

imperial-era epistolography, see, for instance: Bauer, *Paulus und die Kaiserzeitliche Epistolographie*; Klauck, *Ancient Letters and the New Testament*; the collected essay book *Paul and the Ancient Letter Form* (eds. S. E. Porter and S. A. Adams); Hose, *Kleine griechische Literaturgeschichte*; Rosenmeyer, *Ancient Epistolary Fictions*.

45. See 1 Cor 3:10–11; 4:15; 11:17.

46. On the reconstruction of the Corinthian correspondence, see Schnelle, *Einleitung in das Neue Testament*, 251–53 and Th. Schmeller, "Der zweite Korintherbrief," 337–38.

47. Whitmarsh, *The Second Sophistic*, Ch. "Education, Elitism, and Hellenism," talks about "the 'educated' (*pepaideumenoi*)" (p. 15).

48. Whitmarsh, in his excellent article *The Second Sophistic*, Ch. "Sophistry in Action" (pp. 19–22), points out an affinity of the upper class with rhetorical education.

49. See Guido O. Kirner, "Apostolat und Patronage (II). Darstellungsteil: Weisheit, Rhetorik und Ruhm im Konflikt um die apostolische Praxis des Paulus," 27–72. On "political" word choice in 1 Cor see Weissenrieder, "Contested Spaces in 1 Corinthians 11:17–34 and 14:30."

50. VS 578–580 found in Korenjak, *Publikum und Redner*; on Philostratus, see pages 142–47. See also many references in Whitmarsh, *The Second Sophistic*.

seems clear that the opponents were not primarily distinguished by having a different theological profile; rather, the comments suggest that it was Paul himself, his speeches, his rhetoric and his physical presence that were subject to criticism, first by one Apollos of Alexandria (1 Cor 1:12; 3:4,22; 4:4; 16:12), but then also by foreign missionaries about whose theological profile we learn almost nothing (1 Cor 2:17; 11:5,12–17).[51] His visit was a disaster, meeting with mockery and ridicule due to his personal appearance and his physical weakness (2 Cor 2:9; 7:12), and Paul left Corinth precipitously—but not without sending out another letter, known as the tearful letter (2 Cor 10–13).[52] It is primarily this part of the correspondence, particularly 12:5–9, that will be briefly described in the context of this essay.

As in the correspondence between Fronto and Marcus Aurelius, in Chapter 10 Paul also takes up the common motif of bridging distance through a letter, which according to Thraede[53] is normally represented by the motif ἀπών—παρών, by the participles ἀπάντες and παρόντες: as a rule, ἄπειμι means physical absence[54] and πάρειμι means being (physically) close to someone. This connotation can be transferred to physical presence: being

---

51. According to Whitmarsh, *The Second Sophistic*, describing how space and time can fundamentally influence the course of a rhetorical analysis. Nonetheless, we cannot make any concise statements about this with regard to the analysis of Paul.

52. In my opinion, this is clearly explained by Klauck, *Der 2. Korintherbrief*, 29: "Der Vorfall steht in Zusammenhang mit dem Eindringen von Paulusgegnern in Korinth. Ein ortsansässiges, einflussreiches Gemeindemitglied, möglicherweise schon seit den Parteistreitigkeiten des 1 Kor dem Paulus nicht sonderlich gut gesonnen, macht sich die Position der neuen Paulusgegner zu eigen und geht beim Zwischenbesuch vor der Gemeinde gegen Paulus vor. Die Gemeinde unternimmt nichts dagegen. Ihr Stillhalten muss Paulus als Zustimmung interpretieren. Ihm bleibt nur die eilige Abreise." ["This incident is associated with the infiltration of Paul's opponents in Corinth. A local influential member of the community, possibly one who has not been in a particularly good mood since the partisan debates of Paul's 1 Cor, becomes one of Paul's new opponents, and rails against Paul during a visit to the community. The community does nothing about it. Paul is forced to interpret their silence as agreement. His only option is a quick departure."]

The scope of the tearful letter is by no means standardized: while Vielhauer still considers Section 2:14–7:4 (without 6:14–7:1) to be part of the letter, numerous scholars argue for a version that only includes 2 Cor 10–13 [see also Klauck, *2. Korintherbrief*, 9, but also Gräßer, *Der zweite Brief an die Korinther*, 31–33; Marxsen, *Einleitung in das Neue Testament*, 73–77; a different argument comes from Betz, *Galatians*, 1–9, 12–13, who considers the tearful letter to be lost, since 1 Cor 10–13 does not include the semantic field of tears and sorrow.

53. Thraede, *Grundzüge griechisch-römischer Brieftopik*, 95–106; for an extensive discussion of ancient examples, see Koskenniemi, *Studien zur Idee und Phraseologie des griechischen Briefes*, 172–200, who primarily concentrates on Cicero *fam.* 2.4.1, 3.11.2; 12.30.1, 16.16.2; Seneca *Epist.* 75.1.

54. *OGD*: "to be away or absent."

physically close to someone through words, ἐν λόγῳ.⁵⁵ Thus Paul is referring here to the ancient topos of presence by using the word τῷ λόγῳ; in Ch. 12 he then interprets this presence with "hearing" and "seeing." This argument is further supported by the fact that βαρύς is used as a tone of voice in ancient rhetoric, and the tone of voice in the Pauline letters is appropriately powerful.⁵⁶ Since the word becomes alive as a spoken word that wants to be read, it is not so much a sign of his absence as it is a sign of his presence, as is abundantly demonstrated in Cicero, for instance.

Cicero is also the one who writes, in his second letter to his wife and his daughter Tullia, "*Vale, mea Terentia, quam ego videre videor, itaque debelitior lacrimis*—Fare well, my Terentia, because I seem to see [you], and I am disheartened by my tears."⁵⁷ According to Thraede, this is the oldest evidence of the παρουσία motif, which can be interpreted either as ὡς παρών—*quasi adesse* and correspondingly as a motif of absence, or else as "(fictive) actual seeing."⁵⁸ It is certainly worth mentioning that Cicero was overwhelmed by the force of his tears. In the *Epistula familiares*, Cicero expresses sorrow over his spatial distance from close family members. The παρουσία motif is also associated with the situation of mourning, at least in Cicero, in which tears are a visible, outward emotion and thus a topos used in letters that describes a real, internal sorrow.⁵⁹ This example does reinforce the motif of absence by showing that it can also potentially be associated with a real, internal sorrow. If we relate this to the Pauline communication, it provides further insight into the absence motif through the reference to writing in tears as seen in 2 Cor 2:4.⁶⁰ Thus it is significant that the semantic field

---

55. As for instance in Ar. Ach. 513.

56. Arist. *Rhet.* 1403b 30. Classen, "Paulus und die antike Rhetorik," 1–33, by contrast, considers it unlikely that Paul is consciously using rhetorical topoi.

57. Cicero 14.3.5.

58. Thraede, *Grundzüge griechisch-römischer Brieftopik*, 17.

59. See also the article by Eve-Marie Becker, "Die Tränen des Paulus (2 Kor 2,4; Phil 3,18). Emotion oder Topos?," 8–9, who writes, "Das Tränen-Motiv erweist sich also geradezu als ein Grundelement ciceronischer Epistolographie, das in großer Variation begegnet. Es steht für vielfältige Emotionen des Briefschreibers, die er seinen Adressaten mitzuteilen sucht. Mit dem Tränen-Motiv wird gleichsam die emotionale Verfasstheit des Briefschreibers visualisiert." ["The motif of tears is thus shown to be a downright fundamental element of Ciceronic epistolography, and is found in many variations. It stands for a wide range of emotions in the letter writer, which he attempts to convey to the addressee. The motif of tears also serves to illustrate the writer's emotional condition."]

60. Thraede, *Grundzüge griechisch-römischer Brieftopik*, 22; See also Bauer, "Einen missglückten Auftritt retten," 98.

of *infirmus* (weak, physically compromised, sick [the opposite of *valens*])[61] and *infirmitas* (the weakness of the body, particularly in relation to health, exhaustion and illness)[62] particularly comes into play in these letters from Cicero to his family and his friend Atticus, though of course with its own emphasis: the weakness and physical exhaustion come from the absence of the beloved people, and the letter attempts to overcome these feelings. The semantic field of *infirmus* and *infirmitas* is also significant in Seneca's letters to Lucilius, particularly when Seneca discusses the proper attitude toward life and death. The 70th letter is particularly important—it begins with a personal address to Lucilius and describes the goal of a happy life as being ethical goodness. In his "fool's speech," Seneca describes the superiority of the wise man who faces death. As an example, Seneca tells of a wise man who demonstrates both a scorn for death and a longing for death: "This may be true; but life is not to be purchased at any price. No matter how great or how well-assured certain rewards may be I shall not strive to attain them at the price of a shameful confession of weakness." Tearful rhetoric is clearly not excluded here. While it is impossible to say whether the letter-writer Paul wanted his statements in chapters 10–13 to be interpreted "emotionally" in this sense, it cannot be ruled out—particularly when we consider his defensive statements in 2 Cor 12:5–9. Here, the collection of personal pronouns in 5b and 6b and 7b–9 is worth noting: ἐμαυτοῦ, ἐμέ, ἐμοῦ, μέ—μοι, με, ἐμοῦ, μοι, σοι, μοῦ, ἐμέ.[63] These can be read as part of a rhetorical strategy that Paul is able to articulate and visualize for his addressees.

In 2 Cor 12:5–9, Paul explains his rhetorical argument in these verses in greater Christological and revelatory depth. Here he says, "On behalf of ὑπέρ this man I will boast καυχήσομαι, but on my own behalf ὑπέρ I will not boast καυχήσομαι, except of my weaknesses ἀσθενείαις—though if I should wish to boast, I would not be a fool, for I would be speaking the truth; but I refrain from it, so that no one may think more of me than he sees in me or hears from me. 7 So to keep me from becoming conceited because of the surpassing greatness of the revelations, a thorn was given me in the flesh, a messenger of Satan to harass me, to keep me from becoming conceited. Three times I pleaded with the Lord about this, that it should leave me. But he said to me, 'My grace is sufficient for you, for my power is made perfect in weakness [illness].' Therefore I will boast all the more gladly of my weaknesses [illness], so that the power of Christ may rest upon me."

---

61. See *Der Neue Georges*, Vol. 2, 2577–78.
62. See ibid., 2577.
63. Heckel, *Kraft in Schwachheit*, 77.

This passage contains a complex structure with parallel and chiastic syntax: verse 5 shows parallelism through the double use of ὑπέρ and the parallel use of καυχήσομαι, though it is differentiated at the content level by the differing subjects, in one case the object of revelation that cannot boast of itself (5a) and in the other case Paul, who boasts of his illness (5b; as litotes). Syntactically, this creates a contrast between the subjects. To be sure, the structural parallel is again antithetically reinforced between verses 5 and 6–7a. While in verses 6b and 7a Paul refuses to boast about receiving the revelations and distinguishes between two forms of boasting in verse 5—boasting about the revelation and about weakness—in 6a he goes into more detail about receiving the revelation. As the recipient of the revelation (v. 5a), Paul would have had every reason to boast, and this certainty is expressed in v. 6a in the conditional form. Both in v. 5b and in v. 6b, the possibility of boasting is prevented by an adversative "but" δέ, and "not" οὐ is reinforced by the refrain of φείδομαι: no boasting, unless it be due to weakness.[64] In 5b and 6b, Paul describes his situation with a negated final sentence. Naturally, the pronouns and negations in 5b and 6b are central: in 5b "but on my own behalf . . . except (ὑπέρ ἐμαυτοῦ—οὐ εἰ μή)" and in 6b "of me—than (εἰς ἐμέ—μή . . . ὑπέρ)." With these formulations (especially the personal pronouns), Paul places himself at the center while simultaneously distancing himself from the person who received the revelation ("to keep me from being too elated"). Through the dual negation, he also shifts the focus to a positive message, namely the praise of physical weakness. Through this complex syntactical structure of parallelism and antithesis, Paul thus ultimately succeeds in equating the revelatory experience (vv. 2–4) and (physical) weakness. Physical weakness or illness is thus not a stopgap of which he needs to assure himself, but something he can boast about as much as about his revelations (plural). However, this also means that the out-of-body experiences described in vv. 2–4 refer to his own person (7a with reference to verse 1: τῇ ὑπερβολῇ τῶν ἀποκαλύψεων). Even if he claims in verse 5 that he does not want to boast about his revelation, he follows this by positioning his weakness in seeing and hearing as a sign from God. Heckel points out that this was associated with a dual message; in addition to his physical weakness, Paul reminds the Corinthians that he created the community (10:11–18).[65] Certainly the reason for the weakness, the "thorn in the flesh," that can be understood as a *Passivum divinum* ἐδόθη, is central; thus pain is linked with God, while the duration of the weakness is linked

---

64. Black, *Weakness*, 156, pointed out that it should be "because of" and not "in weakness."

65. Heckel, *Kraft in Schwachheit*, 74.

with the angel of Satan, who defeats Paul again and again, through the durative aorist *to keep me from becoming conceited* ὑπραίρωμαι. In contrast to 10:10f., Paul does not speak of the weakness of the body σῶμα here, but rather of a weakness in the flesh σάρξ.

Paul's weakness has been the subject of much speculation. If we look at the occurrence of *weakness*—ἀσθένεια in the *Corpus Hippocraticum*, a body of more than sixty texts from the fifth century BCE, we can see that the concept of weakness is not mentioned in conjunction with a mental illness, such as "epilepsy." Even a (congenital) malformation of the limbs seems unlikely to me given this context. When ἀσθένεια / ἀσθενής appears, it is used to indicate either a temporary physical weakening of the bodily constitution, often in conjunction with fever and feebleness,[66] or a gender-specific weakness of the female sex or seed.[67] A weakness that is expressed in the flesh σάρξ, however, is assigned either a positive or a neutral value in ancient medicine and philosophy.[68] Ancient natural philosophical texts return to σάρξ in the singular as well as the plural form (σαρκές), for instance in the Hippocratic text *De carnibus* (περὶ σαρκῶν), which includes all of the body parts, even the organs (a perspective that is certainly rejected by Aristotle and Plato). The exegetic literature often notes that flesh σάρξ refers only to the muscular parts of the body. Within the context of ancient literature, however, this would be unusual since it is never mentioned alone with this connotation, but always in relation to other body parts, for instance bones (see Arist. *De historia animalium* III 2 646 b 25; *De partibus animalium* II 9 655 b 23 and Alexander of Aphrodisias *De anima* 98.10), sinews (νεῦρα Plato *Tim.* 74 b; 82c; 84a; Arist. *De partibus animalium* I 5 645 a 29; II 1 646 b 25; Alexander of Aphrodisias *De mixtione* 15) or blood (Euripides *fr.* 687,1f.). Aristotle, who particularly focuses on the flesh in his second book *De partibus animalium*, equates flesh with the bodily tissue found between the bones and the skin.[69] Thus he considers the flesh to be more of an "external" body part, like the hair, nails and other characteristics that are central to the body's appearance. Flesh, then, makes weakness outwardly visible! Through his reference to the flesh, Paul makes it clear that anyone can see his weakness.

66. See CH *Epid.* V 18.12; *Loc.Hom.* 43.1; *Morb* 2.39.3; 2.51.8; *Aphor.* 2.28; *Vict.* 1.27.15; *Vict.* 2.54.25; *Vict.* 5.90.40. See Weissenrieder and Dolle, *Körper und Verkörperung*, Ch. 13.

67. See, e.g., in CH *Nat.Mul.* 12.4; *Mul.* 1.21.6; 1.63.7; 2.112.5; 2.119.4; 2.119.42; 2.174.15; *Steril.* 213.66; *Nat.Puer.* 22.3.

68. See CH *Morb.* I 22.12–33; Aristotle, *De partibus animalium* II 8 653 b 19–35; II 9 654 b 27–32; and CH *Oss.* 11.

69. See Arist. *De historia animalium* III 16 519 b26–28.

This result corresponds to Pauline statements to the extent that Paul shows, in the 2nd letter to the Corinthians, that Christ's life and death are manifested in our mortal flesh.[70] Christ's death on the cross is outwardly visible in the flesh; in fact, it is even manifested through physical weakness.

This assertion is in turn made clear by God's mysterious response to Paul's prayer, which Paul cites verbatim: "My grace is sufficient for you, for my power is made perfect in weakness—ἀρκεῖσοιη χάρις μου, ἡ γὰρ δύναμις ἐν ἀσθενείᾳ τελεῖται." Here Paul formulates a principle that he introduces with γάρ and the perfect form εἴρηκεν (and now it applies), and he himself is the one who becomes the subject of a theological revelation. Here, too, he uses a chiastic formulation: "(my) grace and power" and "sufficient" (3. Sg. Act.) and "made perfect" require one another. God's response is not a rejection of the Pauline prayer; rather, God provides grace that is sufficient, as Heckel convincingly argued.[71] Thus the non-fulfillment of the prayer is interpreted not as a rejection by God, but rather as a promise of grace in the power of weakness and illness, and thus a fulfillment of the Pauline prayers. This interpretation is once again suggested by the verb τελεῖσθαι, "to reach fulfillment,"[72] which often indicates the fulfillment of divine will; in this case, it is a reference to John 19:30, Jesus' last words on the cross: "it is finished!" This once again takes up the Apostle's weakness in a Christological sense: just as God's power becomes apparent at the moment of Christ's death, the power of God's grace is revealed through Paul's weakness and illness. Thus weakness and illness are seen as signs of renown.[73] They cannot and do not need to be overcome. Just as God reveals himself at the cross, according to Paul, he also reveals himself through physical weakness and illness.

Thus, like Seneca and Fronto before him, Paul demonstrates a clear connection between rhetoric and illness, though with his own emphasis. Here, illness is the subject of boasting, for it is here that Christ particularly reveals himself and makes God's attending to Paul, the hearing of his prayer, clear. However, rhetoric, emotional engagement and communications about illness are not mutually exclusive here—on the contrary. The polished rhetoric, using the ancient topos of the tearful letter, is an expression of this same emotionality. The power of the rhetoric with which Paul draws on the

---

70. See explicitly 2 Cor 4:11; 5:16.
71. Heckel, *Kraft in Schwachheit*, 88.
72. Ibid., 93 with reference to Bauer.
73. Due to space limitations, it is unfortunately not possible to investigate here how this interpretation relates to the Pauline statements on the Last Supper in 1 Cor 11:29ff. On this, see my remarks in "Darum sind viele körperlich und seelisch Kranke unter euch" (1 Cor 11,29ff.). Die korinthischen Überlegungen zum Abendmahl im Spiegel antiker Diätetik und der Patristik," 239–68.

topoi of the tearful letter, and the physical presence of the read word, open up the emotionality of his statements. This is true even if one does not read chapters 10–13 of the 2nd letter to the Corinthians together with 2 Cor 2:4, where Paul refers directly to his tears. For as in Seneca and Fronto, here it is also true that physical weakness becomes part of the epistolary communication and writing strategy, and is shown through more than a single motif.

CONCLUSION

The three authors—Seneca, Fronto with Marcus Aurelius, and Paul—provide us with internal views of a patient through the act of writing. The patient himself is the author. Rhetoric, emotional investment and physical weakness are closely interwoven. The author makes public his physical weakness, which would not have been immediately noticeable, and clearly expects to meet with a certain level of public interest. However, the writings of the three authors are not homogeneous, either in their choice of genre or in the way in which they deal with physical weakness. They include the form of a teaching letter as well as a friendship letter and the ancient genre of the tearful letter. The diverse literary genres also reflect a non-homogeneous relationship with illness. While Seneca's teaching letters are intended to communicate something about existence and the philosophy of positive thinking, Fronto and Marcus Aurelius communicate a deep bond in their friendship letters that goes beyond the power of the physical as well as the ephemeral nature of human life; finally, Paul attempts to show that his physical weakness is a visible sign that God's power is fulfilled in his physical existence.

In the ancient world, care and sympathy relating to health is thus always more than just an empty formulaic phrase at the beginning or end of a letter. It is an expression of the extent to which rhetoric, emotional investment and physical weakness or health are functionalized and reflected through writing.

BIBLIOGRAPHY

Bauer, Thomas Johann. *Paulus und die Kaiserzeitliche Epistolographie: Kontextualisierung und Analyse der Briefe an Philemon und an de Galater*. Wissenschaftliche Untersuchungen zum Neuen Testament 276. Tübingen: Mohr/Siebeck, 2011.

———. "Einen missglückten Auftritt retten. 2 Kor 10,10f. und die rhetorische Kultur der frühen Kaiserzeit," In: *Logos des Glaubens – Logos der Vernunft*. Festschrift für Edgar Früchtel (F.R. Prostmeier/H.E. Lona eds., Berlin/New York: de Gruyter, 2010, 77–108.

Betz, Hans Dieter. *Galatians: A Commentary on Paul's Letter to the Churches on Galatia.* Hermeneia. Philadelphia: Fortress, 1979.
Bien, Christian G. *Erklärungen zur Entstehung von Mißbildungen im physiologischen und medizinischen Schrifttum der Antike.* ZWG Beihefte 38. Stuttgart: Steiner, 1997.
Bompaire, Jacques. "Quatre styles d'autobiographie au IIe siècle après J.-C.: Aelius Aristide, Lucien, Marc-Aurèle, Galien." In *L'invention de l'autobiographie d'Hesiode à Saint Augustin, École normale supérieure, 14-16 juin 1990,* edited by Marie-Françoise Baslez et al., 199-209. Paris: Les Belles Lettres, 1993.
Cancik, Hildegard. *Untersuchungen zu Senecas Epistulae morales.* Spudasmata 18. Hildesheim: Olms, 1967.
Champlin, Edward. *Fronto and Antonine Rome.* Cambridge: Harvard University Press, 1980.
Classen, C. J. "Paulus und die antike Rhetorik." *Zeitschrift für die neutestamentliche Wissenschaft* 82 (1991) 1-33.
Costa, C. D. N. *Seneca. 17 Letters with Translation and Commentary.* Classical Texts. Warminster, UK: Aris & Phillips, 1988.
Cugusi, Paolo. *Evoluzione de Forme dell'Epistolografia Latina nelle tarda Repubblica e nei primi due secoli dell'Impero con cenni sull'epistolografia Preciceroniana.* Rome: Herder, 1983.
Farquharson, A. S. L. *The Meditations of the Emperor Marcus Aurelius Antoninus.* Vol. 1. 2nd ed. Oxford: Clarendon, 1968.
Garland, Robert. *The Eye of the Beholder: Deformity and Disablity in the Graeco-Roman World.* Bristol Classical Paperbacks. London: Bristol Classical Press, 2010.
Goodwin, James. *Autobiography: The Self Made Text.* Studies in Literary Themes and Genres. New York: Twayne, 1993.
Grässer, Erich. *Der zweite Brief an die Korinther. Band 1: Kap 1,1—7,16.* ÖTBK 8,1. Gütersloh: Güterloher, 2002.
Heckel, Ulrich. *Kraft in Schwachheit: Untersuchungen zu 2 Korinther 10-13 und Gal.* Wissenschaftliche Untersuchungen zum Neuen Testament 2/56. Tübingen: Mohr/Siebeck, 1993.
Hose, Martin. *Kleine griechische Literaturgeschichte: Von Homer bis zum Ende der Antike.* Beck'sche Reihe 1326. Munich: Beck, 1999.
Hout, M. P. J. van den. *A Commentary on the Letters of M. Cornelius Fronto.* Mnemosyne Supplements 190. Leiden: Brill, 1999.
http://www.zedis.uni-hamburg.de/wp-content/uploads/2007/01/intersectionality_raab.pdf
Jäkel, Siegfried. *Marcus Aurelius's Concept of Life.* Turku: Turun Yliopisto, 1991.
Jungck, Christoph. *Gregor von Nazianz: De Vita Sua. Einleitung, Text, Übersetzung, Kommentar.* Wissenschaftliche Kommentare zu griechischen und lateinischen Schriftstellern. Heidelberg: Winter, 1974.
Kirner, Guido O. "Apostolat und Patronage (II). Darstellungsteil: Weisheit, Rhetorik und Ruhm im Konflikt um die apostolische Praxis des Paulus in der frühchristlichen Gemeinde in Korinth (1 Kor 1-4 u. 9; 2 Kor 10-13." *Zeitschrift für Antikes Christentum* 7 (2003) 27-72.
Klauck, Hans-Josef. *Ancient Letters and the New Testament: A Guide to Context and Exegesis.* Translated and edited by Daniel P. Bailey. Waco, TX: Baylor University

Press, 2006 = *Die antike Briefliteratur und das Neue Testament: Ein Lehr- und Arbeitsbuch.* Paderborn: Schönigh, 1998.

———. *Der 2. Korintherbrief.* NEB.NT 8. 3rd ed. Würzburg: Echter, 1994.

Korenjak, Martin. *Publikum und Redner: Ihre Interaktion n der sophistischen Rhetorik der Kaiserzeit.* Zetema 104. Munich: Beck, 2002.

Koskenniemi, Heikki. *Studien zur Idee und Phraseologie des griechischen Briefes bis 400 n. Chr.* Suomalaisen Tiedeakatemian Toimituksia B/102.2. Helsinki: Suomalaisen Tiedeakatemia, 1956.

Leeman, Anton Daniël. "Das Todeserlebnis im Denken Senecas." *Gymnasium* 78 (1971) 322–33.

Lewis, R. G. "Imperial Autobiography. Augustus to Hadrian." In *ANRW* II.34.1 (1993) 629–706.

Luchner, K. *Philiatroi. Studien zum Thema Krankheit in der griechischen Literatur der Kaiserzeit.* Göttingen: Vandenhoeck, 2004

Marcus Cornelius Fronto. Epistulae. Edited by Michael P. J. van den Hout. Bibliotheca scriptorum Graecorum et Romanorum Teubneriana. Leipzig: Teubner, 1988.

Marxsen, Willi. *Einleitung in das Neue Testament: Einführung in die Probleme.* Gütersloh: Gütersloher, 1978.

Mazzoli, Giancarlo. "Le ,epistulae Morales ad Lucilium' di Seneca: Valore letterario e filosofico." In *ANRW* II.36.3 (1989) 1823–77.

Misch, G. *Geschichte der Autobiographie.* Vol. 1.1, *Das Altertum.* 3rd widely distributed ed. Frankfurt: Schulte-Bulmke, 1949/1950.

Möller, Melanie. *Talis oratio, qualis vita: Zu Theorie und Praxis mimetischer Verfahren in der griechisch-römischen Literaturkritik.* Bibliothek der klassischen Altertumswissenschaften 2/113. Heidelberg: Winter, 2004.

Momigliano, Arnaldo. *The Development of Greek Biography.* Cambridge: Harvard University Press, 1971.

Niggl, Günter, ed. *Die Autobiographie: Zu Form und Geschichte einer literarischen Gattung.* 2nd ed. expanded with a postscript on the new edition and a bibliographical addendum. Wege der Forschung 565. Darmstadt: Wissenschaftliche Buchgesellschaft, 1998.

Pittet, Armand. *Vocabulaire Philosophique de Sénèque.* Collection d'études anciennes. Paris: Les Belles Lettres, 1937.

Porter, Stanley E., and Sean A. Adams, eds. *Paul and the Ancient Letter Form.* Pauline Studies 6. Leiden: Brill, 2006.

Reardon, B. P. "L'autobiographie à l'époche de la Seconde Sophistique: Quelques conclusions." In *L'invention de l'autobiographie d'Hesiode à Saint Augustin, École normale supérieure, 14–16 juin 1990,* edited by Marie-Françoise Baslez et al., 279–84. Etudes de littérature ancienne 5. Paris: Les Belles Lettres, 1993.

Rosenmeyer, Patricia A. *Ancient Epistolary Fictions: The Letter in Greek Literature.* Cambridge: Cambridge University Press, 2004.

Rutherford, R. B. *The Meditations of Marcus Aurelius: A Study.* Oxford Classical Monographs. Oxford: University Press, 1989.

Schmeller, Thomas. "Der zweite Korintherbrief." In *Einleitung in das Neue Testament,* edited by Martin Ebner and Stefan Schreiber, 337–38. KStTh 6. Stuttgart: Kohlhammer, 2008.

Schnelle, Udo. *Einleitung in das Neue Testament.* 6th ed. Uni-Taschenbücher 1830. Göttingen: Vandenhoeck & Ruprecht, 2007.

Seneca. *Ad Lucilium. Epistolae Morales.* Vol. 1. Translated by R. M. Gummere. Loeb Classical Library. New York: Putnam, 1917.
Stowers, Stanley K. *Letter Writing in Greco-Roman Antiquity.* Library of Early Christianity 5. Philadelphia: Westminster, 1986.
Fronto, Marcus Cornelius. *The Correspondence of Marcus Cornelius Fronto.* Translated by C. R. Haines. 2 vols. Loeb Classical Library. New York: Putnam, 1919-1920.
Thraede, Klaus. *Grundzüge griechisch-römischer Brieftopik.* Zetemata 48. Munich: Beck, 1970.
Weissenrieder, Annette. "Contested Spaces in 1 Corinthians 11:17-34 and 14:30: Sitting or Reclining in Ancient Houses, Associations and the Ancient Ekklesia." In *Contested Spaces: Houses and Temples in Roman Antiquity and New Testament*, edited by David L. Balch and Annette Weissenrieder, 59-107. Wissenschaftliche Untersuchungen zum Neuen Testament 285. Tübingen: Mohr/Siebeck, 2012.
———. "Innenansichten eines Kranken. Krankheit in der Briefliteratur (L. Annaeus Seneca, Markus Cornelius Fronto und Paulus)" In: *Rezeption biblischer Heilungserzählungen als Konstruktion von dis/ability*, edited by W. Grünstäudl et al., 65-92. Leuven: Brill, 2017.
———. "Darum sind viele körperlich und seelisch Kranke unter euch" (1 Cor 11,29ff.). Die korinthischen Überlegungen zum Abendmahl im Spiegel antiker Diätetik und der Patristik." In *"Eine gewöhnliche und harmlose Speise?" Von den Entwicklungen frühchristlicher Abendmahlstraditionen*, edited by Judith Hartenstein et al., 239-68. Gütersloh: Gütersloher, 2008.
———, Dolle, Katrin. *Körper und Verkörperung. Neutestamentliche Anthropologie im Kontext antiker Medizin und Philosophie. Ein Quellenbuch* (forthcoming 2017).
Whitehorne, J. E. G. "Was Marcus Aurelius a Hypochondriac?" *Latomus* 36 (1977): 413-421.
Whitmarsh, Tim. *The Second Sophistic.* Greece & Rome. New Surveys in the Classics 35. Cambridge: Cambridge University Press, 2005.

16

The Numinous Dimension in New Testament Narratives

Reorienting Miracle Research

—Werner Kahl

Nicht müde werden
sondern dem Wunder
leise
wie einem Vogel
die Hand hinhalten.

—Hilde Domin

INTRODUCTION

THE EXEGETICAL DISCOURSE ON New Testament miracles in the past century has largely been dominated by scholars of the West who do not believe in miracles and who have been quick in denouncing such a belief as an expression of a primitive understanding of the world. In this perspective, Jesus could be presented predominantly as ethical teacher or revolutionary leader. If the term "miracle worker" was still applied to Jesus, then it was with the understanding that *in reality* of course he did not perform miracles, because miracles in the strict sense of the word do not happen, have never happened and will never happen. They are an *absolute* impossibility since they would contradict the rules of the laws of nature as well as everyday experience. Therefore, people of antiquity only misunderstood and portrayed Jesus as miracle worker.[1]

During the past generation, a shift of the centre of gravity in worldwide Christianity has occurred, from the North to the South. In this process, a different kind of Christianity has emerged which is no longer dependent on Western interpretations of reality, the Bible, and the Christian faith. Today a vast majority of Christians worldwide believe in miracles, in works of the Holy Spirit, and in the existence of demonic forces. And theologians and exegetes in the Global South tend to share this belief, rejecting, e.g., the program of demythologizing as implausible within their frames of reference and as irrelevant for their living contexts. Due to processes of global migration, African and Asian versions of Pentecostal and Charismatic Christianity have become domestic also in the Western world. In these churches, members read the Bible as a direct portrayal of their own world. Healing miracles and deliverance from demonic forces hindering a successful life feature prominently as themes in their church services. And the believers are convinced, as the saying goes: "God is the same—yesterday, today, and tomorrow." Therefore, miracles can happen today as they happened in Biblical times.[2]

But also in Western academia the subject "myth" has been revisited and narrations of miracles have been rehabilitated.[3] Slowly these insights are beginning to be reflected also in the exegetical discourse.[4]

The exegetical discourse of the West on miracles in the New Testament is still, however, widely continuing on the exegetical and hermeneutical pathways set out by scholars from Rudolf Bultmann to Gerd Theißen. The concept underlying the recent publication of the *Kompendium der frühchristlichen Wundererzählungen* is a case in point.[5] Here a modern understanding of reality is superimposed onto the New Testament narra-

---

1. Cf. the discussion by Alkier and Moffitt, "Miracles Revisited," 321–24.

2. Cf. Kahl, "Geisterfahrung als Empowerment," 21–29; Fischer, *Pfingstbewegung*.

3. Cf. especially the contribution of the philosopher Hübner, *Die Wahrheit des Mythos*.

4. Cf. for the German exegetical discourse, esp. Klumbies, *Der Mythos bei Markus*; idem, Wunderexegese; Alkier, *Wunder*; idem, "Wen wundert was?"

5. Zimmermann, ed., *Kompendium*. For a critical discussion of the concept laid out by Zimmermann, cf. note 45 below.

tives. What is needed instead, however, is an assessment of New Testament miracle traditions strictly "within *their* concepts of reality."[6]

This present contribution is dedicated to developing an *emic* approach to New Testament *miracle traditions*,[7] taking seriously essentials of ancient Mediterranean concepts of reality.[8] I will focus this investigation on miracles pertaining to a restoration of health or life. Categories long taken for granted such as "miracle story" and "miracle worker" will be deconstructed in the course of this presentation.[9]

---

6. Cf. for this alternative approach taking different conceptions of reality into serious account, the contributions in Alkier and Weissenrieder, *Miracles Revisited*.

7. /Miracle traditions/ refers here generally to *all* episodes in which a *miracle motif* occurs, regardless of its function. Throughout this paper I put between quotation marks "miracle story" and "miracle worker" to indicate the problematic nature of this designation, cf. the discussion and proposal below under 5.

8. Some parts of this paper are an elaboration of my contribution "New Testament Healing," 337–48.

9. This article to a certain degree summarizes and actualizes my research into the New Testament miracle traditions over the past twenty years. In the course of this time, the recognition of the importance of taking different world-knowledge systems into account, including the one shared by the researcher, has become a central concern of my work. This was stimulated by experiences and reflections during fieldwork and life in West Africa. Remarkably, I re-encountered the etic/emic debate which I had introduced into the analysis of "miracle healing stories" on the level of literature, in my ethnologically informed studies regarding West African cultural interpretations of the New Testament. The terminology was coined in the 1950s by the American linguist and anthropologist Kenneth L. Pike in his ground-breaking work *Language in Relation to a Unified Theory* and applied to the study of folklore and texts by his student Alan Dundes, "From Etic to Emic," 95–105, and *Morphology*. Dundes connected the etic/emic distinction with the motif/function distinction which was developed and introduced into the field of the study of folktales in 1928 by the Russian folklorist Propp in his *Morphology of the Folktale*, cf. the introduction to the second edition of 1968 by Dundes (xi–xvii) and especially his "Study of Folklore," 136–142: "The basic methodology of studying folklore in literature and studying folklore in culture is almost exactly the same; in other words, the discipline of folklore has its own methodology applying equally to literary and cultural problems" (136). Interestingly, the analysis of Propp with respect to the morphology of folktales (published in the Russian original in 1928) coincided with similar observations described by Pike's teacher, the American linguist and anthropologist Edward Sapir with respect to the study of native American culture, published in 1927: "Unconscious Patterning," 156–172. For the significance of the etic/emic distinction for the study of miracles in antiquity, cf. below under 4.

THE NUMINOUS—
THE UNPREDICTABLE CAREER OF A CATEGORY

Rudolf Otto introduced the category "das Numinose"—the numinous—into the fields of theology and religious studies. According to Otto, the numinous is the *essence* of all religion. The term denotes "holiness minus moralistic and rationalistic aspects."[10] Not only did Otto identify and write about this new category; even the expressionistic writing style of his influential work *Das Heilige*, 1917, seems shaped by the author's own encounter with numinous realities. After a few decades of thriving amongst some phenomenologists of religion (including van Leuw, Heiler, Mensching, and Eliade), the term was categorically rejected in Germany. Around the middle of the 20th century, the term lost appeal amongst international scholars of theology and of history of religion, the critical study of religion.[11] According to critics from the field of the study of religion, Otto's work demonstrated "the radical decontextualization and deprocessualization of religious data"[12]; it came to be regarded as an expression of "anti-historicism." On the one hand, the numinous appeared devoid of any concern for questions of religious identity and the role of social contexts favouring an irrational emotional dimension of religious experience; on the other hand, it was indicted for its ontologized transcendence.[13] For these reasons, and others, the category became increasingly stigmatised as un-scientific in the study of religion field. Most scholars abandoned the category numinous. Also theologians likewise disregarded the category as being problematic.

The logic behind this rejection is quite telling. I quote from Friedrich Feigel's critique of Otto's work: "Otto's Numinosum erweist sich für die Begründung der *Wahrheit* der Religion als ungeeignet, weil es noch nicht einmal eine Möglichkeit an die Hand gibt, Gott vom Teufel zu unterscheiden."[14]

Ironically, it is this very ambivalence of the term *Das Numinose* which might account for its value as a means to compare religious narratives in more "neutral" terms.[15] This appealed to researchers like Robert Levy,

---

10. Otto, *Das Heilige*, 6: "... das Heilige *minus* seines sittlichen Momentes und ... minus seines rationalen Momentes überhaupt."

11. For an overview on the history of the category on which I rely here, cf. Johannsen, *Das Numinose*, 11–96.

12. Grotanelli and Lincoln, "History of Religions," 317.

13. Kippenberg and von Stuckrad, *Einführung in die Religionswissenschaft*, 142–43.

14. Feigel, *Das Heilige*, 133 (translation: Kahl): "Otto's Numinosum is useless for establishing the *truth* of religion, since it does not even allow to distinguish God from the devil."

15. Cf. Johannsen, *Das Numinose*, 90.

Jeanette Mageo, and Alan Howard who shied away from referring to the "spiritual," "supernatural" or "to a non-empirical reality" because such vocabulary tended to reinforce ethno-centricism. It is therefore no coincidence that Otto's category survived in the fields of ethnology, folklore studies, and comparative literature. In their methodological introduction, the editors of the volume *Spirits in Culture, History, and Mind*—a collection of ethnological papers from 1996[16]—defended their preference for the term "numinous." "Numinous" from this perspective denotes a realm different from everyday experiences within the visible world, without superimposing the interpretation of reality dominant in a particular culture; instead of using the term "spiritual beings" cross-culturally, they prefer the term *numinals* as a more neutral category.

"NUMINOUS POWER" AS USEFUL CATEGORY

In the past generation, the problematic of terminology and categorization has been critically reflected upon in New Testament studies. This pertains especially to terms such as "Spätjudentum" (late Judaism), "Jewish legalism," and the like. With respect to understanding New Testament references to miracles in the Gospel narratives, Rudolf Bultmann, e.g., disregards these traditions as unacceptable expressions of an immature faith. Accordingly he refers to them as "mirakulös." In this perspective, the belief in miracles is due to a magical understanding of the world. A faith that is dependent on the word of God in Christ alone represents the proper Christian attitude. This faith constitutes, for Bultmann, the real Christian miracle.[17]

Especially with regard to understanding the miracles narrated in the Gospels, the question is: Given the fact that Western exegetes generally do not share a belief in miracles and demonic activity, how can we represent in *emically*[18] sensitive and methodologically controlled ways ancient belief systems such as come to expression in New Testament "miracle stories"? The very category "miracle story" might be a problematic designation of particular episodes in the narrative sections of the New Testament. This category might be an expression of an *etic* approach to the material with the potential to cloud, rather than to illumine the meaning dimensions of New Testament texts.[19]

---

16. Levy, Mageo and Howard, "Gods, Spirits, and History," 13.
17. Bultmann, *Mythologie*.
18. As for the emic/etic terminology, cf. the discussion below in section 4.
19. Cf. the discussion below in section 5.

Definition of Miracle

"Miracle" in the context of the academic study of ancient religion is a term referring to the *interpretation and characterization of an event as the manifestation of an activity of a numinous power*, i.e. of a personalized spiritual being with an ability—miracle power—that exceeds human abilities.[20]

The English word miracle—the same applies to the German word *Wunder*—is an imprecise "umbrella term" compared to a whole variety of words available in ancient Greek which highlight distinct features of such an event: *thaûma* (the wonder aspect), *dynámeis* (the power aspect), *érga* (the performative aspect), *parádoxa* (the unexpected and strange aspect), *semeîa* (the signifying aspect), *térata* (the dreadful aspect), to name only the most significant of terms. This variety in terminology reflects a differentiated knowledge of miracles in antiquity.[21]

The Narrative Schema and the Description of "Miracle Healing Stories"

In my book *New Testament Miracle Stories* I tried to compare *neutrally* New Testament *episodes narrating a miraculous healing* with narratives actualizing the same motif in the *Tanakh*, Qumran literature, writings of Hellenistic and Rabbinic Judaism, as well as with narratives from Greco-Roman traditions. The challenge was to avoid *methodologically* the ever luring temptation of elevating the New Testament narratives over against those of other traditions, as had been common in some of New Testament scholarship.[22] Searching for a solution I turned to the study of method with respect to the analysis and comparison of narratives from different cultures: methods that had been developed and tested in the fields of folklore studies, ethnology, and semiotics, esp. structuralism. I adopted the *Narrative Schema* derived from Algirdas J. Greimas' reorganization[23] of Vladimir Propp's thirty one narrative functions[24] which had been introduced into the field of New Testament studies by Hendrikus Boers[25] and I applied it to the analysis and comparison of approximately 150 narratives of "miracle healing stories" from Mediterranean antiquity.[26]

---

20. For the definition, cf. Kahl, "Verständigung," 99.
21. Cf. Kahl, "Wunder," 1966–1977; Alkier, "Wunder—Neues Testament," 1719–20.
22. Cf. the overview in Kahl, *Miracle Stories*, 19ff.
23. Cf. Greimas and Courtés, *Sémiotique*, 244–47.
24. Propp, *Morphology of the Folktale*.
25. Boers, "Introduction," xxxvii–lxix, lxv; Boers, *A Study of John 4, 9–14*.
26. Kahl, *Miracle Stories*, 44–62.

A. NEED	B. PREPAREDNESS	C. PERFORMANCE	D. SANCTION
A subject of a circumstance disjoined from a desirable object or con-joined with an undesirable object.	An active subject, willing or obliged, and able (having the power) to overcome the need, specified in A, by a performance.	The active subject performing the action to transform the circumstance specified in A into the opposite.	Recognition of the success or failure of the performance, or of the achievement of a desired value.

The Narrative Schema

This model proved useful in reducing the risk of favouring one tradition over the other. I simply analysed the sequence of narrative moves, strictly confined to the syntagmatic unfolding of events, in order to distinguish structural features from the level of motif. In so doing, I arrived at the following structuralistically informed *description* of "miracle healing stories" as narratives with a particular thematic actualisation. This is, however, *not* to be mistaken for an attempt at constituting a "genre"—on the contrary:[27]

A so-called "miracle healing story" shares the same morphology with other narratives. It describes the move from a need to the fulfilment of that need by means of a performance of an active subject specially prepared for the task. The difference between *miracle healing* stories and other narratives lies in the way structural features ("motifemic slots") are realised, i.e. the difference is located on the level of *motif*. The initial need belongs to the topic of *health*. This need can only be fulfilled by the involvement of a *bearer of numinous power* in the phase of the preparedness and / or performance,

---

[27] It should be noted that in my *New Testament Miracle Stories* I presupposed, and made use of the category "miracle stories," which was also retained in the title of the book. My structuralist analyses of these stories, however, lead to the realization that this category is problematic and should *not* be regarded as a "genre," and that the same applies to sub-categories. Here the critique of K. Berger has been fully supported by my research. I proposed a *re-classification* of these stories according to *inner-narrative function* together with a similar analysis of the whole narrative, and eventually of non-narrative material of the New Testament, cf. Kahl, *Miracle Stories*, 173–215, 237: "Further studies call for a reassessment of all the narrative material of the NT from a structural perspective." In a recent critique of the form-critical approach to the narrative material in question, Klumbies interprets my analysis in line with former form-critical attempts at circumscribing a "Gattungsschema" for these stories, only "in lediglich modifizierter Nomenklatur," cf. Klumbies, "Grenze," 27. He completely misses the point that by structural analysis, I arrived at the conclusion clearly communicated even in the German summary at the end of the book, "dass die Kategorie 'Wundererzählung' eine zweifelhafte Klassifikation ist" (Kahl, *Miracle Stories*, 239). This was a significant *result* of my analyses.

either directly or through a mediator. The reversal of the initial circumstance depends on the involvement of some numinous power, since—from the perspective of normal human ability—the initial lack is irreversible: "Consequently, the involvement of a *bearer of numinous power* (BNP) in the narrative process, its activation for and its engagement in a NP (narrative program, W.K.) aimed at the reversal of the initial circumstance, plays a crucial role in miracle stories."[28] In consequence, "miracle healing stories" could be described as narratives in which "the initial lack belongs to the category of *health* and a bearer of *numinous power* is involved in the narrative development at the phase of the preparedness and/or performance, either directly or through a mediator."[29]

Differentiating the Term "Miracle Worker"

Comparing about 150 "miracle healing stories" and analyzing the functions of active subjects, I realized that the widely used term *miracle worker* was misleading when it was applied to figures like Abraham, Moses, Elijah, Elisha, Tobit, Hanina ben Dosa, Jesus of Nazareth, Peter, Paul, Asclepios, the God of Israel, Vespasian, Apollonius of Tyana, and others, alike. Those figures function in *different roles* within "miracle healing narratives." Therefore I introduced three types of figures which are actively involved in the miracle healing performance: *bearer of numinous power* (BNP: like the God of Israel, Jesus, Asclepios, and Apollonius), *petitioner of numinous power* (PNP: like Moses, Hanina ben Dosa, Peter, and Paul), and *mediator of numinous power* (MNP: like Tobit and Vespasian). Figures of the latter two types do *not incorporate constantly* numinous healing power. Often PNPs can also function as MNPs in one and the same narrative, as is the case with Moses, Elijah, Elisha, Peter, and Paul. This distinction has proved useful. It helps to understand more precisely than possible before the distinct functions of various figures featured in these narratives.[30]

---

28. Kahl, *Miracle Stories*, 63–64.

29. Ibid., 233.

30. Exegesis from a history of religion and genre point of view has made plausible that New Testament stories narrating a miraculous healing have to be understood in comparison with similar stories which abound in Mediterranean antiquity. While *not* presupposing a general "genre" of "miracle healing stories," it can nevertheless be of heuristic value to compare stories with a common theme or with common motifs. This however can constitute only the *first step* in an attempt at understanding the New Testament narratives. *On the basis of religionsgeschichtliche* comparison and structural and narrative analysis, the stories have then to be interpreted within the given micro- and macro-contexts of a gospel in order to come close to an *emically* appropriate understanding of their particular functions and meaning dimensions; here I am in agreement with Klumbies, "Grenze."

Analyzing narratives from Mediterranean antiquity is an exercise in cross-cultural understanding. Our modes of conceiving of reality and of manipulating "world" in the modern West are markedly different from those presupposed as conventional knowledge in the New Testament writings. Given this difference, the modern interpretation of these writings originating in cultures distant in location and time is a complex endeavour. This problematic is all too often not reflected in depth in New Testament studies. In this respect, much could be learned from insights gained in the field of ethnology, pertaining especially to the problematic of cross-cultural representation and translation as discussed with reference to the etic/emic terminology in the insider/outsider debate.[31]

Comparing narratives from *various* distinct traditions of antiquity, as is necessary in the context of history of religions of "miracle healing stories," how could justice be done to each and every one of them? Terms like magical, miraculous, supernatural, occult, or mythical have problematic and derogatory undertones. "Numinous" as an attribute of "power," however, might be a neutral and broad enough term to denote the competence and activity of such diverse figures as gods, angels, unclean spirits, demons, ancestors, Satan, and so on. In Latin, "numen" at times denotes a deity, and at times the effects of its activity. I propose the use of "numinous" in a more general sense, and give the following *definition of numinous power*: It denotes a power effecting changes beyond human ability which is attributed to the competence and activity of spiritual or divine beings.

The involvement of such figures clearly comes to expression in "miracle healing narratives." It should be noted that "numinous power" in the above definition is considered neutral—simply signifying the activities of figures connected to a numinous sphere. Only in actual healing narratives are the involved powers qualified as good or evil, life enhancing or destructive—depending on the value system of the narrator. It should also be noted that in the New Testament, God and Christ's power can also cause death and destruction, miracles can be attributed to Satan (Rev 13:11–15; 2Thess 2:3–10; Matt 24:24), and critics ascribed Jesus' healing activity to demonic forces (cf. Mark 3:22).

As for the presentation of Jesus in the Synoptic Gospels, the records describe the Holy Spirit descending into (Mark 1:10: εἰς) or onto him (Matt 3:16 and Luke 3:22: ἐπ' αὐτόν). For example, this happens at the occasion of his baptism when the Spirit bestows Jesus with *constant* divine power (cf. Mark 1:22: ὡς ἐξουσίαν ἔχων; 1:27: διδαχὴ καινὴ κατ' ἐξουσίαν; Luke 4:36: ἐν ἐξουσίᾳ καὶ δυνάμει; cf. 4:14: ἐν τῇ δυνάμει τοῦ πνεύματος). Due to this

---

31. Kahl, *Jesus als Lebensretter*, 153–183.

divine preparedness he is enabled to overcome Satan resp. the Devil and to drive out "unclean spirits" from people, healing them, and restoring their personal and communal integrity.³² Like God in the Jewish tradition, angels or other, "unclean spirits" or demons belong to the numinous sphere. As such, however, their activities may have effects within the visible world.

Due to their numinous power, the unclean spirits can overpower human beings, causing illness and social ostracism, among other circumstances that are not desired from a regular human perspective. These spirits recognize that the numinous power of Jesus surpasses theirs. Within the Markan narrative they, and only they, know who Jesus is immediately upon encountering him: Jesus as the Holy one of God: οἶδά σε τίς εἶ, ὁ ἅγιος τοῦ θεοῦ (Mark 1:24; cf. 5:7: Τί ἐμοὶ καὶ σοί, Ἰησοῦ υἱὲ τοῦ θεοῦ τοῦ ὑψίστου;). As such, Jesus was declared by a heavenly voice after the spirit had descended onto him as: "You are my beloved son" (1:11: Σὺ εἶ ὁ υἱός μου ὁ ἀγαπητός, ἐν σοὶ εὐδόκησα). By implication, the narrative informs its readers that Jesus is the "son of God." Whatever the precise meaning of the designation "son of God" might have been in the matrix of ancient Judaism within which the term has to be located,³³ it signifies from an early Christian perspective that Jesus is different from OT prophets, certain rabbinic figures, early Christian apostles, or shamans past and present: He *constantly incorporates divine power* by means of which he is able, inter alia, to restore health and life. This is brought to expression in the numerous miracle healing stories of all the Gospels: God's healing power extends to Jesus. He, as an *innerworldy* figure, is presented as a constant *bearer of numinous power*. This is—apart from the historically later figure of Apollonios of Tyana—a unique attribution in ancient miracle healing stories. Other figures indiscriminately designated as "miracle workers" in New Testament scholarship are either transcendent gods that might appear on earth for a particular performance, or they are human beings who are being used by a god or who might be endowed temporarily with numinous ability for a particular performance. The latter may function as *mediators of numinous power* or they may appear as figures that are able to motivate, persuade, or force a transcendent being to engage in a miracle healing. As such they function as *petitioners of numinous power* like Hanina ben Dosa, who in Rabbinic literature is portrayed as a rabbi with the special ability to successfully reach God with prayer requests. But he is *not* a miracle worker in the strict sense of the word. The same applies to Paul

---

32. Cf. Kahl, "Neutestamentliche Verfahren," 19–29.
33. Cf. the study by Boyarin, *The Jewish Gospels*.

according to Acts[34] and according to his epistles.[35] With respect to Rabbinic literature, the miracle worker is *God* as transcendent *bearer of numinous power.*

NUMINOUS POWER AND CONCEPTS OF REALITY

We try to make sense of the ambiguities of life as members of communities within distinct cultures. We cannot escape being bound to traditions of conventionalized knowledge within which we experience and conceptualize, communicate, manipulate, and forecast reality. This also holds true for discourses on concepts of reality. The very terms "reality" and "existence" open up whole universes of meaning, and at the same time, they also limit our understanding.

Around the turn of the century, I spent three years in West Africa doing field research on the interpretation of the Bible in Ghana. I tried to understand the cultural frame of reference—the encyclopaedia in and through which people make sense of the world and of the Bible in West Africa. My experiences and reflections in Ghana allowed for a fresh view on the "miracle healing stories" of the New Testament, and I became aware of meaning dimensions in these narratives previously hidden from me.[36]

Classicists working in West Africa in the fifties and sixties of the last century had already observed that a West African cultural perspective might be helpful in gaining insights with respect to life in antiquity, as, e.g., John Ferguson claimed 1967 while teaching in Nigeria:

> Our Classics department is set in one of the few parts of the world where you can still consult oracles, where there are tonal languages (as Classical Greek was tonal), where there is a living tradition of religious dance-drama (what is Greek tragedy in origin but that?), where sacrifice is understood, where contemporary society offers many fascinating parallels to ancient Greek

---

34. The story in Acts 14:8–18 is striking since this is the only miracle healing story in Acts where an apostle *seems* to cause miracle healing himself, i.e. without any reference to prayer, to laying on of hands or a reference to the "name of Jesus." The people in Lystra witnessing the healing cannot but interpret it in the following way: The gods Zeus and Hermes have appeared in the human forms of Barnabas and Paul respectively. This is also clear evidence that *human miracle workers* in the sense of humans possessing miracle power *constantly*, i.e. functioning as bearers of numinous power, were not believed to be a realistic possibility.

35. With respect to the Pauline epistles, this has been convincingly pointed out by Alkier, *Wunder.*

36. The results of this research have been published in Kahl, *Jesus als Lebensretter.*

and Roman society. Nigerian scholars, if they will look at the classics with Nigerian and not European eyes, can interpret the classics to us in ways no European scholar can do.[37]

A note of caution is in order here: It would be problematic to *identify* concepts of reality or cultural features of contemporary West Africa with corresponding concepts of societies in Mediterranean antiquity, but certainly the former often exhibit certain degrees of closeness to the latter, esp. when compared with perspectives of the modern West.[38] With respect to the subject of the miraculous and the numinous in New Testament "healing narratives," it is obvious that certain affinities do exist between West African and ancient Mediterranean experiences of life and the construction of reality. This applies first and foremost to the ever present reality of untimely death and the unpredictable occurrence of disease, and secondly to sickness aetiologies which reckon with the possibility of the involvement of evil spirits as root-cause for the predicament of an individual. At the same time, quite a number of people interpret and communicate an experienced healing in terms of miracle. The realities of ever threatening incurable diseases, of disease causing spirits and of miracle healings are to be presupposed as self-evident in antiquity in general and in early Christianity in particular. Against this background, Martin Dibelius' rationalistic and romanticized verdict that New Testament "miracle healing stories" were an expression of a "Lust am Mirakel"—a delight taken in miraculous events—seems to miss the point:[39] New Testament "healing stories" make transparent, inter alia, the struggle of survival or the struggle to (re)gain health in life-threatening circumstances that were common in antiquity. These stories contain a narrative expression of the early Christian belief that God might assist them in overcoming sickness and help ward off potentially fatal attacks of evil spirits. The Lord's Prayer, e.g., asks to deliver us from evil, which most likely refers to saving and protecting from evil forces. What is at stake in the "miracle healing traditions" is a matter of life and death. According to the general concept of reality in antiquity, an individual is *not* the master of his or her life and death; he or she is rather *sub-iectus* to both the family or the community and to the powers of the numinous sphere. Regarding the latter, the visible world is experienced and thought of as *embedded* in a wider

---

37. Quoted in Bediako, *Christianity in Africa*, 252.

38. Cf. the references to African examples in Fortes, *West African Religion*; Burkert, *Creation of the Sacred*.

39. Dibelius, *Formgeschichte*, 171. Dibelius seems to apply an observation made by Aristotle in his Poetics to the New Testament: "The miraculous is pleasant" (*Poetics* 1460a). Aristotle's observation, drawn from everyday experience, refers to tragedies for stage performance and to epic writing, not to quasi historical writings like the Gospels.

net of activities of various spiritual beings including gods, angels, demons, ancestors, etc. belonging to the invisible, numinous sphere.[40] The seen world is always intermingled with the unseen world of spiritual forces.[41]

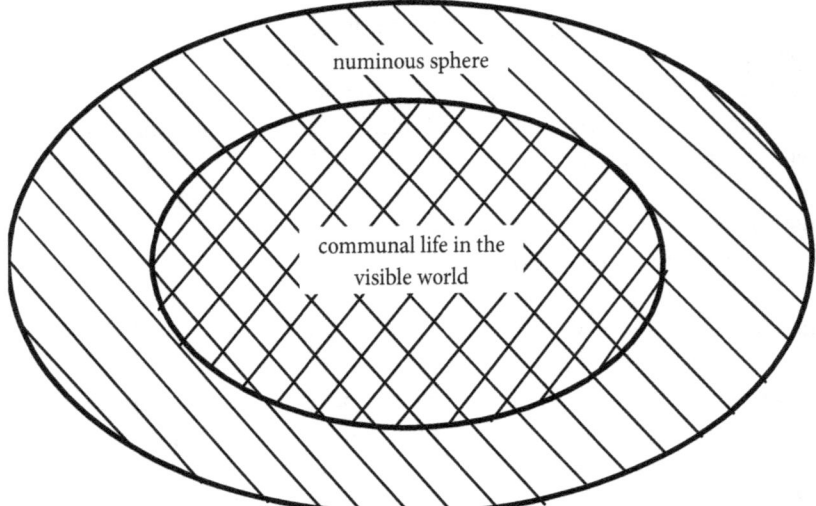

Ancient Mediterranean World Knowledge Systems

With this knowledge of the world, it was of utmost importance to avoid the wrath of gods or fall prey to the spell of an evil spirit in order to avoid disasters such as grave illness.[42] Getting infected or possessed by such a spirit is a problem that is not to be limited to the affairs of the

40. Cf. Kahl, *Lebensretter*, 181–201.

41. Cf. the apt statement by Klumbies in his recent article "Wunderexegese" (31) drawing here on philosophical insights of the philosophers Kurt Hübner and Ernst Cassirer: "Seither hat die Einsicht in die Rationalität des Mythos an Boden gewonnen. Als Konsequenz wird die wechselseitige Durchdringung von Diesseitigem und Jenseitigem, von Menschlichem und Göttlichem, von natürlichen Vorgängen und numinosen Ereignissen, von Materialität und Immaterialität neu wahrgenommen. Spirituelles und Körperliches bilden nach mythischer Weltanschauung eine Einheit. Die auslösenden Ursachen für körperliche Defekte liegen auf spiritueller Ebene. Numinose Mächte nehmen Einfluss auf die empirisch vorfindlichen Welt. Durchweg führt der Erkenntnisweg von den Ursachen im spirituell-numinosen Bereich zu den Wirkungen in materiell-körperlicher Hinsicht." This is supported by the investigation of ancient Greco-Roman medical traditions of, e.g., Weissenrieder ("Stories Just Under the Skin," 73–100); and Tieleman, "Miracle and Natural Cause in Galen," 112: For Galen, "god(s) and nature belong to one and the same continuous reality, in which universal rules obtain."

42. Cf. the following works of classicists and historians: Graf, *Gottesnähe*; Burkert, *Creation of the Sacred*; Rüpke, *Religion der Römer*; Gehrke, *Hellenismus*, 78–85; Dahlheim, *Kaiserzeit*, 273–279.

subject involved. In communal societies which were the norm in Mediterranean antiquity, such a condition would have repercussions for the whole community, transgressing even the bounds of the extended family. Warding off attacks of life threatening spirits could only be achieved by securing the help of a friendly numinous power.[43] Taking this conception into account, I propose a more radical understanding of the significance of the numinous sphere in antiquity compared with positions long taken for granted in New Testament scholarship, according to which numinous powers or evil spirits in antiquity including the New Testament writings played a less dramatic role. Susan Garrett, e.g., in a recent publication speaks of a mere "influence of invisible powers in affairs of the visible world."[44] I propose that this "influence," perceived in antiquity as *all-pervasive* and ever threatening, should be taken more seriously. In this scenario, it is human beings who hope to counter and "influence" the invisible powers. Thus, humans tried to exercise power through their behaviour, by performing sacrifices or magic, or through intermediaries like priests, healers, or shamans.

It should be noted that this ancient concept of reality is *not* irrational[45] and it was also *not* an expression of simple minded and uneducated popula-

---

43. As in Mediterranean antiquity, similar strategies to explain and to address misfortune have been described for traditional societies, e.g., in West Africa. With regard to the Dagomba people in Northern Ghana, cf. the ethnological observation by Kirby, *Northern Ghana*, 237: "Although people believe in the natural causation of various difficulties and problems like illness, victims normally also seek out the root cause and the personal cause—not just how the problem came about but also what was the unseen force behind the visible causes and 'why the thing came to me and not to you.' Thus, in seeking a solution, recourse will usually be made to the unseen world through various shrines and sacrifices, offerings and libations, exorcisms, incantations and invocations, as well as through prayers and supplications to the ancestors, the divinities and finally, after all else fails, to God."

44. Garrett, "Jesus als Befreier," 19.

45. Cf. Zimmermann, "Grundfragen," 7–67, with respect to early Christian "miracle stories" (31): "Die erzählte Veränderung am *realistischen* Inventar (Menschen, Sachen, Natur) überschreitet dabei die Grenze zwischen gewohnter Weltordnung und dem *Irrealen*. Die Erzählung erzeugt hierbei bewusst eine Spannung, inszeniert gerade das *Gegenrationale* und *Unmögliche*" (italics W.K.). Early Christian "miracle stories" are here understood within the reference system of modernity, according to which belief in miracle is irrational since, from the perspective of this conventionalized knowledge of the world, neither miracles in the true sense of the word nor numinous beings were real. The contrary, however, holds true for Mediterranean antiquity in general and for early Christianity in particular. Here, miracles are *not* absolutely "impossible." They are impossible only for human beings who have not been endowed with numinous power. They *are* possible, however, for numinous beings, cf. Luke 1:37: "Nothing will be impossible with God" (cf. for the biblical tradition: Gen 18:14; Job 42:2; Mark 10:27 par.; cf. also Alkier, "Feeding," 5–22). This is common knowledge in antiquity as it is in much of the contemporary world in the Global South. Zimmermann's assessment of

New Testament "miracle stories" is therefore an example of an *etic* perspective which fails to sense and communicate essential meaning dimensions of these narratives. This unsatisfactory approach generates a number of cross-cultural misunderstandings and problematic decisions. A fundamental flaw of this encyclopedia is, e.g., constituted by the decision to consider only "miracle stories" attached to "human miracle workers" (50–51). In consequence, the essential miracle presupposed in early Christianity, i.e. God's resurrection of Jesus is excluded from consideration.

But to what extent is Jesus a "*human* miracle worker"?—a question that Zimmermann himself raises (50–51). He brushes it aside, however, by claiming an avoidance of the application of a "anachronistische(n) Vorstellung der späteren Trinitätslehre" (51) to the New Testament presentations of Jesus. While it would indeed be problematic exegetically to read back into the New Testament later Trinitarian concepts, this is not a sufficient reason to treat Jesus as a "human miracle worker" within the context of the Gospel narratives, which in fact vary in their presentation of Jesus with respect to the relationship of human and divine aspects. The bottom line in the Gospels is that Jesus is *not* just like any other human being, and this comes to expression especially in the narratives that portray him as a miracle worker in the strict sense of the word, i.e. as a *bearer of numinous power*!

Zimmermann himself reads into the New Testament narratives anachronistically a modern concept of reality. Consequently, those early Christian witnesses are not taken seriously within their frames of reference. In their perspective, the human being Jesus *did incorporate divine healing power* (*dynamis* and *exousia*) *permanently*. In antiquity, this had inevitably to lead to the question of the relationship between God and Jesus, and this problematic is already reflected in the Gospels and in other New Testament writings (cf. also the same problematic with respect to Paul in Acts 14:8–18). In the strict sense of the word, a "human miracle worker" is, *from an ancient perspective*, an oxymoron. As I have shown in my *New Testament Miracle Stories*, in order to do justice to the interpretation and communication of reality in antiquity, "miracle worker" in the strict sense of the word should be reserved for figures that incorporate healing power permanently, and this holds true for gods especially—with Jesus and Apollonios of Tyana as remarkable exceptions, both of them being later divinized. The apostles Peter and Paul were clearly not regarded as "miracle workers" on the same level with Jesus. They functioned as *mediators of numinous power* in both directions, but they did not possess miracle power. Rather, God as *transcendent miracle worker* worked through them the same way as God— according to Luke only!—wrought miracles *through* Jesus (cf. Acts 2:22; 5:12; 19:12). It is in the presentation of Jesus as miracle worker in the *Qur'an* that Jesus is portrayed strictly as a human being. Therefore it is repeatedly made clear in the Qur'an that Jesus performed miracles "by the permission of God" (cf. Sura 3:49). In the Qur'an, a tendency that can be found in Luke-Acts (cf. Kahl, *Miracle Stories*, 226–227) appears radicalized.

Due to the afore-mentioned problematic pre-decisions in the *Kompendium*, several narratives with evident miracle motifs (cf. only Luke 1:5–25) are left out of consideration, even though, from an emic perspective, they make transparent the presence of the numinous power of God like any other "miracle story." The concept of the *Kompendium* is severely impaired by the superimposition of a modern understanding of the world in general and of miracles in particular, onto the New Testament narratives. Insights from the academic study of religion—Religionswissenschaft—help to come closer to an emically appropriate understanding of miracles in texts from antiquity, cf., e.g., Mensching, *Wunder*, 39: "Jesus ist in den Evangelien sowohl Objekt wie Subjekt von 'Wundern' . . ."

tions, even though such judgment has been passed by exegetes[46]—a typical attitude that frequently occurs in cross-cultural studies: "People of one nation (or class or society, etc.) may sometimes appear to another to be 'illogical' or 'stupid' or 'incomprehensible' simply because the observer is over a long period of time taking an alien standpoint from which to view their activity, instead to learn their emic patterns of overt and covert behaviour."[47]

This system of world-knowledge was shared by the educated strata of ancient societies. As we learn from Plutarch, there were varying degrees or intensities in reckoning with numinous powers, and only the *extremes* seemed problematic to Plutarch.[48] The reality of the potential involvement of numinous powers in everyday life affairs was self-evident to philosophers from Socrates via Aristotle to Plutarch. Reality was perceived to be more than its reduction to the visible and measurable world. Ancient concepts of the world *extended* reality into the invisible sphere of potent numinous powers or spiritual beings. Their activities could be regarded as spiritual root causes of experiences in the visible world interpreted as direct effects of these activities.

In order to come to a more appropriate, i.e. *emic* understanding of New Testament "miracle healing stories," it is necessary to constantly keep in mind the implications of ancient knowledge systems when interpreting these narratives. Since an understanding of the world in terms of the numinous was regarded as self-evident, its implications are at times only presupposed or alluded to in "miracle stories," so that the modern reader might have difficulty in grasping what is actually at stake in a particular story. The American anthropologist and linguist Edward Sapir described this dilemma in cross-cultural communication back in 1927 when he maintained that untrained observers in a foreign culture are constantly tempted to attribute weight to cultural items which might be of rather secondary importance to the cultural insiders while he or she might totally fail to notice or ignore the essential significance of, let us say, a ritual:

"Let anyone who doubts this try the experiment of making a painstaking report [i.e. an etic one] of the actions of a group of natives engaged in some activity, say religious, to which he has not the cultural key [i.e. a knowledge of the emic system]. If he is a skilful writer, he may succeed in giving a picturesque account of what he sees and hears, or thinks he sees and

---

46. With respect to exegetes like Rudolf Bultmann or Gerd Theißen declaring people who believe in miracles as naïve, primitive, or psychologically unstable, cf. Alkier, *Wunder und Wirklichkeit*, 4 and 28; Kahl, *Jesus als Lebensretter*, 167–68, esp. note 450.

47. Pike, *Language*, 51.

48. Plutarch, *Moralia*, 171E-F; cf. Xenophon, *Memorabilia*, 1:1:6–9. Cf. Kahl, "Gott und göttliche Wesen," 88–91.

hears, but the chances of his being able to give a relation of what happens, in terms that would be intelligible and acceptable to the natives themselves, are practically nil. He will be guilty of all manner of distortion; his emphasis will be constantly askew. *He will find interesting what the natives take for granted as a casual kind of behaviour worthy of no particular comment, and he will utterly fail to observe the crucial turning points* in the course of action that give formal significance to the whole in the minds of those who do possess the key to its understanding."[49]

Sapir's research prepared the etic-emic or insider-outsider debate in ethnology and folklore studies in the USA which was developed by his student Kenneth Pike in the fifties, and from the sixties onward, by Pike's student Alan Dundes.[50] The same dynamics described here are at play in the cross-cultural encounter of exegetes and classicists with ancient texts.

One example is the interpretation of Mark 1:29–31 (The mother-in-law of Simon is lying down feverish): "After Jesus approached her he raised her up after he took her hand. And the fever left her, and she served them" (v. 31). A modern reader might overlook the implication of the following phrase: καὶ ἀφῆκεν αὐτὴν ὁ πυρετός. The fever functions grammatically as active subject of the narrative move that immediately brings about healing, or to put it in terms of the Narrative Schema: The activity of the fever *effectuates* the disjunction from the undesirable object that the woman was previously conjoined with—undesirable from the perspective of the woman and her relatives as well as from the perspective of the Gospel writer. It seems to be implied that the fever is actually forced out of the woman by the physical connection brought about by Jesus: he takes her by the hand. In short, what is being described involves an *exorcism*. Luke's rendering of the story in 4:38–39 strongly reinforces the presupposition of a numinous power struggle in this case. Here we have Jesus ἐπετίμησεν τῷ πυρετῷ (v. 39) resulting in the fever's withdrawal from the woman. ἐπιτιμάω is a *terminus technicus* in ancient "exorcism stories," and we also find the expression in other New Testament "exorcism stories" such as in Mark 1:25 where Jesus commands an unclean spirit to leave a person, or in Mark 4:39 where Jesus commands the storm to calm down. It might not be obvious to a modern reader that an *exorcism* is being narrated in the storm stilling episode, with the storm as a numinous spirit being.

---

49. Pike, *Language*, 39 (italics added).

50. Sapir, "Religion," 134–145; Sapir, "Unconscious Patterning," 156–172; Pike, *Language*; Pike, "On the emics," 28–47; Pike and McKinney, "Understanding Misunderstanding," 39–64; Headland, "Introduction," 13–27; Dundes, "From Etic to Emic Units"; Dundes, *Morphology*.

Concerning Mark 1:29–31 it should be noted that Simon's mother-in-law, after being liberated from the fever, engages in the activity of "serving them," i.e. the visitors. What is the significance of this activity? From a form-critical perspective, this performance would solely signal, i.e. demonstrate the *success* of the miracle performance of Jesus.[51] This is certainly one function of this motif, but there is more to it: If "serving them" implies here—in line with general gender expectations in the Mediterranean world of antiquity—that the woman prepares food, then numinous as well as social-communal dimensions are involved, as would be self-evident, e.g., to the average West African reader of the story: In traditional society nobody would take food from a person regarded as polluted by an evil, i.e. sickness causing spirit. Note that in Mark's Gospel the common attribute of these spirits is *unclean*. This indicates, inter alia,[52] the contagious potential of these spirits resulting in communal stigmatization and separation of an infected or possessed person. People would be afraid to get contaminated, not only with the sickness but—even more dangerous—with the sickness-spirit.[53] Against this background it is remarkable that Jesus establishes *physical* contact with the feverish woman. By means of this touch causing the withdrawal of the fever, the narrator brings out the conviction that *Jesus' purity or divinely bestowed holiness is more contagious and stronger than the impurity of adverse spirits.*[54] Jesus engages here, and at other occasions, in a *spiritual power struggle*. At the same time, his very touching and raising the woman up signify the *reintegration* of the woman into her regular communal and family affairs, so we can come to a deeper understanding of what is being communicated in this short passage: *Jesus' integrative purity overrules the disintegrative impurity of adverse spirits*. From here, we can confirm the results of an anthropological study on James 5:13–16 by M.C. Albl who concludes that in early Christian healing rituals, the levels of the individual, the communal, and the spiritual intermingle.[55]

51. Cf. Lau, "Fieberfrei," 215.

52. Cf. Strecker, "Mächtig," in Zimmermann, *Wunderkompendium*, 205–13.

53. This meaning dimension is completely lost in the Western exegetical discourse, cf. as most recent example, Lau, "Fieberfrei."

54. Cf. Beck, *Nonviolent Story*.

55. Albl, "'Are any among you sick?'" Cf. also Weissenrieder, "Stories Just Under the Skin," who points out the interrelatedness of the—in modern terms—"natural" and the "supernatural" in ancient medical texts in general and in the New Testament episodes which narrate a healing in particular, as she is able to show in an analysis of Luke 17:11–19. It also becomes clear that these New Testament narratives "are often sprinkled with insights of ancient society and politics" (74). Here, the "good news" becomes concrete at the interface between the physical and the spiritual, the individual and the communal including politics and economics.

FROM "MIRACLE STORIES" TO "EPISODES NARRATING MIRACLE EVENTS"

The structuralist analysis of "miracle healing stories" led to the insight that these stories share one and the same fundamental structure with other narratives. The difference is located solely on the level of *motif with a particular theme*: these narratives refer—in one way or another and in a variety of functions—to a restoration of *health* by means of the involvement of a subject possessing *numinous power*.

The diversity of these *episodes*[56] that narrate a numinous move from a need of health or life to the fulfilment of that need, and the fact of the functional variability of the miracle *motif*[57] within episodes, however, strongly suggest that "miracle healing story" neither constitutes a genre nor even a particular "form." The same applies to the more general category "miracle story." All these episodes belong to the genre *narrative* in general and to "short prose" in particular: They could be labelled "short-short stories," "flash stories," "Kürzestgeschichten" or "micronouvelles." Even though these short narratives bear clear markers that justify their demarcation and treatment as episodes or pericopes,[58] their interpretation should never be isolated from their immediate and wider literary contexts. The functions of a particular episode can only be recognized by taking into account their connections with their literary context.[59]

In so-called "miracle stories," the miracle itself might not be located at the center of an episode, cf., e.g., Mark 3:1–6 par.; 7:24–30 par.; Matt 8:5–13 par. In these narratives, the miracle of healing appears only at the periphery of the narrative unfolding of the story. In Mark 3:1–6 par. the miracle healing functions as an *argument* in a debate.[60] The theme of the debate is: Is it allowed to heal on a Sabbath day? In Mark 7:24–30 par. and Matt 8:5–13 par. the miracle healing is mentioned only in passing at the very end of the episode. The theme here and there is the faith and confidence of those approaching Jesus for a healing, in both cases non-Jews. Labelling these episodes "miracle stories" is arbitrary and rather hinders than promotes

---

56. "Episode" signifies the narration of an action. It is demarcated as an enclosed unit of a larger narrative and it is more complex than a single event, cf. Martinez and Scheffel, *Erzähltheorie*, 110.

57. "Motif" or "event" signifies the "smallest elementary unit of an action," cf. Martinez and Scheffel, *Erzähltheorie*, 108.

58. For criteria of demarcating episodes in the Gospel accounts, cf. Patte, *Structural Exegesis*, 9–23.

59. Cf. for example the significance of Mark 8:22–26 in its context, Lang, "Maßarbeit," 115f.; Klumbies, "Wunderexegese," 38–44.

60. Cf. Kahl, "Sabbat," 313–35.

an appropriate understanding of these episodes which are not primarily concerned with the miracle event as such.

Again it becomes obvious: The narratives in question are too diverse to constitute a distinct genre or form of literature. Also, their functions vary significantly, be it with respect to their inner-narrative functions[61] or with respect to the functions these stories assume in their respective literary contexts.[62] Nevertheless, in the common exegetical literature *all* episodes that narrate *somehow* a miraculous move which is—at the same time—*not* attributed to a direct act of God or of numinous beings like angels, are allocated to a genre "miracle story."[63] In the tradition of Gerd Theißen's influential and work on miracles, often the following sub-genres would be delineated: therapies, exorcisms, epiphanies, salvific miracles, provisions and normative miracles.[64] This whole procedure, however, at all its levels is 1. untenable from the perspective of the academic study of literature, and 2. unproductive (at best) from an emic New Testament perspective.

ad 1: It should be noted that in the field of contemporary literary studies a genre "miracle story" is not known.[65] Genre is constituted by structural phenomena, not by content. But even if one were to consider "content," the so-called "miracle stories"—even if we were to limit these stories to the so-called "therapies"—are functionally too diverse to constitute a particular "form," not to speak of genre. The same applies to the other sub-genres suggested by Theißen.[66] Therefore the verdict of Klaus Berger holds: "Miracle story" "ist eine moderne Sammelbezeichnung rein inhaltlicher Art."[67] Not

---

61. Cf. Kahl, *Miracle Stories*, 173–215.

62. Klumbies, "Wunderexegese," is correct in requesting a move away from an isolated and decontextualized analysis of these episodes, favoring an interpretation of these episodes within their respective literary contexts, both on the micro- and macro-levels. This, however, should not lead to the other extreme of a dismissal of a comparison of these episodes with similar ones in Greco-Roman antiquity. Only a careful comparison with comparable *religionsgeschichtliche* material—also in its respective context!—will help to understand both the commonalities and differences between those traditions. Only by means of such comparison, the particular significance attached to Jesus by the Gospel writers in their various ways will become recognizable.

63. Cf. Zimmermann, "Grundfragen," 50–51 where he excludes miracles brought about by non-human "miracle workers" from consideration (cf. my critique of this decision in footnote 45).

64. Theißen, *Urchristliche Wundergeschichten*, 94–120.

65. Cf. Arnold and Detering, eds., *Literaturwissenschaft*; Anz, ed., *Handbuch*.

66. Cf. my critical analysis of several of this typology, in Kahl, *Miracle Stories*, 173–76; and in Kahl, *Jesus als Lebensretter*, 196–97.

67. Berger, "Hellenistische Gattungen," 1218.

surprisingly, in Greek antiquity there was no terminological equivalent to "miracle story."[68]

ad 2: The heuristic value of identifying episodes as "miracle stories" regardless of the specific functions of the miracle motif in particular episodes seems minimal, at best. It is unclear what how such a procedure would contribute to a more appropriate understanding of the meaning dimensions and functions of such diverse episodes, especially when taking into consideration that certain sections of the Gospel narratives most likely were not perceived by readers of antiquity as isolated "miracle stories" as opposed to other episodes any less miraculous. This would certainly apply to Mark 16:1–8 which refers—besides narrating other miracle events—to the basic miracle event in the New Testament, i.e. the resurrection of Jesus by God, by means of *one* verb: ἠγέρθη (16:6).[69] The reaction of the witnessing women corresponds to the experience of a divine miracle: καὶ ἐξελθοῦσαι ἔφυγον ἀπὸ τοῦ μνημείου, εἶχεν γὰρ αὐτὰς τρόμος καὶ ἔκστασις· καὶ οὐδενὶ οὐδὲν εἶπαν, ἐφοβοῦντο γάρ (16:8). Such a fearful reaction has been described as typical feature of "miracle stories" in form-critical exegetical literature. Yet, this episode is usually not counted among the "miracle stories."

Miracles would have been perceived in the Gospels by the ancients also in episodes in which exegetes would not sense any miracle, i.e. with respect to Jesus' *teaching* with authority (ἐξουσία, cf. Mark 1:21–28), including the so-called Sermon on the Mount (cf. Matt 7:28–29: Καὶ ἐγένετο ὅτε ἐτέλεσεν ὁ Ἰησοῦς τοὺς λόγους τούτους ἐξεπλήσσοντο οἱ ὄχλοι ἐπὶ τῇ διδαχῇ αὐτοῦ· ἦν γὰρ διδάσκων αὐτοὺς ὡς ἐξουσίαν ἔχων καὶ οὐχ ὡς οἱ γραμματεῖς αὐτῶν).

By the exegetes' claiming a genre of "miracle story," an emphasis is laid in particular episodes on motifs which are strange and disturbing to the modern mind, i.e. motifs that reflect a miraculous event—but only if the described event stands in *opposition* to what is regarded as possible in reality, from a modern perspective: a healing beyond human ability, an exorcism,

---

68. Also Zimmermann, "Grundfragen," is aware of the fact "dass die frühchristlichen Autoren kein *begriffliches* Gattungssignal im Sinne einer Lektüreanweisung geben, mit der man eine Gruppe von Texten unter eine Überschrift 'Wundererzählung' subsummieren könnte" (25). He nevertheless attributes a "Gattungsbewußtsein" to the Gospel writers, for questionable reasons: In the Gospel accounts, we find 1. summaries of Jesus' miracle activities, and 2. we find collections of particular episodes. These arguments, however, only indicate that the Gospel writers recognized various instances of Jesus' activities as miracles; they fall short of indicating a "Gattungsbewußtsein" in this respect.

69. This would be a "shortest narrative" communicated by one verb which describes—here in the passive voice as *passivum divinum*, cf. also 1Cor 15:5: ὤφθη—a single move from a lack to its liquidation by means of a performance of God, cf. for these minimal forms of narrative Genette, *Erzählung*, 14.

an epiphany, etc. In New Testament exegesis, events like Jesus' teaching are generally *not* regarded as miraculous, even though the reaction of those witnessing his teaching is *identical* with reactions to his exorcisms, indicating that from an emic perspective also the *teaching* of Jesus—and in fact, most if not all of the narrated and remembered expressions of Jesus[70]—could be perceived as miraculous (cf. again Mark 1:21–28 in comparison with Matt 7:28–29, and also Mark 6:2: καὶ γενομένου σαββάτου ἤρξατο διδάσκειν ἐν τῇ συναγωγῇ· καὶ πολλοὶ ἀκούοντες ἐξεπλήσσοντο λέγοντες, Πόθεν τούτῳ ταῦτα, καὶ τίς ἡ σοφία ἡ δοθεῖσα τούτῳ ἵνα καὶ δυνάμεις τοιαῦται διὰ τῶν χειρῶν αὐτοῦ γίνωνται;). The reason for the all-pervasive presence of the miraculous in the Gospel account lies in the fact that—as Stefan Alkier has recently demonstrated for the Gospel of Luke in a meticulous analysis of Luke's discourse universe—"every sign of the Gospel has to be read from (the) perspective" that God has been and still is at work in and through Jesus,[71] who "is the fleshly presence of God."[72]

The exegetical invention and application of the "genre" "miracle story" signifies an undue preoccupation with *some* New Testament miracle motifs. This focus clouds meaning dimensions in New Testament episodes that were essential for readers in antiquity, e.g., the miraculous dimension of Jesus' teaching, which in an emic perspective "was not from this world." In an emic perspective, the *complete range* of Jesus' activities, both in word and in deed, is understood in the four Gospel accounts as an expression of his particular connection with the numinous sphere.[73] Therefore, miracles abound in great variety during his "ministry," including his teaching, according to the Gospel accounts. This is not surprising, once the numinous dimension in ancient world-knowledge systems is recognised as an *essential* feature that was shared by early Christians.

The simple category "miracle story" falls short in achieving an appropriate representation of what is at stake in the Gospel narratives. In addition, by the identification, isolation and de-contextualization of so-called "miracle stories," references to miracles—*defined from a modern perspective as absolutely impossible*—tend to be eliminated from a serious consideration for informing Christian formation, past and present.[74] A case in point is the

---

70. For more evidence, cf. Kahl, "Wunder," 1969–1970, with respect to the Synoptic Gospels; Kahl, *Jesus als Lebensretter*, 197–198, with respect to the Gospel of Mark. Cf. Berger, *Formen*, 364: "Die Fähigkeit Jesu, Wunder zu wirken, ist allemal vorausgesetzt."

71. Alkier, "For nothing will be impossible," 17.

72. Ibid., 19.

73. Cf. Berger, *Formen*, 363: "Die ältere Formgeschichte hat—unter Betonung des Wortes—Wort und Tat zu stark geschieden."

74. It should be noted that in the nineteenth century it was the embarrassment

form-critical attribution of a certain "Sitz im Leben" to these stories which marked them as later inventions of faith communities for questionable functions like "propaganda" among "simple minded people."[75]

It needs to be emphasized that miracle is an *essential constituent* of early Christian faith that is grounded in the foundational miracle according to New Testament witnesses—the resurrection of Jesus from the dead by God.[76] The undifferentiated use of the category is not helpful as a tool to enhance our understanding of New Testament references to the miraculous within the numinous knowledge of the world in antiquity in general. In consequence, the usefulness of the category "miracle story" needs to be critically examined.

In the Gospel accounts, a whole range of various genres and forms contains references to *miracle motifs*. If one were to analyse the Gospels with an interest in these motifs, one could speak of *episodes narrating miracle events*.[77]

It could be instructive to classify *episodes narrating miracle events* according to the main function of the episode.[78] The following need to be observed: Miracle is a motif, and in the New Testament a variety of *allomotifs*[79] can bring this motif to expression—allomotifs pertaining to healing, teaching, saving, feeding, arguing, behaving etc. In order to come close to understanding the intended significance of a particular episode it would be essential to distinguish motifs and functions of motifs. It should be kept in mind that a particular motif may serve in different contexts to bring

---

caused by the New Testament miracles, which were perceived as contradicting the laws of nature, that gave rise to, and that explains the attraction of the Two-Source-Theory—with the *Logienquelle* as a possibility to regain the essentials of Jesus, located in his teachings, cf. Kahl, "Zweiquellentheorie," esp. 408–409.

75. Besides the classic contribution by Dibelius, *Formgeschichte*, cf. Kollmann, *Christen als Wundertäter*, 42–44, 355–362, and Reinbold, *Propaganda*. Cf. also Kahl, "Wunder und Mission," 35–43; Stenschke a.o., "Apologetik," 244ff.

76. Cf. only Paul in 1Cor 15; Alkier, *Auferweckung*. It is puzzling, and telling, that this miracle is usually not discussed in the exegetical contributions concerning "miracle stories" of the New Testament. My *New Testament Miracle Stories* is no exception. Mk 16:1–8 par. even shows a number of miracle motifs, and the reaction of the witnesses attests to that.

77. Berger, *Formen*, 362, speaks of "wunderhaltige Erzählabschnitte" with respect to narrative sections containing miracle motifs.

78. In my *Miracle Stories*, 173–215, I analyzed and typified "miracle healing stories" according to inner-narrative function. This, of course, should be balanced by a consideration of the function of an episode *within its context*.

79. Cf. Kahl, *Miracle Stories*, 38–41.

different functions to expression or that one function may be realized by a variety of motifs.[80]

Episodes narrating miracle events can be differentiated into the following types, depending on the *function* of a narrated miracle event in relation to the function of other narrative moves within that episode, in order to come to a closer understanding of the function and meaning of a particular episode:[81]

a) *Proper miracle stories*: The miracle event constitutes the *main* narrative move (narrative program)—the move that is requested for the fulfilment of a need—at *center* stage of the episode. Other narrative moves are subordinated to that narrative program (e.g., Mark 1:29–31; 7:31–37; 8:22–26).[82]

b) *Improper miracle stories of a first order*: The main narrative move is located at the *periphery* of the episode. Other events take place at center stage (e.g., Mark 7:24–30; Matt 8:5–13)

c) *Improper miracle stories of a second order*: The miracle event is subordinated functionally to another main narrative move (e.g., Mark 3:1–6).

d) *Episodes reflecting the presence of the numinous sphere in an unspecified manner*: This can be achieved either explicitly (e.g., Matt 7:28f. with respect to 5:3—7:27) or by implication (Mark 1:16–20; 12:13–17).

The intensity of the manifestation of the numinous sphere in an episode decreases from a to d.

NEW TESTAMENT MIRACLES OF HEALING AS MERCIFUL ACTS OF DIVINE LIBERATION— KARL BARTH'S THEOLOGICAL HERMENEUTICS

It has long been recognized in New Testament studies that the healing and exorcism stories of the Gospels function as narrative expressions of the closeness of God's kingdom. This is certainly correct, but more can be

---

80. The disregard of this structuralist insight accounts for a serious weakness in Theißen's proposed list of a inventory of 33 motifs, cf. his *Urchristliche Wundergeschichten*, 57–83.

81. Klumbies, "Wunderexegese," 45, has recently proposed to replace "Wundererzählung" with "mythische Sequenz." Since in the Gospel narratives the spiritual-numinous and the material-physical dimensions are potentially *always* intermingled, it does not make sense to demarcate particular episodes as "mythical sequence" in an undifferentiated manner.

82. For the term *narrative program*, cf. Kahl, *Miracle Stories*, 41–44.

said—here I come back to an insight shared by Rudolf Otto. According to him, the announcement of the kingdom by Jesus was first and foremost a "proclamation of the most numinous subject of all, that is, the good news of the kingdom ... The kingdom however is the *absolute* miracle."[83] Inherent in this statement is a polemic against the reduction of Jesus to a moral teacher and preacher, as was widespread in liberal theology.[84]

It was, however, Karl Barth, who presented in great detail and precision an exegetically founded theological interpretation of the miracles of Jesus that might serve as stimulus for future investigation into the miracles of the New Testament—helpful for an exegesis that is interested in understanding the *theological* significance of these miracles. Barth's contribution to the interpretation of the miraculous in the Jesus-presentations of the New Testament is found on about 40 pages—with the exegetical parts in the German original in small print—in volume IV,2 of his *Church Dogmatics* (*CD*),[85] in the context of paragraph 64,3: "The royal man," which is a sub-chapter of paragraph 64: "The exaltation of the Son of Man." Interestingly, Barth's contribution of 1955 has never been discussed in the exegetical discourse on miracles. However, much of what has been suggested above concerning a reorientation of miracle research in New Testament studies had been anticipated in Barth's careful analyses of the Synoptics. Since his valuable research is basically unknown in the exegetical discourse, I will summarize the most significant results of his investigation on miracles below. Barth's interpretation of the miracles of Jesus—both as genitivus objectivus and subjectivus—needs to be understood in the context of the theological foundation of the *Church Dogmatics* according to which God's gracious election of humanity in Christ constitutes the "sum of the Gospel." In *CD* IV Barth expounds the *doctrine of reconciliation*. The Gospel brings to expression that "God is with us human beings" in and through Christ. God is faithful to his covenant with His—universal—people. To Barth, this constitutes the very "center of the Christian message." After he has described in *CD* IV/1 God's humble descent into humanity in Christ ("Jesus Christ, the Lord as servant"), he sets out in *CD* IV/2 to describe the elevation of humanity in Christ towards God ("Jesus Christ, the servant as Lord"). It needs to be understood that Barth does not refer to particular Biblical proof texts to support a theological insight as is otherwise common practice among systematic theologians; rather Barth always develops his argumentation on a broad exegetical basis.[86] This

---

83. Otto, *Das Heilige*, 102.
84. Cf. v. Harnack, *Wesen*; v. Harnack, *Reden*, especially 173.
85. Barth, *The Doctrine of Reconciliation*, 209–247.
86. For an appreciation and assessment of Barth's deep exegetical concern and

holds true also for his treatment of the miracles of Jesus where Barth argues on the basis of the *complete* Synoptic tradition with occasional references to Acts and to the Gospel of John.

After Barth discussed Jesus' resurrection from the dead and his ascension into heaven as miracles of God, he prepares theologically the depiction and interpretation of Jesus as miracle worker in the Synoptic Gospels: Jesus is the "the royal man," who is the true, new human being in whom the sanctification of all men and women took place and has become a reality. His existence as man is analogous to God's existence. Jesus is the one who was overlooked, forgotten, disregarded, and despised by men. As such, God in Jesus shows a preference for the low, the little ones, the weak ones, the poor, and also the sinners and the pagans. He is the *crisis* of this world, including religion, economy, and politics. As the "divine Yes" to man, the love and loyalty of God is reflected in everything that Jesus did, as presented in the Gospel accounts in great variety:

- Both the words and the deeds of Jesus make God's will *transparent*. His deeds correspond to his words in the realm of the physical and the material. They are signs of the kingdom that has drawn near. As such, these deeds are extraordinary and paradoxical in character (reference to Luke 5:26).[87]

- From the perspective of the miracle works of Jesus, his *words and deeds* are not to be separated; both reflect the kingdom of God. Barth refers here explicitly to the "Sermon on the Mount" (reference to Matt 7:29).[88]

---

expertise, cf. Marquardt, "Exegese," 651–676.

87. Barth, *CD* IV,2 211.

88. Ibid.: "The Sermon on the Mount—we have only to recall the concluding words of the Evangelist (Mt. 7:29)—was no less a miraculous Word, the irruption and occurrence of something incomprehensible to man, than the raising of the young man at Nain (Lk. 7:11f.) was a miraculous act ... Those who try to throw doubt on the distinctive action of Jesus, as recorded in the Gospels, by referring it to the sphere of mythology must ask themselves whether in the first instance it is not His teaching, as recorded in the same Gospels, that must be referred to this sphere. For it leaves no less to be desired—and perhaps much more—in terms of normal apprehension." 215: "According to the proclamation in the Word of Jesus the alien and miraculous and inconceivable thing that takes place in His actions in the world, and in defiance of all human being and perception and understanding, is nothing other than the kingdom of God." 217: "There is an indissoluble connexion of proclamation, miracle and faith." Cf. the statement by Otto concerning the kingdom above.

- The miracle works of Jesus are neither to be reduced to the dimension of factuality nor to the dimension of symbolism. The narratives describing these acts imply *both*.[89]
- The designation *dynámeis* for these powerful miracle deeds indicates that they are beyond human ability and attributed to the *free grace* of God's authority alone.[90]
- The *addressees* of the miracle deeds: "It is the man with whom things are going badly; who is needy and frightened and harassed. He is one who is in every sense 'unfortunate.'"[91] In general terms, Jesus searches out and sees man "in the shadow of death," and "the miracle consists" in his liberation: "He unburdens man; He releases him."[92]
- Theologically speaking, the miracles make transparent that *God is interested* beneficially in the human being as his creature–"beyond or above or through his sin He is interested in man himself..."[93]
- The *beneficial* aspect of this liberation consists in the fact that "that oppressed and therefore anxious and harassed men can breathe and live again, can again be men."[94] God "does not will the destruction of man, but his salvation. And He wills this in the basic and elemental sense that he should be whole."[95]
- As much as God's "Yes" to man is a fundamentally joyful Yes, his "No" is a fundamentally uncompromising, wrathful "No" ready to fight. *God takes sides* against "nothingness" ("das Nichtige") which wants to destroy ("zunichte machen") man.[96]

89. Ibid., 218: "It belongs to the connexion between proclamation, miracle and faith that there is probably no account of any such action in the Gospels which (quite apart from its factuality and concrete content) does not also have what we may boldly describe as a symbolical quality."

90. Barth, *CD* IV/2 219.

91. Ibid., 221.

92. Ibid., 222.

93. Ibid., 224.

94. Ibid., 224.

95. Ibid., 225.

96. Ibid., 225. Barth in his *Church Dogmatics* decided to replace designations such as Devil, Satan or demons with "das Nichtige," by means of which he intended terminologically to diminish their importance and potency while at the same indicating their very intention, i.e. to destroy, for people to become "nothing." This, to Barth is the anthropological predicament of human beings that they are "possessed" or captivated by "nothingness" in one or the other of its expressions. This subject is therefore not to be delegated to a so-called mythical world-view (228). In this context he refers to Acts 10:36–38: "In the summarised account in Ac. 10:36f. the whole action of Jesus is stated

- Against this background, the miracle acts of Jesus are *pronounced deeds of combat* ("ausgesprochene Kampfhandlungen"), as becomes especially evident in resurrections of the dead and the exorcisms. God's power is neither a neutral nor a complacent power, "but the omnipotence of mercy—not quiet and passive mercy, but a mercy which is active, and therefore hostile to that power on behalf of poor man. It is with this that we have to do in the miracles of Jesus. And it is because we have to do with this that they are miracles."[97]

- An *excursus* into typical tendencies of miracle interpretation in *Protestantism* from its beginnings: It has failed to see "this dimension of the Gospel which is so clearly attested in the New Testament—its power as a message of mercifully omnipotent and unconditionally complete liberation from φθορά, death and wrong as the power of evil."[98] "How could Protestantism as a whole, only too faithful to Augustine, the 'father of the West,' orientate itself in a way which was so one-sidedly anthropological (by the problem of repentance instead of by its presupposition—the kingdom of God)? In other words, how could it become such a moralistic affair-so dull, so indifferent to the question of man himself, and therefore so lacking in joy?"[99]

The *miracle faith* of the believers: "The distinctive feature of the New Testament faith in miracles is that it was faith in Jesus and therefore in God as the faithful and merciful God of the covenant with Israel; and that in this way and as such it was this confidence in His power."[100] Barth defines this faith which is qualified in a double sense: "To sum up, it is faith qualified in this twofold sense-man's turning to Jesus and His power upon the basis of the fact that Jesus has turned to man in His power. When all this is borne in

---

in the words: "Who went about doing good, and healing all that were oppressed of the devil; for God was with him (v. 38)."

97. Ibid., 232.
98. Ibid., 233.
99. Ibid., 233.

100. Ibid., 236. To Barth, the belief in the miracle power of God is an extension of the belief in the merciful God who is loyal to his covenant with Israel. Barth makes clear that the miracles are the result of the free and gracious mercy of God: "He was under no compulsion to do this. But He could do it . . . There was no question, of course, of His having to do this, of their having a right to demand it, for in relation to Him they had no right to assert, no claim to anything. But they had the freedom to trust Him for this overflow of His mercy, to be absolutely certain that in the power of His free grace He could also do this." Such a belief in miracle power is not to be isolated and made absolute. This, of course, has been a tendency in so-called "power-ministry" which is dominating much of contemporary West African Christianity.

mind, faith in miracles as the New Testament sees it cannot possibly be confused with the monstrosity of an acceptance of the possibility and actuality of all kinds of miracles of omnipotence."[101]

- A faith that corresponds to Gospel is a *faith that is focused on Jesus*, not on his miracles.[102] The miracle functions to point to Jesus as Lord of mercy and compassion. The incomprehensibility and the paradox of the miracles only reflect the deeper incomprehensibility paradox of Jesus. The believer comprehends, by means of the miracles, the nature and function of Jesus.[103] This is their particular significance.

- Since all the expressions of Jesus—his words and his works—are incomprehensible and paradoxical, i.e. miraculous, it can be said that faith always originates from experiencing a miracle, in this concrete sense, grounded in *Jesus as miracle worker*.[104] Even a faith that claims to be derived from listening to the word of Jesus needs to be attentive to the dimension of the miraculous: "It is decisive, however, for the true hearing of the Word of Jesus that it, too, should belong to this dimension, that the faith which is based on a hearing of His Word should have this dimension, that it should therefore be faith in the One who in the mercy and power of God can also work miracles."[105] Otherwise Jesus' word would be reduced to "moral teaching and religious instruction" that would not have been different from the practice of the scribes.[106]

Conclusion with respect to the significance of the miracles of Jesus: "(T)he free grace of God [is] the meaning and power of these actions of Jesus . . ."[107] The free grace of God *can* become concrete in particular saving acts in the here and now. This insight, together with the Gospel accounts of Jesus' miracles, is an offense to "normal Christianity."[108] It could and should

---

101. Ibid., 238.

102. Ibid., 239: "It is to Him and not to the miracle that the believer gives his attention and interest. It is to Him and not to the miracle that he gives the glory."

103. Ibid., 239: "What is learned from the miracle is who and what He is—the Lord."

104. Ibid., 239: "Even the Word of Jesus is an incomprehensible act. It has the dimension of miracle. It has the character of *an act of divine mercy and power*" (italics added).

105. Ibid., 239.

106. Ibid., 240.

107. Ibid., 243.

108. Ibid., 247.

be, however, a source of constant joy for the church.[109] Jesus "was the man who put His proclamation into practice in these acts, thus characterising it as the proclamation of the kingdom, or—and it comes to the same thing—of the superabounding free grace of God."[110]

Karl Barth has developed a theological hermeneutics that helps to locate the particularity of the miracles of Jesus in their reflection of the grace of God. In this context, the New Testament miracles can be understood generally as *merciful acts of divine liberation*.[111] As such, they point to, and they reflect the basic miracle of the New Testament—the resurrection of Jesus by God.[112] Barth's hermeneutics successfully provides an approach to the New Testament miracles beyond rationalistic and supra-naturalistic avenues of interpretation. He brings this concern to expression, e.g., when he discusses the subject of *Angelology*: "How are we to steer a way between this Scylla and Charybdis, between the far too interesting mythology of the ancients and the far too uninteresting 'demythologisation' of most of the moderns?"[113]

This approach seems particularly promising in present times where the South meets the North, due to global processes of migration: Christians from Nigerian and Ghana, from India and the Philippines, representing to a large degree Pentecostal versions of Christianity, meet Christians in Germany and in the Netherlands, in Sweden and in Great Britain, who to a large degree represent rationalistic Protestant versions of Christianity. The deeply Biblically grounded theological hermeneutics as developed and presented

---

109. Ibid., 247. From the perspective of the *free grace of God* that Barth sees at the center of the miracles in the New Testament, it is interesting to note that both enlightened Protestant Christianity and Neo-Pentecostal power Christianity—from different angles—tend to limit the freedom of God: Western Protestants deny that God could cause particular miracles, while Neo-Pentecostals in, and from, West Africa and elsewhere try to force God into miracle activity. Both are equally problematic.

110. Ibid., 247.

111. Recent attempts at understanding the New Testament miracles in new perspectives unknowingly reflect a theological hermeneutics similar to the one developed by Barth, cf. Kahl, "Neutestamentliche Wunder als Verfahren des In-Ordnung-Bringens," and "New Testament Healing Narratives and the Category of Numinous Power," esp. 348–49; cf. also Alkier, "For nothing will be impossible," 21: "(O)ne needs a theological hermeneutic that considers the intertextual connections among texts that focus on the God of Israel as the god who is merciful, just, and who desires to communicate with his creatures."

112. The connection between the Gospel accounts of the miracles of Jesus and the reflection and interpretation of the main resurrection miracle in the Pauline epistles, is provided in Acts 10:34–43 (cf. 2:22–24), where Luke is in line with the interpretation of the Christ event by Paul (universal de-limitation of salvation with a particular view on the weak, the despised and excluded ones, cf. 1Cor 1:18–31; Gal 3:26–29; Rom 3:21–31).

113. Barth, *The Doctrine of Creation*, 369.

by Karl Barth might provide a common basis for Christians of various confessional backgrounds to communicate in general and to exchange views on the miracles in particular.

Barth clearly saw the limitation of the common Western theological approach to the understanding of the world in general and to the New Testament miracles in particular. He tried to counter-balance this strong position by appreciative, although not uncritical, references to perspectives of peoples of the global South:

> In this matter we have one of the not infrequent cases in which it has to be said that not all people, but some to whom a so-called magical view of the world is now ascribed, have in fact, apart from occasional hocuspocus, seen *more*, seen more *clearly*, and come [much] *closer* to the reality in their thought and speech [Sprache: language, W.K.], than those of us who are happy possessors of a rational and scientific view of things, for whom the resultant clear (but perhaps not wholly clear) distinction between truth and illusion has become almost unconsciously the criterion of all that is possible and real.[114]

Quite amazingly, Barth even envisioned a time when Christians from the global South might assist Christians in the North in understanding the world, the Bible, and the Gospel—around 1960, i.e. one generation before the first churches of Africans or Asians were actually founded in continental Europe!

"A magical picture of the world? Might it be that our fellow Christians from the younger churches of Asia and Africa, who come with a fresher outlook in this regard, can help us here? We hope at least that they will not be too impressed by our view of the world and thus be afflicted by the eye disease from which we ourselves suffer in this matter."[115]

Barth did not embrace uncritically pre-critical approaches to the miracles of the New Testament. His hermeneutics challenges both sides to move away from problematic notions of the miraculous that stand in opposition to the *Gospel as the good news of the free grace of God which manifests itself in merciful acts of divine liberation.*[116]

---

114. Barth, *The Christian Life*, 216. I have slightly corrected the official English translation after consulting the German original: the italics are in the original. It should be noted that according to the original Barth does not have "much" before "closer."

115. Barth, *The Christian Life*, 219.

116. Much of what can be observed in the miracle-discourse especially in neo-pentecostal Mega-Churches in West Africa and elsewhere amounts to a *merciless exploitation of the poor and suffering by so-called "powerful men of God."* This is the direct opposite to the meaning of Gospel as it has been so clearly brought to expression by Karl Barth.

CONCLUSION:
REORIENTING NEW TESTAMENT MIRACLE RESEARCH

This paper is an attempt at resetting investigations into New Testament miracle traditions. I suggest approaches to New Testament references to miracles that take seriously the conventionalized knowledge of the world in Mediterranean antiquity as it was shared in early Christianity.

In order to come close to an *appropriate* interpretation of New Testament miracle references—aiming at a reliable representation of the meaning dimensions of these texts *and* at understanding their possible significance for the formation of faith in present times—i propose, as summary of the most significant results of my research for a *reorientation* of miracle research, the following suggestions and notions:

1. World-knowledge systems and contexts

- The miracle references in the New Testament are to be studied within their literary micro- and macro-contexts (*universe of discourse*) on the one hand, and within the systems of conventionalized knowledge (*encyclopedia*) in Mediterranean antiquity, on the other hand.

- The encyclopedia of the researcher—in its relationship to encyclopedias presupposed in studied text—is to be reflected upon, in order to prevent unnoticed anachronistic readings into the texts. This requires especially a critical reflection of the terms and categories used traditionally to represent and classify texts from another culture and time, into the language of a modern culture. Here, the ethnological emic/etic debate becomes important for New Testament studies.

- World-knowledge in Mediterranean antiquity: the visible world is embedded in a net of activities of numinous powers of the invisible world to the effect that the causes for conditions in the visible world can be attributed to those powers.

2. Categories and definitions

Miracle, miracle-worker, and miracle story are terms that fall short of representing appropriately early Christian understandings of the miraculous dimension of Jesus' existence. All three exegetically used terms are imprecise umbrella terms that need to be redefined and differentiated.

- *Miracle*

Miracle is an *interpretive category* ("Deutekategorie"). "Miracle"—in German "Wunder"—is an umbrella term that covers a whole range of meanings communicated in antiquity by a number of terms by means of which different aspects of a miraculous event could be accentuated. Miracle in the context of the academic study of ancient religion is a term referring to the *interpretation and characterization of an event as the manifestation of an activity of a numinous power*, i.e. of a personalized spiritual being with an ability—miracle power—that exceeds human abilities.

- *Miracle Worker*

The category *miracle worker* has to be differentiated into three categories:

a) *bearer of numinous power* (BNP: miracle worker proper)[117]

b) *petitioner of numinous power* (PNP)[118]

c) *mediator of numinous power* (MNP).[119]

- *Miracle Story*

The category *miracle story* is not the designation of a genre. The category should not be used in an undifferentiated manner. One could speak instead of *episodes narrating miracle events*. This category is to be differentiated into the following types—depending on the *function* of a narrated miracle event:

a) *Proper miracle stories*

b) *Improper miracle stories of a first order*

c) *Improper miracle stories of a second order*

d) *Episodes reflecting the presence of the numinous sphere in an unspecified manner.*

The belief in miracles—as witnessed to in the New Testament writings—is not just a cultural feature to be dismissed in exegesis. It is an *essential constituent* of early Christian belief. As such, the early Christian belief in the miracles of Jesus remains a challenge to the understanding of the world and of the Gospel in present times. It is a welcome challenge inasmuch as it invites Christians to reflect critically upon the cultural conventions that have shaped their particular understanding of the world and of the Gospel. Remembering the miracles of Jesus and the cross-cultural and cross-confessional exchange about their possible significance[120] may open up new

---

117. In German: Träger numinoser Macht.

118. In German: Bittsteller numinoser Macht.

119. In German: Mittler numinoser Macht.

120. For the benefits of intercultural hermeneutics, cf. Kahl, "Jesus Power."

ways of perceiving reality and of shaping life[121]—in light of these *merciful acts of divine liberation*.

BIBLIOGRAPHY

Albl, Martin C. "'Are any among you sick?' The Health Care System in the Letter of James." *JBL* 121 (2002) 123–43.

Alkier, Stefan. "'For nothing will be impossible with God'[Luke 1:37]: The Reality of 'The Feeding the Five Thousand' [Luke 9:10–17] in the Universe of Discourse of Luke's Gospel." In *Miracles Revisited: New Testament Miracle Stories and Their Concepts of Reality*, edited by Stefan Alkier and Annette Weissenrieder, 5–22. Studies of the Bible and Its Reception 2. Berlin: de Gruyter, 2013.

———. "Wen wundert was? Einblicke in die Wunderauslegung von der Aufklärung bis zur Gegenwart." *ZNT* 7 (2001) 2–15.

———. "Wunder—Neues Testament." In *RGG4* 8 (2005) 1719–22.

———. *Wunder und Wirklichkeit in den Briefen des Apostels Paulus*. WUNT 134. Tübingen: Mohr/Siebeck, 2000.

Alkier, Stefan, and David Moffitt. "Miracles Revisited: A Short Theological and Historical Survey." In *Miracles Revisited: New Testament Miracle Stories and Their Concepts of Reality*, edited by Stefan Alkier and Annette Weissenrieder, 315–35. Studies of the Bible and Its Reception 2. Berlin: de Gruyter, 2013.

Anz, Thomas, ed. *Handbuch Literaturwissenschaft*. 3 vols. Stuttgart: Metzler, 2007.

Arnold, Heinz Ludwig, and Heinrich Detering, eds. *Grundzüge der Literaturwissenschaft*. Munich: DTV, 1996.

Barth, Karl. *Church Dogmatics*. Vol. III/3, *The Doctrine of Creation*. Edited by Geoffrey W. Bromiley and Thomas F. Torrance. Edinburgh: T. & T. Clark 1960.

———. *Church Dogmatics*. Vol. IV/2, *The Doctrine of Reconciliation*. Edited by Geoffrey W. Bromiley and Thomas F. Torrance. Edinburgh: T. & T. Clark 1958.

———. *Church Dogmatics*. Vol. IV/4, *The Christian Life: Lecture Fragments*. Edited by Geoffrey W. Bromiley. Grand Rapids: Eerdmans, 1981.

Beck, Robert R. *Nonviolent Story: Narrative Conflict Resolution in the Gospel of Mark*. Maryknoll, NY: Orbis, 1996.

Bediako, Kwame. *Christianity in Africa: The Renewal of a Non-Western Religion*. Maryknoll, NY: Orbis, 1995.

Berger, Klaus. *Formen und Gattungen im Neuen Testament*. UTB 2532. Tübingen: Francke, 2005.

———. "Hellenistische Gattungen im Neuen Testament." In *ANRW* II.25.2 (1984) 1031–432.

Boers, Hendrikus. "Introduction." In W. Egger, *How to Read the New Testament. An Introduction to Linguistic and Historical-Critical Methodology*. Edited by Hendrikus. Boers. Peabody, MA: Hendrickson, 1996.

---

121. Alkier, "Wunder III. Neues Testament," 1722: "Die Wunderfrage als notwendig offene Frage hält das Nachdenken über Gott und die Welt, d.h. über die Wirkweisen des trinitarischen Gottes, die Beschaffenheit der Realität und den Grund christl. Hoffnung wach."

———. *Neither on This Mountain nor in Jerusalem: A Study of John 4.* SBL Monograph Series 35. Atlanta: Society of Biblical Literature, 1988.

Boyarin, Daniel. *The Jewish Gospels: The Story of the Jewish Christ.* New York: New Press, 2012.

Bultmann, Rudolf. *Neues Testament und Mythologie: Das Problem der Entmythologisierung der neutestamentlichen Verkündigung.* Munich: Kaiser, 1941. Reprinted, 1985.

Burkert, Walter. *Creation of the Sacred: Tracks of Biology in Early Religions.* Cambridge: Harvard University Press, 1996.

Dahlheim, Werner. *Geschichte der römischen Kaiserzeit.* 3rd ed. Oldenbourg Grundriss der Geschichte 3. Munich: Oldenbourg, 2003.

Dibelius, Martin. *Die Formgeschichte des Evangeliums.* 6th ed. Tübingen: Mohr/Siebeck, 1971.

Dundes, Alan. "From Etic to Emic Units in the Structural Study of Folktales." *JAF* 75 (1962) 95–105.

———. *The Morphology of North American Indian Folktales.* Helsinki: Academia Scientiarum Fennica, 1964.

Feigel, Friedrich Karl. *"Das Heilige": Kritische Abhandlung über Rudolf Ottos gleichnamiges Buch.* 2nd ed. Tübingen: Mohr/Siebeck, 1948.

Fischer, Moritz. *Pfingstbewegung zwischen Fragilität und Empowerment: Beobachtungen zur Pfingstkirche 'Nzambe Malamu' mit ihren transnationalen Vepflechtungen.* Kirche-Konfession-Religion 57. Göttingen: V&R Unipress, 2011.

Fortes, Meyer. *Oedipus and Job in West African Religion.* Cambridge: Cambridge University Press, 1959.

Garrett, Susan R. "Jesus als Befreier vom Satan und den Mächten." *ZNT* 28 (2011) 14–23.

Gehrke, Hans-Joachim. *Geschichte des Hellenismus.* 4th ed. Oldenbourg Grundriss der Geschichte 1B. Munich: Oldenbourg, 2008.

Genette, Gérard. *Die Erzählung.* Munich: Beck, 1994.

Graf, Fritz. *Gottesnähe und Schadenzauber: Die Magie in der griechisch-römischen Antike.* C.H. Beck Kulturwissenschaft. Munich: Beck, 1996.

Greimas, Algirdas Julien, and Joseph Courtés. *Sémiotique: Dictionnaire raisonné de la théorie du langage.* 2 vols. Classiques Hachette. Paris: Hachette, 1993.

Grotanelli, Cristiano, and Bruce Lincoln. "A Brief Note on (Future) Research in the History of Religions." *Method & Theory in the Study of Religion* 10 (1998) 311–25.

Harnack, Adolf von. *Sprüche und Reden Jesu: Die zweite Quelle des Matthäus und Lukas.* Leipzig: Hinrichs, 1907.

———. *Das Wesen des Christentums.* Leipzig: Hinrichs, 1900.

Headland, Thomas N. "Introduction: A Dialogue between Kenneth Pike and Marvin Harris on Emics and Etics." In *Emics and Etics*, edited by Thomas N. Headland, Kenneth L. Pike, and Marvin Harris, 13–27. Frontiers of Anthropology 7. Newbury Park, CA: Sage, 1990.

Hübner, Kurt. *Die Wahrheit des Mythos.* Munich: Beck, 1985.

Johannsen, Dirk. *Das Numinose als kulturwissenschaftliche Kategorie: Norwegische Sagenwelt in religionswissenschaftlicher Deutung.* Stuttgart: Kohlhammer, 2008.

Kahl, W. "Geisterfahrung als Empowerment angesichts der Zerbrechlichkeit menschlicher Existenz. Zur pneumatischen Hermeneutik der Pfingstbewegung am Beispiel des charismatischen Christentums afrikanischer Herkunft." *ZNT* 25 (2010) 21–29.

———. "Gott und göttliche Wesen." In *Neues Testament und Antike Kultur*. Vol. 3, *Weltauffassung, Kult, Ethos*, edited by Jürgen Zangenberg, 88–109. Neukirchen-Vluyn: Neukirchener, 2005.

———. "Ist es erlaubt, am Sabbat Gutes zu tun?—Jesu Sabbatheilungen im Kontext der Schriften vom Toten Meer und der Mischna." *Novum Testamentum* 40 (1998) 313–35.

———. *Jesus als Lebensretter: Westafrikanische Bibelinterpretationen und ihre Relevanz für die neutestamentliche Wissenschaft*. New Testament Studies in Contextual Exegesis 2. Frankfurt: Lang, 2007.

———. "Jesus Power, Super Power: Productive Frictions in Intercultural Hermeneutics—A German Perspective." *Journal of Mothertongue-theology* 1 (2014) 78–109.

———. "Neutestamentliche Verfahren des In-Ordnung-Bringens." *Interkulturelle Theologie* 37 (2011) 19–29.

———. "New Testament Healing Narratives and the Category of Numinous Power." In *Miracles Revisited: New Testament Miracle Stories and their Concepts of Reality*, edited by Stefan Alkier and Annette Weissenrieder, 337–48. Studies of the Bible and Its Reception 2. Berlin: de Gruyter, 2013.

———. *New Testament Miracle Stories in their Religious-Historical Setting: A Religionsgeschichtliche Comparison from a Structural Perspective*. FRLANT 163. Göttingen: Vandenhoeck & Ruprecht, 1994.

———. "Überlegungen zu einer interkulturellen Verständigung über neutestamentliche Wunder." *Zeitschrift für Missionswissenschaft und Religionswissenschaft* 82 (1998) 98–106.

———. "Vom Ende der Zweiquellentheorie oder Zur Klärung des synoptischen Problems." In *Kontexte der Schrift*. Vol. 2, *Kultur. Politik. Religion. Sprache—Text (FS Wolfgang Stegemann)*, edited by Christian Strecker, 404–42. Stuttgart: Kohlhammer, 2005.

———. "Wunder." In *ThBNT* 2 (1999).

———. "Wunder und Mission in ethnologischer Perspektive." *ZNT* 15 (2005) 35–43.

Kippenberg, Hans G., and Kocku von Stuckrad, K. *Einführung in die Religionswissenschaft—Gegenstände und Begriffe*. C. H. Beck Studium. Munich: Beck, 2003.

Kirby, Jon P. *The Power and the Glory: Popular Christianity in Northern Ghana*. Trends in African Christianity. Akropon-Akuapem: Regnum Africa, 2012.

Klumbies, Paul-Gerhard. "Die Grenze form- und redaktionsgeschichtlicher Wunderexegese." *BZ* 58 (2014) 21–45.

———. *Der Mythos bei Markus*. Berlin: de Gruyter, 2001.

Kollmann, Bernd. *Jesus und die Christen als Wundertäter: Studien zu Magie, Medizin und Schamanismus in Antike und Christentum*. FRLANT 170. Göttingen: Vandenhoeck & Ruprecht, 1996.

Lang, Friedrich Gustav. "Massarbeit im Markus-Aufbau: Stichometrische Analyse und theologische Interpretation. Teil 1." *Biblische Notizen* 140 (2009) 101–34.

Lau, Markus. "Fieberfrei auf dem Weg Jesu (Die Heilung der Schwiegermutter des Petrus) Mk 1,29–31 (Mt 8,14f)." In *Kompendium der frühchristlichen Wundererzählungen, Bd. 1, Die Wunder Jesu*, edited by Ruben Zimmerman, 214–20. Gütersloh: Gütersloher, 2013.

Levy, Robert I., Jeannette Marie Mageo, and Alan Howard. "Gods, Spirits, and History: A Theoretical Perspective." In *Spirits in Culture, History, and Mind*, edited by Jeannette Marie Mageo and Alan Howard, 11–28. New York: Routledge, 1996.

Marquardt, Friedrich-Wilhelm. "Exegese und Dogmatik in Karl Barths Theologie: Was meint: 'Kritischer müßten mir die Historisch-Kritischen sein!'?" In Karl Barth, *Die Kirchliche Dogmatik. Registerband*, 651–76. Zurich: EVZ, 1970.

Mensching, Gustav. *Das Wunder im Glauben und Aberglauben der Völker*. Leiden: Brill, 1957.

Otto, Rudolf. *Das Heilige: Über das Irrationale in der Idee des Göttlichen und sein Verhältnis zum Rationalen*. Munich: Beck, 1963.

Patte, Daniel. *Structural Exegesis for New Testament Critics*. Guides to Biblical Scholarship. Minneapolis: Fortress, 1990.

Pike, Kenneth L. *Language in Relation to a Unified Theory of the Structure of Human Behavior*. 2nd ed. The Hague: Mouton, 1967.

———. "On the Emics and Etics of Pike and Harris." In *Emics and Etics. The Insider/Outsider Debate*, edited by Thomas N. Headland, Kenneth L. Pike, and Marvin Harris, 28–47. Newbury Park, CA: Sage, 1990.

Pike, Kenneth L. and Carol L. McKinney. "Understanding Misunderstanding as Cross-cultural Emic Clash." In *The Mystery of Culture Contacts, Historical Reconstruction, and Text Analysis: An Emic Approach*, edited by K. R. Jankowsky, 39–64. Washington, DC: Georgetown University Press, 1996.

Propp, V. *Morphology of the Folktale*. Translated by Laurence Scott. 2nd ed. Austin: University of Texas Press, 1968.

———. "The Study of Folklore in Literature and Culture: Identification and Interpretation." *Journal of American Folktales* 78 (1965) 136–42.

Reinbold, Wolfgang. *Propaganda und Mission im ältesten Christentum: Eine Untersuchung zu den Modalitäten der Ausbreitung der frühen Kirche*. FRLANT 188. Göttingen: Vandenhoeck & Ruprecht, 2000.

Rüpke, Jörg. *Die Religion der Römer*. Munich: Beck, 2001.

Sapir, Edward. "The Meaning of Religion." In *The Collected Works of Edward Sapir*, 134–45.

———. "The Unconscious Patterning of Behavior in Society." In *The Collected Works of Edward Sapir*, Vol. 3, *Culture*, edited by R. Darnell et al., 156–72. Berlin: de Gruyter, 1999.

Scheffel, Michael. *Einführung in die Erzähltheorie*. 8th ed. Munich: Beck, 2009.

Stenschke, Christoph W. et al. "Apologetik, Polemik und Mission: Der Umgang mit der Religiosi-tät der 'anderen.'" In *Neues Testament und Antike Kultur*, Vol. 3, edited by Jürgen Zangenberg. Neukirchen-Vluyn: Neukirchener, 2005.

Strecker, C. "Mächtig in Wort und Tat (Exorzismus in Kafernaum) Mk 1,21–28." In *Kompendium der frühchristlichen Wundererzählungen*. Vol. 1, *Die Wunder Jesu*, edited by Ruben Zimmerman, 205–13. Gütersloh: Gütersloher.

Theissen, Gerd. *Urchristliche Wundergeschichten: Ein Beitrag zur formgeschichtlichen Erforschung der synoptischen Evangelien*. 5th ed. StNT 8. Gütersloh: Mohn, 1987.

Tieleman, Teun. "Miracle and Natural Cause in Galen." In *Miracles Revisited: New Testa-ment Miracle Stories and their Concepts of Reality*, edited by Stefan Alkier and Annette Weissenrieder, 101–13. Studies of the Bible and Its Reception 2. Berlin: de Gruyter, 2013.

Weissenrieder, Annette. "Stories Just under the Skin: *Lepra* in the Gospel of Luke." In *Miracles Revisited: New Testament Miracle Stories and their Concepts of Reality*, edited by Stefan Alkier and Annette Weissenrieder, 73–100. Studies of the Bible and Its Reception 2. Berlin: de Gruyter, 2013.

Zimmermann, Ruben. "Grundfragen zu den frühchristlichen Wundererzählungen." In *Kompendium der frühchristlichen Wundererzählungen.* Vol. 1, *Die Wunder Jesu*, edited by Ruben Zimmerman, 7–67. Gütersloh: Gütersloher.

———, ed. *Kompendium der frühchristlichen Wundererzählungen.* Vol. 1, *Die Wunder Jesu.* Gütersloh: Gütersloher, 2013.

17

Word and Touch:
Ritualizing Experiences of Illness and Healing in Christian Liturgical Traditions

—Andrea Bieler

INTRODUCTION

"DISEASE OCCURS NOT ONLY in the body—in the sense of an ontological order in the great chain of being—but in time, in place, in history, and in the context of lived experience and the social world. Its effect is on the body in the world."[1] A biocultural understanding of medicine[2] will thus perceive illness not exclusively as a physiological malfunction of the mechanics of the body but rather as a biological and social phenomenon that is embedded in interactive processes of meaning making. Such an understanding will pursue an inquiry into various realms of the body: besides the external medical view of the body the individual body-self of lived experience will come to the foreground. From a biocultural perspective the social body of symbolic representation as well as the body politic of power will come into focus as well.[3] A deeper perception of illness seeks to understand the means and the processes that mediate the interactions and exchanges between these

---

1. Good, *Medicine*, 133.
2. With regard to the biocultural model see further Morris, *Illness*.
3. Kirmayer, "The Body's Insistence," 324.

realms. It is my assertion that narration and ritualization[4] of illness experiences are two basic means that serve the act of mediation. Rituals as well as narration are grounded in the lived experiences of body selves as well as in social symbolism.

The following essay seeks to unfold the claim that Christian liturgical traditions as well as emerging practices hold the potential to create liminal spaces in which illness narratives and body images can be reordered *coram deo* in life enhancing ways. This claim will be unfolded in three movements: I begin with a few historical highlights regarding rituals of healing as they have developed in Christian liturgical traditions. What follows are some insights from a survey of about a hundred contemporary liturgical texts drawn from North American Protestant liberal mainline resources. This essay will be concluded by introducing a case study in which narrative, metaphor and ritual enter into a powerful synergy which reshapes the body image and interpretation of self for a person who lives with an HIV infection.

HISTORICAL HIGHLIGHTS

From the days of the early church Christians have developed ritual practices that respond to experiences of illness. These rituals were geared towards reorienting the infirm in regard to their relationship with God, their place within the community, and their interpretation of being embodied selves. They were embedded in rich symbolic webs of ritual actions, objects, words and prayers through which divine intervention towards healing and in some cases forgiveness of sins were evoked. The meanings that arose from such webs shifted over time and they were multilayered within a single era. This is noticeable if we differentiate and pay attention to official interpretations generated from clerical bodies or if we focus on the piety of the people, which often was syncretistic.

Three texts from the New Testament have been critical in the development of Christian ritual regarding the sick. Mark 7:12–13 describes

---

4. I borrow the concept of ritualization from Catherine Bell who defines it as a strategic practice: "Viewed as practice, ritualization involves the very drawing, in and through the activity itself, of a privileged distinction between ways of acting, specifically between those acts being performed and those being contrasted, mimed or implicated somehow. That is, intrinsic to ritualization are strategies for differentiating itself—to various degrees and in various ways—from other ways of acting within any particular culture. At a basic level, ritualization is the production of this differentiation. At a more complex level, ritualization is a way of acting that specifically establishes a privileged contrast, differentiating itself as more important or powerful." (Bell, *Ritual Theory*, 91). Acts of ritualization happen not only in the realm of religious ritual but in all kinds of every day life situations, in formalized as well as informal environments.

anointing of the sick as part of the calling of the disciples as they were sent out by Jesus; Mark 16:18 references the laying hands on the sick in the name of Jesus. In James 5:14–16 two main ritual actions are mentioned: the elders of the church are supposed to pray over the sick and they are instructed to anoint them with oil in the name of the Lord. What follows is the description of two major effects of these actions: the prayer of faith will save and heal the sick (the Lord will raise them up) and secondly, their sins are forgiven. A variety of problems were discussed within liturgical history as these texts were used to legitimize particular liturgical practices, e.g.: What does anointing in the name of the Lord mean? Does it refer to the first person of the Trinity or to Christ? Who is authorized to say those prayers? What kind of oil should be used? What is the efficacy of the ritual action? How is divine agency understood? Which body parts ought to be anointed? What is the connection between sin and sickness? How seriously ill does one have to be in order to receive anointing? These rites inspired a variety of theological debates which were accompanied by power negotiations between clergy and laity.

Praying over the sick, anointing, and laying on of hands were three foundational practices for ritualizing experiences of illness in the East as well as in the West.

If we focus on the ritual action of anointing of the sick we can already see how a complex world of meaning making unfolds on the textual level. For instance, in the Egyptian Prayer Book attributed to Sarapion, water, bread and also oil are regarded as possessing therapeutic value:

> We call upon you who have all authority and power, the Saviour of all people, Father of our Lord and Saviour Jesus Christ. And we pray that you send forth a healing power of the Only-Begotten upon this oil, that it may become those who are anointed with it or partake of these your created elements, for a throwing off of every disease and every sickness, for a remedy against every demon, for a banishment of every unclean spirit, for a casting out of every evil spirit, for a driving out of every fever and shivering fit and every illness, for good grace and forgiveness of sins, for a medicine of life and salvation, for health and wholeness of soul, body and spirit and for complete bodily strength.[5]

This prayer is remarkable in its multidimensional assumption about the healing power of the oil imbued through divine action: God the Father is asked to send forth Christ's healing power right into the oil which then makes it an efficacious remedy. There is no hierarchical dualism between

---

5. Barrett, *Sacramentary*, Prayer 17, 47–49.

the spiritual and the physical at work here. Health of the body and wholeness of soul belong together; bodily health is not disconnected from grace and forgiveness of sin, although the question of how these are related is not made explicit in this prayer. Anointing is conceived to be a remedy against fever and other illnesses, but it has also exorcising power—it can cast out demons. Anointing of the body conveys grace and forgiveness of sins.

It is not before the ninth century that we find detailed instructions, e.g., in the Gallican sacramentaries about how anointing should be practiced. "In general we can assume a diversity of practices during this time period. In most instances, the Gallican formularies show that sanctified oil could be applied in the sign of the cross to the nape of the neck, the throat, the breast and the back, and places most stricken with pain or injuries."[6] These body parts were simply anointed in the name of the Trinity. Another formula explicitly mentions anointing of the sick in connection with committed offenses as they relate to certain body parts: "I anoint your eyes with sanctified oil, that whatever offense you have committed by your sight may be expiated by unction of this oil." Other anointing practices would limit the anointing to the five senses with an accompanying depreciative formula such as "may the Lord remit."[7] Usually the oil was applied to the skin, and in some cases the sick were instructed to taste it. The usage and application of the oil could be administered by presbyters and lay people as well, while the preceding blessing of the oil was reserved for the clerical hierarchy. "A primordial importance was attached to the epicletic blessing of the oil whereby the oil was imbued with divine efficacy placing it in the category of a *sacramentum* (Innocent I)."[8]

If we look further into the Middle Ages we find that a shift takes place from anointing the sick as medicine for healing and forgiveness of sin and recovery to anointing the sick for penance in anticipation of death. The connection between penance in light of one's own death became the narrow focus of anointing. Extreme unction became a sacrament in the thirteenth century, which could only be administered by an ordained priest. Scholastic doctors of the thirteenth century, for instance, understood unction "as a preparation for the glory of the beatific vision as a point of departure for determining the principal effect of the sacrament—be this the forgiveness of venial sins (Bonaventure, Scotus and the Franciscan school) or the

---

6. Westerfield-Tucker, "Christian Rituals," 160.
7. Westerfield-Tucker, "Christian Rituals," 160.
8. Gusmer, "Liturgical Traditions," 532.

remission of the remnants of sin (Albert the Great, Thomas Aquinas and the Dominican school)."[9]

The reformers responded to this development in the sixteenth century by refuting such restrictions of anointing to the dying alone and by challenging the status of healing as a sacrament. John Calvin focused on the power of the preached word and thought the gift of healing had vanished away.[10] He also urged the Christian community to consider its social responsibility regarding the promotion of public health, the building of hospitals and further advancements of the public medical systems.[11] By doing so he expanded the debate about how Christians ought to attend to the sick and the dying in the public realm of social responsibility. For Martin Luther, however, anointing remained a means for encouraging faith for those bearing illness with impatience.[12] He also refused to understand the rite of extreme unction as a sacrament. Especially in his later writings he emphasized the visiting of the sick and the prayer of faith as essential with regard to caring for the sick within the Christian community as well as preaching about death and eternal life.[13] Over time the rite of anointing of the sick became more and more marginalized in Protestant mainline churches.

A major shift occurred within the Roman Catholic Church when the Second Vatican Council expanded the narrow focus on extreme unction by reclaiming the anointing of the sick beyond the context of death.[14]

RITUALIZING EXPERIENCES OF ILLNESS: CONTEMPORARY PROTESTANT LITURGICAL TEXTS

Since the 1980s however we can recognize in North America as well as in Germany a growing interest in the development of healing rituals. Books

---

9. Ibid., 534.

10. "...the gift of healing like the rest of the miracles, which the Lord willed to be brought forth for a time, has vanished away in order to make the preaching of the gospel marvelous for ever." (Calvin, *Institutes*, Book 4:19.18).

11. See further Weissenrieder/Etzelmüller in this volume.

12. See Luther, *The Babylonian Captivity*, 121.

13. In 1528 Luther states: "If anointing were practiced in accordance with the gospel, Mark 6: (13) and James 5: (14), I would let it pass. But to make a sacrament out of it is nonsense. Just as, in place of vigils and masses for the dead, one might well deliver a sermon on death and eternal life, and also pray during the obsequies and meditate on our own end, as it seems was the practice of the ancients, so it would also be good to visit the sick, pray and admonish, and if anyone wished in addition to anoint him with oil, he should be free to do so in the name of God." (Luther, Confession, 370).

14. See Larson-Miller, *Anointing*.

of Worship, liturgical literature, worship aids, the Stephen Ministry movement, emerging rituals that have responded to the AIDS epidemic, and the feminist ritual movement within Christianity and beyond all show a keen interest in ritualizing experiences of illness. Currently the Evangelical Lutheran Church in America is working on a new worship resource that attends specifically to different experiences of illness. The resource will entail extensive material that addresses various stages of a disease and all sorts of illness crises.[15]

I reviewed about 100 liturgical texts that can be situated within the liberal spectrum of North American mainline Protestantism and were published in the last 20 years.[16] The examined rituals of healing can be found in the official worship books of the Presbyterians, Methodists, Lutherans, and United Church of Christ as well as in more informal worship aids that have been published by individuals or church bodies such as the Metropolitan Community Church. It is interesting to see that the basic ritual actions we have discussed above—laying on of hands and praying over the sick as well as anointing with oil—can be found in many of those liturgies. Depending on the liturgical and political context they are framed in particular ways. In addition many texts propose prayers of intercession as a practice of reorientation with regard to the communal web. Praying for someone who is ill is perceived as a way of almost mystical connection among the members of the body of Christ.

The following questions provide a lens for the analysis of such texts: How are healing and illness understood in those liturgical texts? How is God addressed in prayers, music, confessions, meditations, etc? What are the body images that are evoked? How do those liturgies address sin and forgiveness in relation to experiences of illness?

Regarding the understanding of illness and health in relation to the divine we can recognize a vital interest in overcoming a dualism that privileges the soul and the mind over the body by identifying the first with the spiritual realm and the latter with the somewhat devalued material world. It is rather stressed that God is present to all kinds of bodily, mental and spiritual crises. Most of these liturgical texts are based on the distinction

---

15. See Evangelical Lutheran Worship Pastoral Care. Provisional Draft for Review October 2007. In the table of contents the following situations are listed under chapter 5, which deals with healing and health: before and after a medical procedure and surgery, the beginning of an extended course of treatment, the difficult choices regarding treatment, the diagnosis of terminal illness.

16. See the books of common worship for the major Protestant mainline churches in the US as well as Wagner, *Healing Services*; Peterman, *Speaking*; Evans, *Healing Liturgies*; Kavar, *To Celebrate*.

between cure and healing. While cure pertains to the transformation of physical illness in scientifically measurable terms, the term healing is used to describe a sense of holistic integration. A typical statement in this vein can be found in the United Methodist Book of Worship: "A Service of Healing is not necessarily a service of curing, but it provides an atmosphere in which curing can happen. The greatest healing of all is the reunion or reconciliation of a human being with God. When this happens, physical healing sometimes occurs, mental and emotional balance is often restored, spiritual health is enhanced, and relationships are healed. For the Christian the basic purpose of spiritual healing is to renew and strengthen one's relationship with the living Christ."[17] The Presbyterian Book of Common Worship avoids the notion of healing and rather speaks of services for wholeness, which is probably another way to express the distinction between cure and healing. The Book of Worship of the United Church of Christ frames its theological understanding as follows: "Healing, in the Christian sense, is the reintegration of body, mind, emotions, and spirit that permits people, in community, to live life fully in a creation honored by prudent and respectful use."[18] This reintegration flows out of God's reconciling work among human beings, which touches the places of physical and spiritual distortion, broken relationships, and alienation.

In most liturgies, God is addressed as the one who restores and mends broken relationships. Divine efficacy is envisioned not in manipulative or causal forms but in more open ways that honor the diverse and unexpected ways God touches human lives.

The human-divine relationship, although it does not necessarily encompass physical cure, nevertheless has a bodily dimension. Besides the aforementioned dimension of healing with regard to the restoration or affirmation of divine-human relationship in which God's graciousness and goodness are revealed, we can identify a desire for integration that relates to communities, such as the church, the life-world environment and to planet earth.

God is often addressed in these liturgies as healer, creator, or divine physician. It is thus assumed that God is able to affect the human body-self. Restoration and affirmation of the human-divine relationship is prayed for.

Especially with regard to actual anointing we find formulae which indicate the anointing in the name of the Trinity: "I anoint you with oil in the name of the Father, and of the Son, and of the Holy Spirit."[19] Like in the

---

17. Methodist BOW, 613 ff.
18. United Church of Christ BOW, 296.
19. Presbyterian BOW, 1021.

case of the Trinitarian baptismal formula it might be suggested that this formula carries a spatial connotation, which draws the one who is anointed into the space of divine relationality. The connection of words and touch thus evoke intimate communion between the Triune God and the person seeking healing.

I could hardly find any liturgies which deeply struggled with the question of theodicy in the face of illness or which lamented the experience of divine absence. The voices that are raised in psalms of lament as well as the voice of Job who is involved in a fierce struggle with God while he is facing deep suffering are pretty much absent. Some of these liturgies give space for lament, the aching of the body, the fear of being isolated. God however is addressed in relation to these experiences as comforter and as a source of bodily and spiritual healing: "Our healing and saving Christ, we place each of these precious ones into your hands, the Great Physician."[20]

With regard to the body images that are evoked two major strands can be highlighted. The suffering body is perceived as being surrounded by and wrapped in God's presence. The following prayer reflects this sentiment as it addresses God: "Live-giving God, your love surrounded each of us in our mothers' wombs, and from the secret place you called us forth to life."[21]

The second strand articulates the desire for integration with regard to experiences of alienation from one's own body. Thus a naive affirmation of physical wholeness is at least implicitly questioned. The loss of body parts is grieved, as in the case of a ritual before or after a mastectomy. Janet Peterman writes in her meditation: "Making love. Nursing a baby. Holding a child. Hugging a friend. Standing in a bathing suit at the pool. It's my life with others that I have such trouble imagining if I were to be without a breast."[22] Or in Judy Hart's voice: "And when [the doctor] touched the area, I felt my flatness."[23] Audre Lorde's reflection gives room for the agony: "Between the telling and the actual surgery, there was a three week period of the agony of an involuntary reorganization of my entire life . . . within those three weeks, I was forced to look upon myself and my living with a harsh and urgent clarity that has left me still shaken but much stronger."[24]

Many liturgies do not give much room for lamenting the aching and fragile body, nor do we find many places where we find the struggle with the body that contains self-destructive processes.

20. Wagner, *Healing Services*, 32.
21. Methodist BOW, 624.
22. Peterman, *Speaking*, 142.
23. Ibid., 143.
24. Ibid., 141.

Confession of sin in the context of healing services provides particular challenges. Although various liturgies contain confession of sin, there is a strong interest not to draw the connection between sin and illness in relation to the sick. It is rather the church and individuals in it who have turned away from caring for the sick who become the center of confession. Confessions call for a reorientation of a particular community.

An example is a service of Healing and Anointing for Persons with AIDS: A litany of confession that prepares the prayer of confession laments:

> Leader: He was dying of AIDS.
> He said to me, "no one touches me."
> People: I did not touch him.
> Leader: Her face was old and worn before its time.
> She told me "I am sick and tired of being sick and tired."
> People: I had no time to stop.
> Leader: His dreams for the future were dimmed.
> He asked: "Where is the welcome I once enjoyed?"
> People: I remained silent.
> Leader: She was angry, with feelings of resentment
> And the unfairness of life.
> She implored: "Where were you when I needed you?"
> People: I turned away from her.
> Leader: In these and in many ways, O God, we are caught in fear, confusion, and anger.
> We have not loved our neighbors or heard their needs.
> Forgive us, we pray, as we reach out with hearts to respond, hands to help, and ears to hear.
> People: Amen.[25]

This litany of confession challenges the ignorance of the community, its fear and silence. The rubrics state explicitly: "When a Prayer of Confession and Act of Pardon are used, the tone should be one of assurance, acceptance, and hope. The emphasis should be on the confession of all the sins of all people present. The confession or pardon should not insinuate in any way that AIDS is either the result of sin or a punishing judgment from God."[26]

Especially liturgies that were created during the first rise of the AIDS epidemic strongly express that people with HIV are members of the body of Christ. The Metropolitan Community Church in North America develops a mantra at the Eucharistic table before the bread is broken: "We are the body

---

25. From Methodist resources, in: Evans, *Healing Liturgies*, 263 ff.
26. Evans, *Healing Liturgies*, 266 ff.

of Christ. The body of Christ has AIDS." Louis F. Kavar published in 1989 a collection of liturgies that were celebrated in the Metropolitan Community Church who had many HIV positive members. Here, the confessions of sin lament a trust in God's comforting and healing presence in the midst of the turmoil of the first stage of the AIDS epidemic: "Yet, confronted by AIDS, we have often failed to remember that your presence is with us. We have allowed the pain we have experienced to keep us from sharing in the goodness you continue to offer us each day."[27]

The official books of worship offer their commonly known confessions of sin which are supposed to be spoken in every ordinary service. They do not mention an explicit connection between illness and sin, but speak in rather general terms about the life of the Christian community and of the individuals entrenched in the realities of sin. How worshippers who participate in such healing services receive these confessions would be an issue for further exploration.

We conclude that the notion of healing in the examined liturgical texts is multilayered. It refers to the sense of embodied self for the sick, the restoration of the human divine relationship and the reorientation of the community, meaning that those who experience themselves as marginalized or invisible due to sudden or chronic illness ought to be included.

If we pay attention to the bigger North American landscape beyond mainline Protestantism regarding issues of religion and healing we can find a similar complex understanding of what healing might be about. Linda Barnes offers the following picture in her attempt to sketch the meaning of healing.

> It can mean the direct, unequivocal, and scientifically measurable cure of physical illnesses. It can mean the alleviation of pain or other symptoms. It can also mean coping, coming to terms with, or learning to live with that which one cannot change (including physical illness and emotional trauma). Healing can mean integration and connection among all the elements of one's being, reestablishment of self worth, connection with one's tradition, or personal empowerment. Healing can be about repairing one's relationships with friends, relations, ancestors, the community, the world, the Earth, and/or God. It can refer to developing a sense of well being or wholeness, whether emotional, social, spiritual, physical, or in relation to other aspects of being that are valued by a particular group. Healing can be about purification, repenting from sin, the cleaning up of one's own

---

27. Kavar, *To Celebrate*, 13.

negative karma, entry into a path of purity, abstinence, or moral daily living, eternal salvation, or submission to God's will.[28]

TRANSFORMING ILLNESS NARRATIVES IN RITUAL

Most of the liturgies I have focused on, especially those that address living with HIV and AIDS as well as various forms of cancer, seek to express the gospel by joining with the general enlightened consensus that such diseases should not be considered the result of divine punishment for committed sins. If the liturgies speak of sin they mainly do so in structural or social terms by shifting the focus from the individual person who suffers to the social environment and the cultural fabric that produces such stigmatisation. These liturgies resist for good reasons a fundamentalist framework, which would consider the AIDS epidemic as divine punishment for the "sin of homosexuality" as well as such strands within the history of Christian liturgy, which focused heavily on the causal connection between sinful behavior and illness. I however claim that such narrow causal focus should not prevent us from reconsidering a theological and liturgical reflection on sin as a profound experience of alienation from God, from one's own embodied self, and from the net of relationships we live in. Such reframing might powerfully shed new light on the illness narratives of people who struggle to make sense of their lives. This understanding of sin encompasses all dimensions of life. The metaphorical field connected with sin as alienation and forgiveness rather than sin and divine punishment holds the potential to transform illness narratives that reflect a sense of stuckness and compulsive reiteration, which theologically speaking might reflect the *homo incurvatus in se ipsum*—the person who is curled in him or herself without a chance to unravel the tragic and hurtful way of narrating illness.

If we consider empirical studies that analyze illness narratives of people who live with illnesses caused by an HIV infection we can recognize that many patients indeed do struggle with feelings of shame, guilt, a sense of sinfulness, archaic expressions of feeling dirty, and being invaded or polluted by the virus.[29] The introjection of such images and metaphors often lead to a strong sense of disorientation with regard to one's life trajectory. Taking these studies into consideration I wonder how effective rituals finally are that do not touch on these self expressions and feelings but rather suppress them in an implicit attitude of: "You should not feel this way . . ."

---

28. Barnes and Sered, *Religion*, 10.
29. See, e.g., Davies, *Interim*; Crossley, "Sense," 284ff.

If we take seriously the lived experience of faith as a crucial layer in the fabric of theological inquiry we need to consider the complexities of meaning making processes: how people narrate and ritualize their lives implicitly or explicitly in relation to divine reality. I would like to know how the ritualization of embodied metaphors and narratives might hold the potential to transform hurtful patterns with regard to a particular sense of body-self, and of community in relation to God. The theological question at stake here is how people envision the ways God affects and is at work in human's lives—most intimately in relation to their embodied existence. The theoretical question that needs to be addressed is how metaphors in the context of ritual might affect processes of reorientation with regard to shattered body and self images.

Regarding the articulation of illness experiences metaphors grounded both in bodily experience as well as in social interaction are pivotal. The bodily grounding of illness metaphors is based on the connection with sensorimotor equivalences; the social grounding is steeped in the pragmatics of language where context and intention are merged in the process of meaning making. "Metaphors allow for inventive play, despite the dual constraints of body and society, by requiring only piecemeal correspondences to the world through ostension. The meaning of metaphors is then to be found not in representation but in presentation—modes of action or ways of life."[30] A patient who struggles for a long time with migraine headaches and who remarks: "My head is made of glass" might capture in this metaphor a variety of things such as the bodily sensation derived from this severe illness, the understanding of migraine as illness. It might also relate to the perceived social environment, to relationships and institutions like the health care system which might be perceived as fragile. Such metaphors also have a relational quality. Expressed in a conversation with a doctor the sentence "my head is made of glass" could convey as well the implicit wish that the patient wishes to be treated with sensitive attention.[31]

Philosophers and linguists, such as Mark Johnson and George Lakoff, who are in conversation with cognitive science make a similar claim that our ways of reasoning and thus our processes of meaning making are deeply entrenched in our bodily experience. They assert that there exists no disembodied mind. "The centrality of human embodiment directly influences what and how things can be meaningful for us, the way in which these meanings can be developed and articulated, the ways we are able to comprehend and reason about our experience, and the actions we take. Our

---

30. Kirmayer, "The Body's Insistence," 323.
31. Ibid., 340.

reality is shaped by the patterns of our bodily movement, the contours of our spatial and temporal orientation, and the forms of our interaction with objects."[32] Embodied meaning is embedded in imaginative structures which have two essential features: image schemata and metaphorical projections. Metaphorical projections derive from bodily sensation; they are the basis for conceptual and abstract thinking. Metaphorical projections such as being flooded, invaded, polluted or attacked by a virus capture, in a nutshell, the embodied sense of self and world of many HIV-positive persons. Such projections potentially integrate the social constructions of this particular infection, the stereotypes as well as a perceived sense of loss of control over one's circumstances.

Metaphors express something that is literally not true: my head is not made of glass, the liturgical assembly is not a body, nor is God a physician or a father. The infected body is not dirty nor does it become a battle field. Yet metaphors express truth that is not graspable in concise scientific terms. They express truth in dense images that capture a universe of experiences, which cannot be pinpointed as a singular event, person or sensual expression. They are like windows thrown open that give us a glimpse into the universe hinted at. Metaphors are connected to sensual and emotional layers; they often have a relational quality. They stimulate our imagination. Paul Ricoeur states that metaphors expand human imagination by layering, in human thought and communication, what is with what is not.[33] We can say that this process of layering happens in ritual all the time. When God is invoked as Great Physician, when Audre Lorde's diary is quoted which holds fragments of her battles of breast cancer, or when the community joins in the old spiritual "There is a Balm in Gilead." Thus lifting up the metaphorical quality of ritual language in connection with ritualized physical actions such as human touch in the context of anointing is a way of expanding our imagination; it holds the potential for the expression of ambiguity and might give participants permission to express what is perceived of as irrational, immature, pre-modern or "wrong" consciousness. Embodied metaphors in the context of ritual might also give room for surprise, dissent and reorientation through symbolic action. Metaphors enfleshed in ritual practice can facilitate the reorientation of an infected or sick person in relation to perceptions of the divine human relationship, body-self and one's place in community. In the anointing of the sick rituals the metaphors used unfold their power through the sensual dimension, e.g., the lavish spending of oil rubbed onto the surface of the skin and onto different areas of the

32. Johnson, *Body*, xix.
33. See Ricoeur, *The Metaphorical Process*.

body. It seems to be the connection of word and human touch that ritual participants experience as powerful.

The medical anthropologist Laurence Kirmayer stresses that prior "to narratization, salient illness experiences are apprehended and extended through metaphors... These metaphors may subvert the project of narrative and come to dominate the sense of self... For many illness episodes, narrative represents an end point not a beginning."[34] Kirmayer asserts that narratives are important for codifying and reconstructing experience in the act of remembering, but other forms of knowledge, for instance that which is conveyed through metaphor, are able to serve the same purpose: "Just as fragments of poetry can be written with no overarching narrative, or the briefest strand hinted at, so can we articulate our suffering without appeal to elaborate stories of origins, motives, obstacles and change. Instead, we may create metaphors that lack the larger temporal structure of narrative but are no less persistent and powerful. Such fragments of poetic thought may be the building blocks of narrative: moments of evocative and potential meaning that serve as turning points, narrative opportunities, irreducible feelings and intuitions that drive the story onward."[35]

In ritual metaphors as fragments of poetic thought become alive in an embodied sense as they are put into conversation with the unfolding illness narratives of the people and with the old liturgical texts and rituals actions that have traveled through time.[36] Metaphors in the context of ritual are

---

34. Kirmayer, "Broken Narratives," 153.

35. Ibid., 154.

36. By stressing the importance of ritualization and metaphor I would like to recall the work of Susan Sontag who made the opposite claim. In 1977 Susan Sontag published her essay *Illness as Metaphor*, which was followed by *AIDS and Its Metaphors* in 1988. The latter received an incredible amount of responses, since the AIDS epidemic had reached its first peak in North America in the late 80s.

In both essays Sontag struggles passionately with the negative effects that the metaphorization of illnesses such as cancer and AIDS might potentially have on patients. She suggests to resist metaphorical thinking in this realm is the healthiest way of dealing with actual illness. Sontag identifies three major dimensions of the metaphorical field she finds problematic: the punitive connotations, images that evoke economic catastrophe, and warfare. She claims that especially punitive notions are attached to cancer. "There is the 'fight' or the 'crusade' against cancer, cancer is a 'killer disease'; people who have cancer are 'cancer victims.'" (57) At the same time she claims the cancer patient is made culpable of his or her disease. Sontag points to cancer metaphors that evoke economic catastrophe of unregulated spending, and abnormal incoherent growth: "The tumor has energy, not the patient; 'it' is out of control... Cancer is described in images that sum up the negative behavior of twentieth century homo economicus. Abnormal growth; repression of energy that is refusal to consume or spend." (62ff.) The most powerful illness metaphor however that Sontag identifies is the warfare metaphor. Cancer cells invade the body, they "colonize" from the original tumor. A patient's body is under

embodied expression. In time and space they are embedded in energy, flow, movement, gesture, and, last but not least, language. Language thus is not to be separated from the body. We think and speak bodily; we are in that sense speaking bodies.

I would like to illustrate this with an example taken from an interview with a German Lutheran pastor who has worked intensively with HIV positive congregants.[37] He told the story of a woman who was working as a prostitute in Hamburg where she finally was infected with HIV by one of her johns. She saw the pastor for counselling sessions for about two years. A firm narrative had developed in their meetings which had two major strands. The first strand consisted of the effort to point to people, circumstances and institutions for her destiny, including the people who disappointed and betrayed her hopes when she came as an immigrant from Poland to Germany and how she got into the prostitution business and into drugs etc. At the same time she employed extremely powerful metaphors about her body-self: "I am dirty," or "I feel like a garbage bin."

Neither strand of her narrative left much room for the perception of agency, her own resources to change her situation. There was not much explicit God talk in their conversations. She was suspicious especially of the Roman Catholic but trusted the pastor and the efforts of this particular congregation. Since the pastor felt stuck in his counseling efforts he proposed to her to develop together a cleansing and anointing ritual in which a liminal space was created. The ritual consisted of the following basic elements: They changed their meeting space and met in the chapel. Both changed their clothing. He came in a robe, which signified his role as ritual leader; she came in a party dress that she would wear only on special occasions. They began listening to a portion from Brahms' Requiem: "Und alles Fleisch es ist wie Gras." Then the pastor greeted her and told her that here in this place everything could be brought before God, and that God would not condemn her but that God has chosen life for her and has said yes to her. In preparation for this meeting they had worked together on a litany in which she offered fragments of her life story which found their dense expression in the

---

attack; the body's defenses are under scrutiny. "Treatment also has a military flavor. Radiotherapy uses the metaphors of aerial warfare, patients are 'bombarded' with toxic rays. And chemotherapy is chemical warfare, using poisons. Treatment aims to 'kill' cancer cells without it is hoped killing the patient." (63) With regard to the discourse about AIDS she sees a premodern experience of illness arising, "before the era of medical triumphalism, when illnesses where innumerable, mysterious, and ther progression from being seriously ill to dying was something normal . . ." (122).

I still find Sontag's essays powerful to read, although I cannot agree with her claims about how such metaphors affect the self-image and the health of those who are sick.

37. See also Bieler, *Written*.

metaphors she had invented for her life. He would interrupt her narration by interspersing metaphors from Psalm 51 and from Psalm 32: "While I kept silence, my body wasted away through my groaning all day long . . . Wash me thoroughly from my iniquity and cleanse me from my sin . . ."

As the litany moved along she repeatedly washed her hands in the flowing waters caught by the baptismal font. Then they sat in silence for a while, she was crying. The pastor broke the silence by quoting again from those psalms: "I said: I will confess my transgressions to the Lord and you forgave the guilt of my sin . . . Happy are those whose transgression is forgiven, whose sin is forgiven." Then he began to anoint her forehead, the eyes, ears, lips, and hands, and feet. He closed with a prayer. He opened the church door. They had agreed beforehand that she would pour the water silently onto the ground outside of the chapel. But instead she took the bowl, ran outside and flung its contents into the streets. The pastor followed her outside puzzled but relieved.

In the following weeks they continued their counseling sessions. He got the sense that the ritual had broken open the stuckness of their conversation. He observed how she slowly began to claim more agency over her life. God-talk did not occur explicitly. The pastor felt, however, the ritual had also reoriented implicitly her religious world view.

This example challenges the claim that articulating a connection between sin and illness must be in all circumstances an oppressing force in the lives of the sick. A broader understanding of sin as encompassing experience of alienation might help to address and transform illness narratives in profound ways.[38]

BIBLIOGRAPHY

Barnes, Linda L., and Susan S. Sered, eds. *Religion and Healing in America*. Oxford: Oxford University Press, 2005.
Barrett-Lennard, R. J. S. *The Sacramentary of Sarapion of Thmuis*. Alcuin/GROW Liturgical Study 25. Nottingham: Groove, 1993.
Bell, Catherine. *Ritual Theory: Ritual Practice*. New York: Oxford University Press, 1992.
Bieler, Andrea. "Written in Their Bodies: On the Significance of Rituals in Caring for AIDS-Patients." In *Transgressors: Towards a Biblical Theology*. Edited by Claudia Janssen, Ute Ochtendung, and Beate When. Translated by Linda M. Maloney. Collegeville, MN: Liturgical, 2002.
Book of Common Worship for the Presbyterian Church (U.S.A.). Louisville: Geneva, 1993.

---

38. I thank Michelle Kate Weber, PhD student in the Liturgical Studies Program at the Graduate Theological Union in Berkeley for the careful reading of this text.

Book of Worship. United Church of Christ, New York United Church of Christ. Office for Church Life and Leadership, 1986.

Calvin, John. *Institutes of the Christian Religion*. Edited by J. T. McNeill. Philadelphia: Westminster, 1960.

Crossley, M. L. "Sense of Place and its Import for Life Transitions: The Case of HIV-Positive Individuals." In *Turns in the Road: Narrative Studies of Life Transitions*, edited by Dan P. McAdams, Ruthellen Josselson and Amia Lieblich. Washington, DC: APA Books, 2001.

Davies, M. L. *Interim and Final Reports to the Directorate DGIV of the European Community*. Luxembourg: European Commission, 1995.

Epperly, Bruce G. *Healing Worship: Purpose & Practice*. Cleveland: Pilgrim, 2006.

Evans, Abigail Rian. *Healing Liturgies for the Seasons of Life*. Louisville: Westminster John Knox, 2004.

Good, Byron J. *Medicine, Rationality and Experience: An Anthropological Perspective*. Lewis Henry Morgan Lectures 1990. Cambridge: Cambridge University Press, 1994.

Gusmer, Charles W. "Liturgical Traditions of Christian Illness." *Worship* 46 (1972) 528–43.

Johnson, Mark. *The Body in the Mind. The Bodily Basis of Meaning, Imagination, and Reason*. Chicago: University of Chicago Press, 1987.

Larson-Miller, Lizette. *The Sacrament of Anointing of the Sick*. Lex Orandi Series. Collegeville, MN: Liturgical, 2005.

Luther, Martin. *The Babylonian Captivity of the Church*. LW 36.

———. *Confession Concerning Christ's Last Supper*. LW 37.

Kavar, L. F. *To Celebrate and to Mourn. Liturgical Resources for Worshiping Communities Living with AIDS*. Gaithersburg: Self Publishing, 1989.

Kirmayer, Laurence J. "The Body's Insistence on Meaning: Metaphor as Presentation and Representation in Illness Experience." *Medical Anthropology Quarterly* 6 (1992) 323–46.

———. "Broken Narratives. Clinical Encounters and the Poetics of Illness Experience." In *Narrative and the Cultural Construction of Illness and Healing*, edited by Cheryl Mattingly and Linda C. Garr, 153–80. Berkeley: University of California Press, 2000.

Morris, David B. *Illness and Culture in the Postmodern Age*. Berkeley: University of California Press, 1998.

Peterman, Janet S. *Speaking to Silence: New Rites for Christian Worship and Healing*. Louisville: Westminster John Knox, 2007.

Ricoeur, Paul. "The Metaphorical Process as Cognition, Imagination and Feeling." *Critical Inquiry* 5 (1978) 143–59.

Sontag, Susan. *AIDS and Its Metaphors*. New York: Picador, 1989.

The United Methodist Book of Worship. Nashville: Cokesbury, 1992.

Wagner, James K. *Healing Services*. Nashville: Abingdon, 2007.

Westerfield-Tucker, K. "Christian Rituals Surrounding Sickness." In *Life Cycles in Jewish and Christian Worship, Two Liturgical Traditions 4*, edited by Paul F. Bradshaw and Lawrence A. Hoffman, 154–72. Notre Dame: University of Notre Dame Press, 1996.

18

Holistic Medicine in Late Modernity
Some Theses on the Efficacy of Spiritual Healing

—Anne Koch and Karin Meissner

INTRODUCTION

RESEARCH DURING THE LAST years has come up with some exciting insights into spiritual healing and what might affect its positive influence on the subjective well-being of many of the participants. This is also the aim of our interdisciplinary approach from cultural studies and placebo research. We aim at better understanding the underlying biopsychosocial mechanisms, rules and dynamics of spiritual healing. We therefore have to bring together our very different and at the same time highly specialized categories and methods of describing and analyzing the healing intervention. Interdisciplinary work in this field means that the relevant contexts of healing performance are multiplied: semantic, interpersonal, chemical, neural, behavioral contexts have to be considered and, as a greater challenge, they have to be related and at best combined. This article therefore will localize the phenomenon of modern spiritual healing in the context of contemporary spirituality and introduce into our findings and assumptions of our work-in-progress on the efficacy of spiritual healing.

One of our goals is to determine *specific* factors for improved well-being as an outcome of participating in healing rituals. This goal is challenging because an interpersonal intervention in healing involves such a huge number of features that range from touching, talking, sharing or teaching wisdom to moving and performing. Further, through regular performance a new bodily and emotional experience may turn into a more permanent attitude. We must not overlook the factors belonging to a ritual community and the highly sensorial environment created by a specific brightness of light, the tactile quality of materials, symbols and the "genius loci." In the meantime it is a well-proven fact of ritual studies that even non-human "participants" of the ritual, like powers, spirits and devotional objects, may take over agency within the happening according to the experience of the participants. We will have to ask how this way of experiencing healing energies also triggers psychophysiological responses on the side of the participants. And this again enlarges the bundle of possibly relevant factors contributing to the benefit of partaking in healing ceremonies. Placebo research[1] along with medical psychology and ritual studies are the reference sciences vital to taking a step towards understanding the crucial factors for the efficacy of spiritual healing. It needs to be stated clearly that with a background in cultural study of religion *and* medicine we are not at all aiming at a physico-reductionist or naturalizing view of spiritual healing.

Effect—Efficacy—Benefit

Let us start with some important clarifications of the concept of efficacy and keep them in mind for the evaluation of the manifold forms of alternative treatments. A common distinction in pharmaceutical research is that between: a) effect, b) efficacy, and c) benefit.[2] First of all, a substance or treatment has to prompt some biochemical response in the human organism: the effect. The underlying mechanisms of the effect may differ widely: blocking neural transmission to alleviate pain, activating enzymes to accelerate metabolic processes etc. Many alternative pharmaceutical substances already fail at this stage since the amount or type of substance is powerless (e.g., homeopathic and anthroposophical remedies, tissue salt ["Schüssler Salz"], Bach flower extracts). Then, the amount of the dose plays a crucial role: increasing the dose increases the effect to a certain degree, after which it can harm; below a certain dose it has no effect. The effect is a precondition for the efficacy that is the sum of all desirable effects. Here some severe problems occur when medication intrudes in a metabolism that is

---

1. Benedetti, *Placebo effects*.
2. For further discussion see: Witt, "Efficacy, Effectiveness, Pragmatic Trials," 292–94.

unimaginably skilled by nature. A small input may have unforeseeable and intertwined consequences. Next, what is desirable for one person may harm another person with a differing pre-existing health condition. The dose of a substance or intensity of treatment also interferes with other biochemical processes and may have side effects that are desirable or not. At this stage clinical studies have to prove the specific efficacy of the dose or treatment. Only then the benefit of a product for patients can be evaluated by its ability to lengthen life expectancy and to mitigate pain. Knee surgeries, for example, in comparison with placebo knee surgeries turned out not to be beneficial[3] like many other interventions, e.g., some cancer screenings.[4]

These distinctions can help us to better conceive of the causality of intervention in types of spiritual healing. In the context of spiritual healing we will have to think of tissue salt, for example, as biochemically non-effective and therefore not efficacious. In this terminology a placebo effect is an effect insofar there is an underlying biochemical process even if this is not triggered by use of a prescribed substance. Nevertheless, a benefit may arise from the general psychic improvement of having a good feeling about taking precautions and being active in dealing with one's illness. The same goes for energy work with *qi* or *prana* that as long as it depresses blood pressure it contributes to better well-being even if this does not heal a severe illness. Psychophysiological processes can be involved even if many of the spiritual healing practices do not prescribe remedies or substances but involve, for example, touching the client and embedding him into specific environments or making him move in a specific way. We want to understand which mechanisms on an autonomic, hormonal, and muscular level are involved in realizing improved well-being.

Holistic Medicine

Spiritual healing may be subsumed under holistic medicine. Therefore our understanding of holistic medicine needs some conceptual explanation, as it denotes a vast field of diverging practices and is not used always in the same sense but often overlaps with complementary and alternative medicine (CAM). Holistic medicine or mind-body-medicine[5] is not only a trend in the CAM sector but also in the fields of alternative spirituality and religion as for example in Christian revivalism where spiritual healing is very common. Some scholars observe the emergence of a service industry of healing

---

3. Moseley et al., "A Controlled Trial of Arthroscopic Surgery."
4. Bleyer and Welch, "Effect of Three Decades of Screening Mammography."
5. Harrington, *The Cure Within: A History of Mind-Body Medicine*.

originating from the many movements and organizations within alternative spirituality. The new profession of a spiritual entrepreneur offers angel healing, aura cleansing, therapeutic touch, touch healing, movement therapies, bioresonance, shamanic and indigenous healings, bioenergetic meditation and many other forms. Holistic medicine encompasses on the one hand complex complementary medical systems like homeopathy, Ayurveda, traditional Western medicines, anthroposophical medicine, and on the other hand secularist treatments. They are called secularist because they stem from various sciences:[6] from psychologies (Neo-Reichian, humanist psychology, human potential movement, self-regulation, self-realization), biology and physiotherapy (cell memory: osteopathy, craniosacral therapy, Rolfing), medicine (immune system: self-healing powers, bio feedback, psychosomatics, placebo research), physics (quantum physics: entanglement, non locality), cybernetics, information theory and so on. Some secularist spiritualties stem from a blending of arts, spirituality and (body) therapies like modern dance (contact dance, 5 rhythms of Gabriel Roth, Biodanza, Qi Dance, Yoga Dance).

The impressive rise of holistic medicine correlates with deep changes in our societies during the last decades. Holistic medicine and spiritual healing in their many facets are part of a self-therapy culture and self-care,[7] the third pillar of health-care besides pharmacological and other medical interventions. Therefore, we will first embed holistic medicine and spiritual healing from the mid-1990's onwards in the context of late modernity.

Future Potential of Integrating Holistic Medicine in Health Service

Our general aim is to recognize the resources for public healthcare that lie within holistic medicine, especially spiritual healing. Fisher et al. talk of "effectiveness gaps" in the context of "an area of clinical practice in which available treatments are not fully effective."[8] Their telephone survey of 22 General Practitioners (GP) in London came up with about 80 clinical problems for which effectiveness gaps were reported, the most important being musculoskeletal problems, followed by depression, eczema, chronic pain, and irritable bowel syndrome. Furthermore, a literature survey by the authors showed that CAM may offer effective interventions in all of these

---

6. Binder and Koch, "Holistic Medicine between Religion and Science."

7. Self-care in the context of salutogenesis should be distinguished from the concept of self-care in the archaeology of knowledge and subject theory (Michel Foucault).

8. Fisher, van Haselen, Hardy, Berkovitz, and McCarney, "Effectiveness Gaps."

clinical areas. One future aim would be a standardized check-up of relevant features of personal beliefs and preferences at the entrance of public health institutions. This idea is that this could predict if some specific type of spiritual healing or holistic medicine may be beneficial for this patient and therefore should complement the mainstream treatment. For patients who are recognized as persons and made to feel part of something bigger or of some plan, the involvement of spiritual healing elements can promise at least a better relationship between patient and healthcare institution. Even if the economizing of cost is not our main concern, it may also emerge from this double supply and make the "spiritual healing type check up" attractive for clinics and health insurance companies. For this far future aim we need to evaluate the efficacy and benefit of spiritual healing. This is not possible in general, but only in view of types of healing and types of person. For this aim we will have to elaborate a taxonomy of spiritual healing and holistic medicine with the criteria of specific factors of efficacy that they include. For such a taxonomy at first we have to know: what are the benefits in spiritual healing?

In this search for a suitable tool for understanding healing, insights from study of religion and medical anthropology concerning local cultural belief systems, sensorial practices, emic narratives, transformation dynamics and ways of exercising power all contribute. Thus, knowledge obtained from the study of religion is indispensable for the shaping of future health-preserving or health-restoring interventions based on the resource of self-healing. Scholars have studied the relations between body and symbolic meaning, somatic manipulation and social purpose, self-regulation and aesthetic regimes, especially form the aesthetics of religion perspective. They pursue the questions: Are coherent beliefs stronger than isolated beliefs? Are embodied and highly sensory coded worldviews more powerful than intellectual beliefs for the efficacy of healing? How important is the overall social integration of healees, the empathy of the healer and the involving of imaginative healing forces? These are some of the questions we aimed to understand in our two interdisciplinary pilot studies of therapeutic touch in a spiritual healing context.

HOLISTIC MEDICINE IN LATE MODERNITY

Modernity is the relevant environment of contemporary holistic medicine. It has been theorized as late or high modernity (Anthony Giddens), multiple modernities (Shmuel Eisenstadt), second or entangled modernity (Ulrich Beck), liquid modernity (Zygmund Bauman), and alternative modernity

(Bruce Knauft), to name just some often discussed theories. Without going into too much detail of these multivariable models, we will summarize some findings and explanations that are relevant for spiritual healing.

Late modern societies underwent a formatting process from production to consumption regimes with economization as the central force. In consumer societies, identity and authenticity widely manifest in specific consumption. Insofar as the consumption of lifestyles is constitutive for identity, this consumption is productive. This phenomenon is named prosumption (from *pro*-duction and con-*sumption*). What a person prosumes is a signaling of what she is and wants to be. A symptom of prosumption is the individual's involvement in production: self-service, user generated content, online-self administering of finance, voting etc. Self-care shows itself against this background as highly economized. For Andrew Dawson[9] spiritual prosumption is linked to a specific subjectivity: the self is autonomous and self-responsible. The location of performing autonomy is the individual's own body. The body has to be kept in a fit, healthy, relaxed and balanced condition. The body is the space where cosmic energies are linked to the challenges of the work life. Embodiment is therefore the spiritual mode *par excellence*, and practices of healing and psychophysical manipulation are the decisive knowledge to realize wholeness. Methods of healing are a knowledge of self-regulation and governance. In view of this logic of affect and action of late modern prosumption, it is evident how important they are insofar as they enable the subject to empower itself and express itself vis-à-vis the community: "The fundamental premises [of spiritual healing] are an advocacy of nature, vitalism, 'science,' and spirituality. These themes offer patients a participatory experience of empowerment, authenticity, and enlarged self-identity when illness threatens their sense of intactness and connection to the world."[10]

Holistic medicine is above all characterized by the presumptions of holism and energies ("vitalism"). Holism is expressed in a philosophical anthropology of mind-body-unity often embedded in a continuum of cosmic and subtle energies. Bodies are not seen in a biological manner but as several bodies or mantles alongside the material body (according to school): the astral, subtle, mental, emotional, ethereal bodies also known as aura. Cosmic elements often correspond to character types, food and spiritual tasks. Balance of energies is the clue to harmonious and healthy being. Therapeutic treatments therefore can follow several ways: energetic body work,

---

9. Dawson, "Entangled Modernity and Commodified Religion."

10. Kaptchuk and Eisenberg, "The Persuasive Appeal of Alternative Medicine," 1061.

meditation, and dietetics are some of them. Holism not only concerns the bodily interaction but the world as such that is penetrated by one principle that is a lived energy, a position named vitalism.

According to many of these doctrines, illness is an imbalance of energies or a blockage of energy channels. The reasons for this condition are various. The sociologists Susan Sered and Amy Agigian explored in a field study in the US "holistic sickening." By this they mean that, for example, CAM-"practitioners" discursive construction of breast cancer transforms it from a discrete physical disease of the breast to a much larger problem potentially involving all areas of a woman's life (and possibly her past lives). "This re-framing is what we call *holistic sickening*; that is, a discursive process through which a discrete corporeal diagnosis (cancer cells clustered in the breast) is widened into a broad assessment of trauma, misfortune, character defects, stunted spirituality, bad food choices, gender trouble, and a degraded environment."[11] In the practitioners' emic etiologies of the illness of their clients *and* of our time are explained by environmental degradation, toxic food, and genetic considerations. In the social dimension typically stress, social alienation, and contemporary lifestyles are said to be responsible for diseases. And as a third group of reasons for a personal illness the CAM-practitioners draw on personal traits like trauma, character defects, negative thoughts, and spiritual stagnation.

Spiritual stagnation is a very common term in the holistic milieu of late modern spirituality. It offers many kinds of self-techniques that help overcome blockages and stagnation. Disease is linked closely together with spiritual transformation. Health and disease are poles of a continuum. The task of staying healthy or recovering from a disease is an open-ended and life-long project. Transformation of the self is an utmost important issue behind holistic medicine besides encountering transcendence.[12] This being said, it is evident that healing will vary widely relative to self-conceptions within western and non-western cultures and within individualist, collective, peer-group or family-oriented social formations.

And this brings us back to our topic of efficacy: for the CAM-practitioners of the breast cancer study the efficacy of their treatment seems not to be a topic: "for the most part the practitioners described efficacy as of marginal relevance to their work. None of our interviewees kept track of success rates or used any sort of systematic means of assessing their own work."[13] Sered

---

11. Sered and Agigian, "Holistic Sickening," 627.

12. Koss-Chioino, "Spiritual Transformation, Relation and Radical Empathy: Core Components of the Ritual Healing Process"; and Kaptchuk, "Placebo Studies and Ritual Theory," 1854.

13. Sered and Agigian, "Holistic Sickening," 626.

and Agigian determine efficacy as "constructs in which a variety of actors have more or less power to shape narratives in which certain outcomes are labeled as successes, a variety of experts have the power to judge success, and a variety of methods are used in those assessments."[14] Efficacy in this constructivist and discursive sense is the result of communication and legitimating processes. In our terminology introduced above what they name efficacy is the "benefit" that can be a positive outcome of a treatment without any underlying effect and efficacy. What is evidently true for the emic understanding leaves unanswered our concern for the correlation of specific and efficacious interventions with improvement of well-being.

TOWARDS AN UNDERSTANDING OF EFFICACY IN SPIRITUAL HEALING

A survey of the academic classification of the vast and heterogeneous alternative healing field uncovers that current propositions for taxonomies do not derive criteria for a taxonomy from the dominant efficacy factors in the different types of healing.[15] This neglect has several reasons: First, many scholars are not interested in efficacy but rather in the historical reconstruction of specific religious traditions and their sources or the type of healing energy assumed. Second, if efficacy and symptom alleviation are taken into account, then they are seen as cultural constructions, as they are—no doubt. But the direction of questioning then is to explain them in their constructiveness instead of giving reasons why some *are* efficacious and others are *not*. One could say that exactly this is the difference between medical and cultural research, that natural sciences explain and cultural studies "understand" aims, feelings, and communal life. But this was part of the pioneering work for the beginning of cultural studies at the end of the nineteenth century and is not tenable any more long-since. The professionalization in psychology, medicine, neuroscience *and* cultural studies means overcoming the rationalist binary bias that divides humans into two parts: One part that has to be understood by hermeneutical means and one that has to be understood by physical laws. Beyond this methodology contemporary research on holistic medicine has a huge field of interest in common with both medical and cultural studies. Understanding the efficacy of spiritual healing has to include the effect of normally non-medical entities like touch, worldview, spatial setting, symbols, ritual pageantry etc. We will start with a very short characterization of the setting of our two pilot studies and the kind of data

---

14. Ibid., 625.
15. Koch, "Alternative Healing as Magical Self-Care."

we were gathering and then explicate our own results, drawing on further insights from research in the field and outlining additional hypotheses.

The Pilot Studies

In two pilot studies on spiritual healing we, a medical doctor working in medical psychology and a scholar in cultural study of religion, elaborated a number of criteria that seem to be relevant for efficacy from the point of view of the performance and meaning-making of the healer and the clients. In our first pilot study[16] (2007–09) we conducted participant fieldwork and took psychophysiological measurements during weekly healing ceremonies of the White Eagle Lodge near Munich/Germany. This small group is located in the hybrid tradition of theosophical-spiritist-Christian chakra-work. In this ritual of therapeutic touch the female healers visualize different-colored light into the chakras of the healee. Other than an opening prayer there is no verbal communication during the healing ceremony. The healee is sitting on a stool, facing altar (Fig. 1). The healer starts from the crown chakra on top of the head of the healee and works her way down the line of the body chakras mostly not touching the healee but stroking along the body outline at a little distance of two inches. She only touches and strokes lightly the shoulders, the back line of the vertebra and lets her hands lie down simultaneously on the belly and the back at the height of the solar plexus. We collected quantitative data with a validated questionnaire on current burden of discomfort and had the participants rate their expectation of benefit before and after the ceremony.[17] In both pilot studies we measured the benefit as an improved subjective well-being of participants. Psycho-physiological measurements of heart rate, gastric activity, breathing frequency and skin conductance levels were taken before, during, and after the 15–20 minutes-long treatments. In guided interviews the 27 group members and test persons were asked about their body image, what they were feeling during the treatment, what illness means to them, why they think that this ritual heals and with whom this ritual will probably be inefficacious.

---

16. Meissner and Koch "Sympathetic Arousal during a Touch-Based Healing Ritual Predicts Increased Well-Being."

17. Short Questionnaire on Current Burden (SQCB) (Müller and Basler, *Kurzfragebogen zur aktuellen Beanspruchung—KAB*. Beltz Test GmbH, Weinheim, 1993).

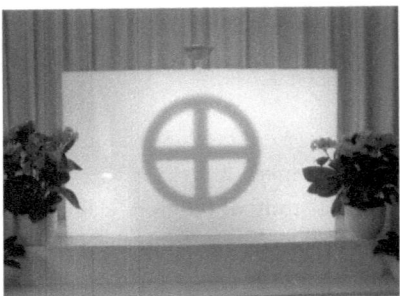 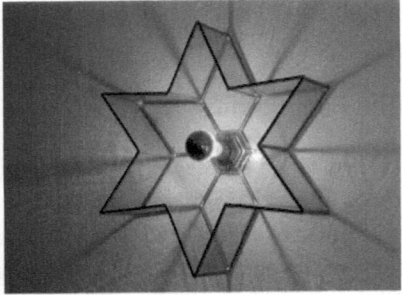

Fig. 1:
The illuminated altar of plastic material in the ceremonial room of the White Eagle Lodge in Germering (near Munich, Germany) with the symbol of a cross in a circle and the goblet of light on top of it, a crystalline bowl with a swimming candle (left side). A wall lamp in the form of a star radiates a pattern over the wall (right side). The aesthetics encodes the significance of light as healing energy and emplaces light-figurations into the setting of healing (photos: A.K.).

In a second pilot study 2009 in Munich we worked with an independent practitioner, a male German healer around 65 years old. This healer applies therapeutic touch and also works energetically with the body sensation of warmth. His self-understanding can be described from a religious-studies-perspective as a combination of chakra-work and modern Western shamanic healing (e.g., the healer feels guided during healing by several inner spirits from the middle ages and antiquity, to some of whom he was related in earlier lives). During the healing ceremony the healer evokes the feeling of warmth in the healee starting at the sacrum bone (he calls the tailbone a chakra) by spinning movements of his hand on the skin of the participant. In our study the participant was lying on his stomach on a couch. Once the participant feels the warmth, the healer "waits" for the feeling to deepen from a superficial to an inner-body warmth, still constantly spinning his hand, and then guides the sensation of warmth with his moving hand through the healee's body. He understands his healing as chakra work, re-energizing the flow and detecting and resolving energetic blockages. We videotaped six study participants during the healing sessions so that we could transcribe the verbal communication between healer and participant and capture the treatment's timeline. The former is important for correlation with the psychophysiological data that were recorded throughout the treatment. Psychophysiological measurements of heart rate, gastric activity, breath frequency and skin conductance levels were taken before, during, and after the one-hour or even longer treatments.

Some Efficacy Factors in Spiritual Touch Healing

Our research focuses on two healing rituals that involve touching the client's body. According to this procedure at least the following dimensions might be relevant for efficacy:

Intensifying Embodied Emotions

The client's amount of sympathetic arousal during the ritual proved to be relevant in both pilot studies. Sympathetic arousal is due to activation of the sympathetic branch of the autonomic nervous system (ANS), which connects the brain with the inner organs of the body.[18] The ANS is made up of two parts: the sympathetic nervous system, which responds to stressful situations, and the parasympathetic nervous system, which generally relaxes the body once the danger has passed. Even pleasant situations, such as a wedding, can be perceived as stressful. Thus, both positive and negative emotions can lead to sympathetic activation, which is perceived as increased heart rate and sweating, for example. The finding that increased sympathetic activation during the healing ritual correlated with increased well-being thereafter may indicate that strong emotions, induced by contextual factors of the ritual, could be important for the benefit of the ritual process. This emotional attitude can be amplified by activating bodily emotions in certain body parts. This can be realized through touch along symbolically meaningful body zones, by applying ointments at body parts, by hiding some body parts under a cover etc. Even negative emotions can be decisive for the outcome of the treatment because they are strong emotions, and strong emotionality seems to be a key factor for experiencing subjective benefits during healing and from healing.[19]

Selective Body Attention

An important technique to trigger emotionality is therefore the reshaping and recalibrating of the body scheme. This is realized by directing selective attention towards body parts and thus the organism of the client over a period of time. Ritual sequencing over time is a vital element here. Frequently,

---

18. Meissner / Anne, "Sympathetic Arousal during a Touch-Based Healing Ritual Predicts Increased Well-Being."

19. The US-American placebo researcher Ted Kaptchuk states this for the feeling of doubt by participants towards the efficacy of the healing, see Kaptchuk, "Placebo Studies and Ritual Theory."

spiritual healing involves a repositioning within the body of sensitive channels, of multiple subtle body envelopes or of energy centers (Fig. 2). For example, the belief of a group may be that the energy centers of a person have to be strengthened. This is carried out by infiltrating energy in the form of light with a specific color into the place where the energy center is said to be localized. In the imagination of the group it is necessary to bring in the light by first opening the energy channel at another specific body part and to close it again at the end of the sequence. The colorful light then is guided through a specific energetic landscape of the body to the energy center in need. On its pathway it may have to overcome blockages, to clean or enervate other spots. The guiding is performed in imagination with a drawing attention along the pathway as well as often with an embodied feeling such as warmth, prickling and tingling. Hence a healing ceremony entails several sequences that contain treatments along particular meaningful body zones and match somatic sensations.

Repositioning is carried out during the ritual and is decisive for the interpretation of what has taken place, usually by both parties, the healer and the client. The sequencing of the treatment makes it possible to build up autonomic arousal, for instance when there is an interaction based on social cognition between the healer and the client, or, on a more somatic level, when an effective third force is involved, the classic example being the healing energy. Often, a specific or unspecific factor in a given performance is that the healer works with the concepts of risk and security, so that the body is opened (e.g., at the site of a chakra) and made penetrable through the creation of a safe healing space. This intensifies the body awareness and feelings and creates an interactive space for the "third force."

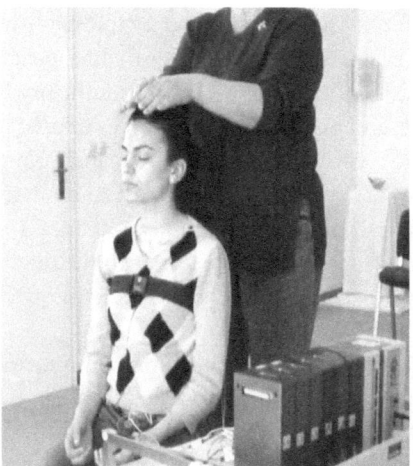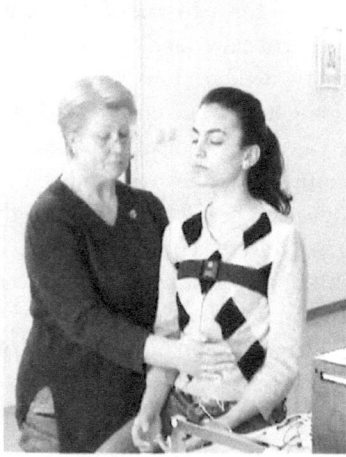

Fig. 2:
A test person is sitting on a stool with the healer holding her hands a few centimeters above her head at the beginning of the sequence "opening the crown chakra" (left side) and later during the treating the healer touches belly and back of the test person with both her hands (right side) (photos A.K.). In the right front corner you see the device used for the recording of physiological signals.

Modes of Performance—Empathy and Congruence

The mode of performance of the ritual also influences the emotional and autonomic effects of the treatment. It has often been noticed that the mode of great empathy by the healer, a very loving touch, or a very careful or slow or long-lasting treatment, creates a positive response and gives rise to certain intensified experiences and better outcomes in clinical trials.[20] The personality of the healer is important because he or she is a partner in the transformation the client goes through. To differing degrees, and depending on the particular relationship, the personality of the healer can significantly raise the level of expectation, supply plausible meanings, or use empathy to increase the client's level of self-esteem, etc.[21] The importance of this dimension can hardly be underestimated. We need to establish fundamental categories with regard to the mode of interaction between client and healer

---

20. See for example Blasi et al., "Influence of Context Effects on Health Outcomes"; and Kaptchuk et al., "Components of Placebo Effect."
21. Lindquist, "Healing Efficacy."

and the way a particular healer communicates with the client, or assesses the client through one of these channels. The healer's capacity to establish a congruent experiencing is an ability that is for Galina Lindquist an aspect of a charismatic personality: "charismatic individuals wield their authority by tapping into the symbolic, discursive, and performative resources offered by the culture".[22] Radical empathy of the healer as introduced by Joan D. Koss-Chioino[23] goes beyond simply a supportive attitude. With radical empathy a wounded healer who has gone through his own psychophysical crisis immerses into the client's situation. This resonance of the healer to the degree of his depersonalization is said to evoke deep memories and feelings on the side of the healee.

In our pilot studies we also observed on the somatic and communicative level a moment of matching between healer and healee we call congruence. In our second pilot study with congruence we address exactly the moment when agency is ascribed to the healing power by the healee, which means that from then on the deepened subcutaneous warmth can be guided through the client's body by the spinning hand of the healer. This congruence in the treatment process was easier and faster to perform with some clients than with others. Congruence might be induced by the constant and thus tiring somatic stimulus of the spinning hand of the healer on the client's naked skin and the repetitive monotonous communication asking every minute about the feeling of the warmth, its intensity, if the warmth is superficial or deepening, if the warmth follows the moving hand or not, if the degree of warmth changes or not etc. We assume that both stimuli—touch and talk, applied in a repetitive manner—induce a relaxed state of consciousness comparable to trance.[24]

Instruments

The instruments used in the ritual as carriers of healing power may also intensify the autonomic arousal and corresponding bio-chemical reactions. Interestingly, sham injections and sham acupuncture induce greater pain reduction than oral placebo pills, and sham surgery is one of the most

22. Lindquist, "Healing Efficacy," 339.
23. Koss-Chioino, "Spiritual Transformation, Relation and Radical Empathy."
24. There is a longstanding debate over the specificity of a state of consciousness in hypnosis. It seems that hypnosis need not be seen as so extraordinary as it sometimes appears in its mise-en-scène. Many scholars in hypnotherapy agree that similar states of consciousness and relaxation can be realized with task motivated instructions like the levitation of body parts, liveliness of sensorial imagination.

potent healing rituals.²⁵ That is, the more complex and emotionally arousing a healing ritual is, the greater the placebo effect seems to be. Thus, the Plexiglas rod or second copper rod used sometimes by the healer in our second pilot study to visualize light will be a more powerful instrument for interiorizing an image of the healing energy in the test person than the healer's placing together of thumb, first finger and middle finger to "fill in" the energy.

Learning Processes—Training the Body Knowledge

Living means to constantly adapt to sensorial and social environments. In this context forms of adaptation and learning are relevant to describe dynamics realized through spiritual healing performances. The (regular) performance of healing, body techniques and body practice in healing is essential for learning and training religious experience and inscribing somatic genres of feeling.

Learning occurs in several contexts, one of which is the socialization process for which habitualization is central. The concept of habitualization in cultural studies has to be distinguished from habituation in medical psychology. The latter means the extinction of a response to a stimulus by repetitive demonstration of the stimulus. On the contrary, the concept of habitualization addresses an enforcement of a behavior through regular performance: We get used to social forms of greeting, talking and expressing our wishes and adapt them mostly implicitly. We learn social forms and ways of communication. Tanya M. Luhrmann has explained the training of feelings and embodied experiences with the example of Christian prayer, especially charismatic ecstatic prayer techniques.²⁶ Social learning can even affect perception. Very much as charismatic Christians come to recognize God's presence in their bodily behavior in ecstatic prayer, participants in spiritual energy healing can recognize the healing power in their body. For an analysis of efficacy in spiritual healing it is important to take into account how habitualization and habituation are performed on the somatic, behavioral and intellectual level. These different types of adapting to contexts—the stimuli or the social context—do not exclude one another but are complementary.

---

25. Meissner et al., "Differential Effectiveness of Placebo Treatments"; Kaptchuk et al., "Sham Device v Inert Pill"; de Craen et al., "Placebo Effect."

26. Luhrman, "Building on William James."

Body Image or Body Scheme

The body image or scheme represents the physiological condition of the body. It is a neural umbrella representation derived from interoception of organs, moving, balance, hunger, temperature, oxygen supply, skin tension, pain and the like. Let us unfold why the body scheme is so central for the bodily manipulation of spiritual healing. In recent times the regulatory mechanisms of the body image are better understood in terms of their pathway:[27] the sensory afferents from the body's tissues and organs are first put together in autonomic and homeostatic centers of the spinal cord and brainstem and from there are processed to the thalamocortical area were they are represented as pain, itch, hunger, air hunger, temperature etc. These body feelings are an aspect of the ongoing homeostasis of the body based on thermoregulation, breathing, congestion etc. Important for us is that the body image or body scheme is a representation of the body as a whole and essentially emotional. Hunger, pain, warmth are felt as comfortable or uncomfortable. The body image is assumed to be the neural location where we feel well and comfortable or not. Ultimately, this basic or holistic feeling of ourselves is at stake in manipulating the body parts and thus activating autonomic afferents and homeostatic circuits. In working with warmth, as here, it is basically thermoregulation that is involved and triggered. Other spiritual techniques work with steering breathing, heart rate or muscle tone. At the bottom of the described procedures of spiritual healing lies the alteration of basic autonomic and homeostatic circuits that are responsible for the emotional body image—our feeling well in our bodies.

Regular participation presumably leads to a bodily reconfiguration of the body image in the direction of the idiosyncratic or indicated treatment narrative. One could assume that the body scheme stores in a bodily memory the ordering in which the organic systems were activated. As a consequence the experience in each section of the ritual and the emic attribution of meaning to this phase can be somatically recalled and re-enacted more quickly. Here a reinforcing role could be played by a combination of body techniques, for instance if the client has experience with a certain type of meditation, or, depending of course on the healing ritual, a coordination sport, autosuggestion, prayer of the heart, breathing techniques, rhythmical or musical synchronization, etc.

---

27. Craig, "Interoception."

The Place of Treatment as a Therapeutic Landscape

Embodied actors interact in and with space in several different ways. In the sense of a "cognitive download" as used in cognitive theory, the spatial scenery and objects in it, or their arrangement, provide information which the actor can use in any given situation. In terms of the aesthetics of religion, aspects of the material environment, including the amount of light, the type of floor, or audible sounds, are part of a whole. They become players in the healing procedure through selective perception, depending on the narrative of meaning and degree of sensory intrusiveness. Therapeutic landscapes[28] may be places of retreat with a deprivation of sensory stimulus like the desert or caves, like Zen-aesthetic places, dark or mono-material places, e.g., with wooden and natural materials. Landscapes and places can be therapeutic through under-regulation or over-regulation. Vision quest with fasting and staying alone during several days as well as Yoga with clearly prescribed moving and breathing within 1,5 square meter over-regulate the practice. Free dancing with unforeseeable contact with co-agents or feasts with alcohol are under-regulated. Therapeutic landscapes are at the interface of real and imagined places and co-constitute the recipient who moves within their framework. Many therapeutic landscapes are not extraordinary but common places that temporarily distinguish themselves as therapeutic. Even then they often are ambivalent as places of breach, violation or injury and of healing. Whether a landscape is seen as therapeutic depends on the recipient. Also which forces are viable within the place is the product of a meaning-making process. Nature can be ascribed a restoring power; disturbing materiality like heat or cold can play a role to steer attention and trigger processes of self-confrontation; the experiencing of a counter world to everyday life can be therapeutic; the experiencing of a diverging setting may have the same effect; through moderation of the healer a perceptive space in relation to the sensorial environment may be opened for somatic-symbolized interaction; the space my offer images for emotions and exteriorize them, thus taking a first step towards psychic distancing etc. There are countless ways in which places might be integrated on a very somatic level into healing. All this may unleash deep and hidden emotions, intensify the feeling and reconfigure the body scheme. Emotional ambivalences may be expressed in the experiencing of stability-instability of a movement or posture. This enables therapeutic landscapes to pass on and access emotions in healing.

---

28. Williams, *Therapeutic Landscapes*.

The Role of Meaning and Reframing of Worldview for Efficacy

According to psychological motivation theories, goal-attainment is connected with positive emotions. The healing ritual can be seen as an interactional form that enables the participant to attain his goals of self-realization and human growth. In this respect the ritual will motivate the person to participate to attain goals. From a more somatic point of view, the bodily self-experiencing during the ritual can serve to explain the motivation to participate in a ritual healing. The more concordant the ritual experience is to the person's worldview the more the person will be motivated to participate and benefit from the performance.[29] Then it is not only the successful outcome of the ritual—the ritual as an instrument to reach a better condition—but the ritual in itself that motivates to participate.

Cognitive schemes, their change and actualization are also relevant to the spiritual healing rituals we are considering. They are debated in ritual theory under the concept of frames and re-framing. Frames are psychological as well as cognitive concepts that structure subjective reality, frames select information and evaluate it by cultural codes. Frames are action orienting devices; they are therefore, like all perception, contextualized in the sense of situated cognition. They bind together different types of knowledge: semantic knowledge, procedural knowledge, practical knowledge, somatic knowledge. Participants in rituals have several sequential frames for ritual sequences that are hierarchically ordered and embedded in the unifying ritual frame. Frames are learned and to some degree habitual, depending on how regularly people activate them through use. Findings suggest that a spiritual framing of healing is higher in positive outcome for spiritual people than a secularist one, whereas expectancy always correlates with a positive outcome.[30] In a study by psychologist Michael P. Hyland et al.[31] high scores in the spirituality variable better predicted the positive outcome of a flower essence self-treatment than expectancy. If spirituality is central in the worldview and attitude of a person, religious coping can be a precious resource in overcoming disease and life crisis.

Specific cues within frames give signals when a sequence starts or ends. These cues may be explicit or implicit as in the case of metacommunication with gestures or mimicry. If features are interpreted as the opener of a new sequence of the ritual then the general program or script of the ritual sequence is actualized for the participant and his experiencing of the

---

29. Hyland and Whalley, "Motivational Concordance."
30. Ibid.
31. Hyland, Geraghty, Joy, and Turner, "Spirituality Predicts Outcome."

action. Since frames are the psychological structures of ritual, they bring together the individual experience with the collective structure of repeated action at a time that is very prone to subjective interpretation. Frames are an important device to decide intentionally or spontaneously what is part of the healing ritual and what does not belong to it. Methodologically frames are current with anthropologists and sociologists because they can relate some conceptual binaries, such as for example individual/collective, active/passive, intentional/unconscious, stable/changing.

Re-framing also takes part in Sered and Agigian's holistic sickening: They discover a congruence on the worldview level between healer and healee: this congruence is the re-framing of the illness as holistic sickening. This reframing is a precondition for personal transformation: "this transformation is experienced positively by many patients, particularly in situations in which there is congruence between the worldviews of the practitioner and the client."[32] Frames make a healee recognize a claim of healing power as authentic. Charismatic healers implicitly or explicitly refer to healing energies, depending on the given framework. The psycho-physiological sense of these energies is their role of affect intensification and of creating this one field of experience. The healing energy or spirit or whatever the image is connects the individual to the source of healing.

The laying on of hands can be performed with imagining energetic life forces going through the bodies or in the belief that God will do a miracle out of his sovereign power. The phenotype and performance of the sequential laying on of hands are very similar if not the same, but the accompanying images and explicit or implicit symbols differ widely. Today they also often intermingle with popcultural symbols since the energetic worldview is so common in public discourse.

An important factor in the efficacy of the treatment is the client's agreement and plausibilization in the cognitive *and* the somatic dimensions. The US-American placebo researcher Ted Kaptchuk (2011) names this "evaluation." He thinks that the evaluation at the end of the ritual, or after and outside the ritual, is decisive for its efficacy as it reframes the experience. On the basis of our pilot studies, we think that somatic meaning-making through the experience of congruence is equally important. This means that throughout the whole duration of the ritual the client has a sustaining and affirmative attitude which constantly recalculates the success of today's ritual. This is shown for instance by that fact that some test persons attribute the occasional shallowness of their healing energy experience to their initial constitution ("I had to rush to get here"), their current need ("I don't

---

32. Sered and Agigian, "Holistic Sickening," 627.

need anything at the moment"), or their spiritual disposition ("I wasn't open today"). The creation of meaning probably is intensified by habitualization. Habitualization as regular attendance and performance of healing ritual fosters the learning process and familiarity with the healing narrative, alters the expectation and builds up a somatic pattern of how it feels.

CONCLUSION

In the sense discussed above, spiritual healing is a highly ambivalent practice situated in late modernity. Most late modern societies practice holistic medicine, spiritual healing, wellness with relaxing, stress relief, well-being and prevention through fitness, singing, dancing and sports, while some of them are mixed practices also offering "meaning (of life) on demand," e.g., in yoga, self-help therapies or martial arts. Spiritual healing offers a self-cure where the self seeks to experience itself and enforces "energies." One could call this understanding magical insofar it tends to belief in the power of consciousness and self-reflexive powers like self-healing forces of the immune system to be manipulated by the respective practices for healing success.[33] This ascription of causality to invisible cultural entities is based on an alternative conception of subtle fields.[34]

For reasons of comparability and to measure the psychophysiological data we choose healing rituals that guide "energy" through the body by touching body parts following a specific sequence. For the type of treatment we studied we could determine at least some features as relevant for a subjective positive outcome of spiritual healing. For some features we still assume hypothetically that the underlying psychophysiological mechanisms could be attached to the action. The healee's affirmative familiarity with certain healing practices including their symbolic meaning or worldview and his emotional congruence with the healer at some specific point of the treatment are relevant, as are the centrality of spirituality in the healee's life (the degree to which spiritual convictions, e.g., of energetic forces are connected to experiencing; Huber and Huber "The centrality of religiosity scale [CRS]"), suggestibility, how a sequential healing treatment steers attention through the body, high emotionality triggered also on the somatic level, and the interaction with the ritual environment as therapeutic landscape. Also the reconfiguration of the body scheme and an evaluative reframing proved to be relevant. They rely on the effect of afferent emotionality and gain efficacy mediated by the regulating circuits of the reframing of emotions,

33. Koch, "Alternative Healing as Magical Self-care."
34. Johnston and Samuel, eds., *Religion and the Subtle Body in Asia and the West.*

cognitive evaluation and the emotional body-image. Efficacy depends to some degree on repeated and even regular practice that can be followed by behavioral change (for example in work load, relationships, sportive profile). Against many descriptions of a singularizing individualization we also found the healer-healee-interaction to be crucial in the healing practices we studied.[35]

There still is great need for further interdisciplinary research to examine the relations between various specialized studies on efficacy and to set up hypotheses regarding the different kinds of healing practice. Due to the complexity of the healing process, it is not yet possible to make a list of scalable factors that influence healing. At the present stage of research, much could be gained on both sides (medical and psychological research, and research by scholars of religion), by comparing the detailed results of dozens of very specific placebo experiments on the relevant level with the comparatively broad concepts used to describe spiritual healing in the cultural sciences.

BIBLIOGRAPHY

Benedetti, F. *Placebo Effects: Understanding the Mechanisms in Health and Disease*. New York: Oxford University Press, 2009.

Binder, S., and A. Koch. "Holistic Medicine between Religion and Science: A Secularist Construction of Spiritual Healing in Medical Literature." *Journal of Religion in Europe* 6 (2013) 1–34.

Blasi, Z. D. et al. "Influence of Context Effects on Health Outcomes: A Systematic Review." *The Lancet* 357.9258 (2001) 757–62.

Bleyer, A., and H. G. Welch. "Effect of Three Decades of Screening Mammography on Breast-Cancer Incidence." *New England Journal of Medicine* 367.21 (2012) 1998–2005.

Craig, A. D. "Interoception: The Sense of the Physiological Condition of the Body." *Current Opinion in Neurobiology* 13 (2003) 500–505.

Dawson, A. "Entangled Modernity and Commodified Religion: Alternative Spirituality and the 'New Middle Class.'" In *Religion and Consumer Culture: Brands, Consumers and Markets*, edited by F. Gauthier and T. Martikainen, 127–42. Aldershot, UK: Ashgate, 2013.

de Craen, A. J. M. et al. "Placebo Effect in the Acute Treatment of Migraine: Subcutaneous Placebos Are Better than Oral Placebos." *Journal of Neurology* 247.3 (2000) 183–88.

Fisher, P., et al. "Effectiveness Gaps: A New Concept for Evaluating Health Service and Research Needs Applied to Complementary and Alternative Medicine." *The Journal of Alternative and Complementary Medicine* 10 (2004) 627–32.

---

35. Ann Taves and Michael Kinsella talk of the "dyadic relationship of healer and patient" as fundamental for the metaphysical healing tradition: "Hiding in Plain Sight."

Harrington, Anne. *The Cure Within: A History of Mind-Body Medicine*. New York: Norton, 2008.
Huber, S. and O. Huber "The Centrality of Religiosity Scale (CRS)." *Religions* 3 (2012) 710–24, http://www.mdpi.com/2077-1444/3/3/710
Hyland, M. E. et al. "Spirituality Predicts Outcome Independently of Expectancy Following Flower Essence Self-treatment." *Journal of Psychosomatic Research* 60 (2006) 53–58.
Hyland, M. E., and B. Whalley. "Motivational Concordance: An Important Mechanism in Self-Help Therapeutic Rituals Involving Inert (Placebo) Substances." *Journal of Psychosomatic Research* 65 (2008) 405–13.
Kaptchuk, T. J. "Placebo Studies and Ritual Theory: A Comparative Analysis of Navajo, Acupuncture and Biomedical Healing." *Phil. Trans. R. Soc. B* 366 (2011) 1849–58.
Kaptchuk, T.J. and D. M. Eisenberg. "The Persuasive Appeal of Alternative Medicine." *Annals of Internal Medicine* 129.12 (1998) 1061–65.
Kaptchuk, T.J. et al., "Components of Placebo Effect: Randomised Controlled Trial in Patients with Irritable Bowel Syndrome." *British Medical Journal* 336.7651 (2008) 999–1003.
———. "Sham Device v Inert Pill: Randomised Controlled Trial of Two Placebo Treatments." *British Medical Journal* 332.7538 (2006) 391–97.
Koch, A. "Alternative Healing as Magical Self-Care in Alternative Modernity." *Numen* 62 (2015) 431–59.
Koss-Chioino, J. D. "Spiritual Transformation, Relation and Radical Empathy: Core Components of the Ritual Healing Process." *Transcultural Psychiatry* 43.4 (2006) 652–70.
Lindquist, G. "Healing Efficacy and the Construction of Charisma: A Family's Journey through the Multiple Medical Field in Russia." *Anthropology and Medicine* 9 (2002) 337–58.
Luhrman, T. M. "Building on William James: The Role of Learning in Religious Experience." In *Mental Culture: Classical Social Theory and the Cognitive Science of Religion*, edited by Dimitris Xygalatas and William W. McCorkle Jr., 145–63. Bristol, CT: Acumen, 2014.
Meissner, K. et al. "Differential Effectiveness of Placebo Treatments. A Systematic Review of Migraine." *JAMA Internal Medicine* 173.21 (2013) 1941–51.
———, Koch, A. "Sympathetic arousal during a touch-based healing ritual predicts increase in well-being," *eCAM. Evidence-based Complementary and Alternative Medicine*, Article ID 641704 (2015), 6 pages.
Moseley, J. B. et al. "A Controlled Trial of Arthroscopic Surgery for Osteoarthritis of the Knee." *New England Journal of Medicine* 347.2 (2002) 81–88.
Samuel, Geoffrey, and Jay Johnston, eds. *Religion and the Subtle Body in Asia and the West: Between Mind and Body*. Routledge Studies in Asian Religion and Philosophy 8. New York: Routledge, 2013.
Sered, S., and Amy. Agigian. "Holistic Sickening: Breast Cancer and the Discursive Worlds of Complementary and Alternative Practitioners." *Sociology of Health & Illness* 30 (2008) 616–31.
Short Questionnaire on Current Burden (SQCB) (Müller B and Basler, HD. *Kurzfragebogen zur aktuellen Beanspruchung—KAB*. Beltz Test GmbH, Weinheim, 1993.
Taves, A., and M. Kinsella. "Hiding in Plain Sight: The Organizational Forms of 'Unorganized Religion.'" In *New Age Spirituality: Rethinking Religion*, edited by

Steven J. Sutcliffe and Ingvild Saelid Gilhus, 84–98. 2013. Reprinted, London: Routledge, 2014.

Williams, A., ed. *Therapeutic Landscapes*. Ashgate's Geographies of Health Series. Aldershot, UK: Ashgate, 2007.

Witt, C. M. "Efficacy, Effectiveness, Pragmatic Trials: Guidance on Terminology and the Advantages of Pragmatic Trials." *Forschende Komplementärmedizin* 16 (2009) 292–94.

www.ingramcontent.com/pod-product-compliance
Lightning Source LLC
Chambersburg PA
CBHW021927290426
44108CB00012B/750